FUNDAMENTALS OF PEDIATRICS

Mary Bayonla Banks

ALLIED HEALTH PRESS

Fundamentals of Pediatrics

Author: **Mary Bayonla Banks**

Allied Health Press
4164 Lakeshore Road
Burlington ON L7L 1A4
Canada
www.alliedhealthpress.com
Email: orders@arclereducation.com

ISBN: 978-1-77956-237-1

ABOUT THE AUTHOR

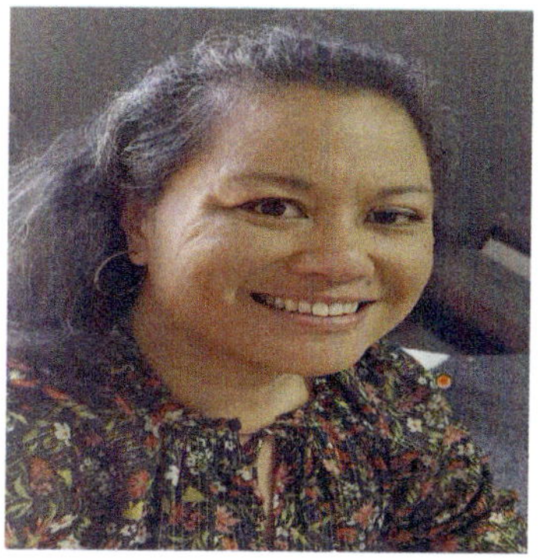

Mary Bayonla Banks is a dedicated physical therapist with a diverse background in pediatrics both school-based and outpatient, geriatrics, and orthopedics. She is also a retired secondary school athletic trainer. She currently works as a staff physical therapist in the Virginia Beach City Public School system where she works with special needs children ranging from ages 2-22 focusing on access to educational program through working on acquisition of gross motor milestones and locomotor skills, as well as attaining and maintaining independent functional mobility. She also works with the geriatric population by providing high quality outpatient orthopedic as well as aquatic physical therapy. Mary attended the Medical Campus of Virginia Commonwealth University in Richmond, VA where she earned her Doctor of Physical Therapy degree in 2004.

Word Roots, Prefixes, and Suffixes by Chapter

Chapter 1 Pediatric Care

chol/e gall, bile
col/o colon
colon/o colon
dys- painful, abnormal, difficult, labored
endo- within, in

Chapter 2 History Elicitation and Physical Examination

abdom- the abdomen
bronch(i)- the lungs
cardi-, coron- the heart
cran- the skull
digit- the fingers

Chapter 3 Newborn Care

ambi- both
bi- two
circum- around
dis- not, apart
inter- between, among
-ac pertaining to

Chapter 4 Growth and Development

abdom- the abdomen
andro- male
axill- armpit region
col-, colo-, colono- the colon/large intestine
cut-, derm- the skin

Chapter 5 Nutrition

-emia related to blood
-algia pain
ante- before
anti- attacks, treats condition
cephal- head

Chapter 6 Immunization and Infectious Diseases

brady Slow
dys- Bad, abnormal, painful, difficult
endo- Within, in
epi- On, upon, over
hyper- Above, excessive
hypo- Below, deficient

Chapter 7 Common Disorders in Children

-ectomy Surgical removal (excision) of a body part
-orrhaphy Surgical repair or suture
-gram record
-graphy process of recording

Chapter 8 Pediatric Surgical Conditions

-anemia related to blood
ante- before
anti- attacks, treats condition
brady- slow
cardio- related to the heart
cephal- head

Chapter 9 Pediatric Emergencies

dys- Bad, abnormal, painful, difficult
endo- Within, in
epi- On, upon, over
hyper- Above, excessive

Chapter 10 Child Health Nursing in PICU

-graphy Process of recording, radiographic imaging
-ion Process
-oma Tumor
-osis Abnormal condition
-scopy Process of viewing
-gram Record, radiographic image

Table of Contents

10 Child Health Nursing in PICU 389

Index 417

LIST OF FIGURES

LIST OF TABLES

PREFACE

Pediatrics is a medical field that deals with the development and healthcare of children, as well as the diagnosis and treatment of childhood illnesses. The practice of pediatrics began to take shape in Europe in the 18th century, with the establishment of specialized children's hospitals like the London Foundling Hospital in 1745. These hospitals became important centers for pediatric training, which became a distinct discipline in medical schools by the mid-19th century.

Early pediatrics focused on treating infectious diseases that affected children, with notable contributions from figures like Thomas Sydenham in the 17th century. Clinical studies of childhood diseases expanded in the 18th and 19th centuries, leading to the publication of one of the first modern pediatric textbooks in France in 1838–43. However, effective treatments for these diseases did not emerge until the late 19th century.

As advances in pediatrics, immunology, and public health helped control childhood diseases, the focus of pediatrics shifted. In the early 20th century, the first well-child clinics were established to monitor normal child growth and development. By the mid-20th century, antibiotics and vaccines had drastically reduced serious childhood infections in developed countries, leading to significant declines in infant and child mortality rates.

In the latter half of the 20th century, pediatrics expanded to include the study of behavioral, social, and medical aspects of child health. Today, pediatric care aims to provide focused medical treatment for children with severe illnesses, emphasizing growth and development, nutrition, disease prevention, and treatment. This book takes a different approach to current pediatric issues, discussing topics such as nutritional infant health and subspecialties like cardiology, hemato-oncology, and infectious diseases.

Pediatrics and society share a deep-rooted connection, dating back to the late 18th century. The earliest European pediatric schools were not only centers for clinical and scientific advancement but also champions of social causes. The founding figures of Pediatrics were not just brilliant scientists but also compassionate humanitarians, dedicating their lives to caring for disadvantaged children and advocating for social welfare programs. Their work focused on studying, preventing, and treating various childhood illnesses, including infectious, nutritional, and neurological diseases, while also addressing issues of abandonment.

The influence and responsibilities of pediatricians grew steadily after the establishment of these first schools. Universities played a significant role by establishing pediatric chairs and journals, which not only advanced the field but also elevated its cultural and academic standing. These efforts quickly spread across Europe, leading to substantial improvements in child healthcare and significant reductions in neonatal and infant mortality rates.

Today, pediatricians continue to play a crucial role in society, advocating for children and their families, bridging social gaps, and serving as credible voices in public discourse. The recent COVID-19 pandemic has underscored existing social inequalities, making the pediatrician's role as a defender of children's rights and well-being more critical than ever.

The aim of the book "Pediatrics" is to provide a comprehensive and up-to-date resource for medical students, residents, practicing pediatricians, and other healthcare professionals involved in the care of children. The book aims to cover a wide range of topics in pediatrics, including developmental milestones, common pediatric illnesses, preventive care, and the management of complex medical conditions in children.

The book is designed to be a practical guide for healthcare professionals, providing essential information on the diagnosis, treatment, and management of pediatric conditions. It includes detailed explanations of key concepts, evidence-based guidelines, and practical tips for managing pediatric patients in various clinical settings.

In addition to covering clinical topics, the book also addresses important issues in pediatric practice, such as ethics, cultural competence, and communication skills. It aims to help healthcare professionals develop the knowledge, skills, and attitudes necessary to provide high-quality care to children and their families. The book is written clearly and concisely, with an emphasis on practicality and relevance to clinical practice. It is supplemented with illustrations, tables, and case studies to enhance understanding and facilitate learning.

Chapter 1

PEDIATRIC CARE

Contents

INTRODUCTION

Pediatric care is specialized medical attention given to kids who have serious illnesses. Pediatric care is concerned with the growth and development of children as well as their diet, illness treatment, and disease prevention. Improving both the child's and the family's quality of life is the goal. Children under the age of 18 can receive medical care from a team of doctors, nurses, and other skilled caregivers who work together to provide pediatric care. Pediatric care includes specialized care for preterm newborns and adolescent children in addition to treating medical diseases, which include abnormalities of many body systems, hereditary conditions, and cancers. It addresses a range of conditions' symptoms, including pain, dyspnea, fatigue, nausea, constipation, lack of appetite, and trouble falling asleep. In conclusion, it gives the child and the family the willpower to carry on with their regular lives.

Family is the main focus of pediatric care. In addition to easing the child's pain, the care gives parents and other caregivers the tools they need to take better care of their child. Families are better able to make decisions that are in line with their characteristics, customs, and culture when they have access to the close communication that pediatric care provides. The family as a whole benefits from this in terms of quality of life. In order to provide the child with the best care possible, pediatric care should start as soon as the child is born and address a variety of concerns. It is best for the experts to handle any potential issues. Cooperating closely with primary care physician (Thomas Moshang, 2005; Sandra, 2007; Wetmore, 2007).

Orientation and Directional Terms

Term	Definition	Illustration
Antenatal	A term that means 'before birth' (alternative terms are 'prenatal' and 'antepartum').	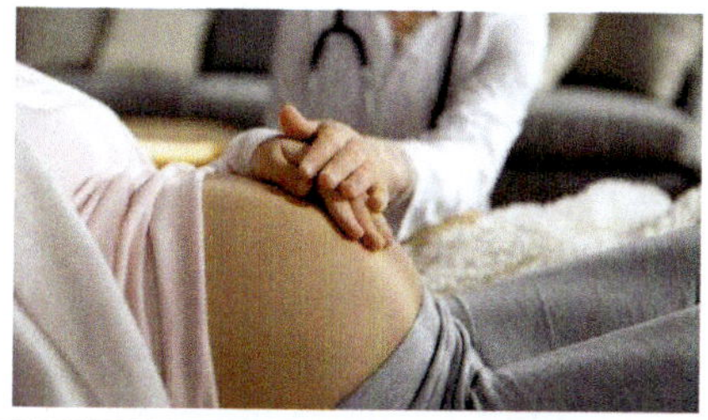
Conception	The process of becoming pregnant, when a sperm and egg join to form a single cell (alternative terms include 'fertilization,' 'impregnation' and 'insemination').	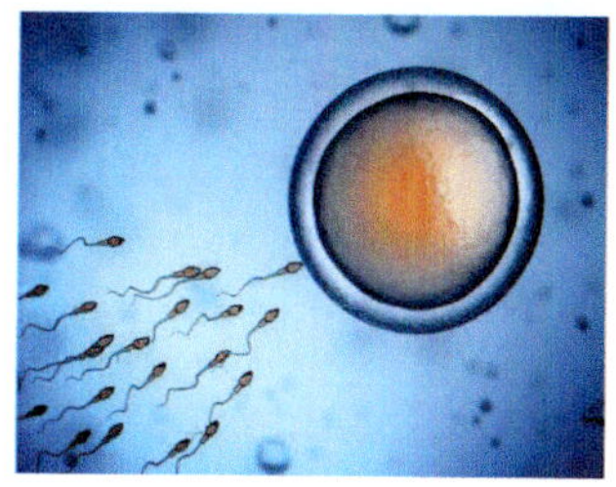
Pregestational Diabetes	Preexisting diabetes (also called pregestational diabetes) means you have diabetes before you get pregnant.	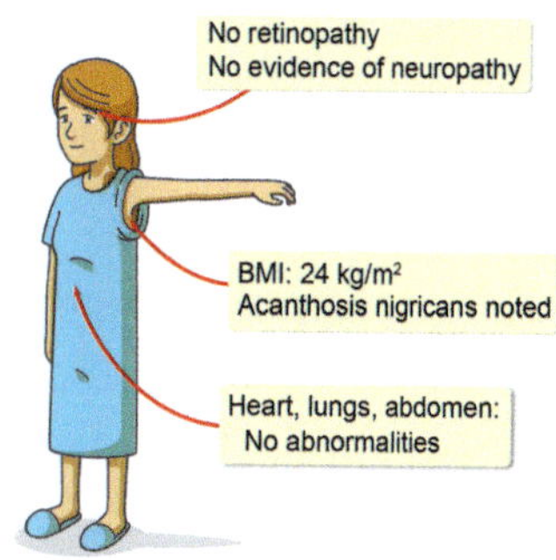
Non-Hodgkin lymphoma	Non-Hodgkin's lymphoma is a type of cancer that begins in your lymphatic system, which is part of the body's germ-fighting immune system.	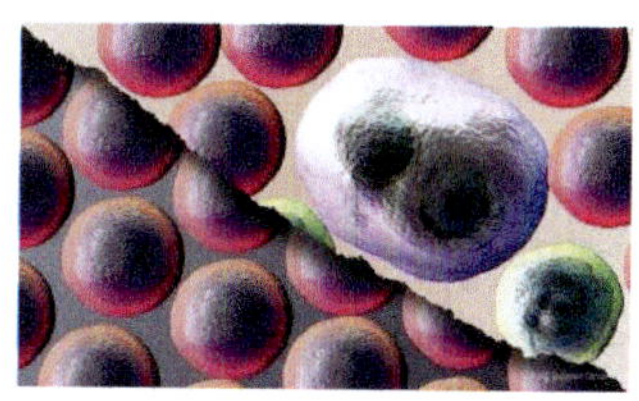

1.1. IMPORTANCE OF PEDIATRICS AND PEDIATRIC CARE

Pediatrics differs from adult medicine in that children are more than just little replicas of adult males and females. Pediatric specialists are educated in expert evaluation with an emphasis on the avoidance, identification, and treatment of a wide range of child-related issues. Pediatric healthcare providers must take into account growth and developmental issues that do not exist in adult patients because children are dynamic beings. These factors can have a big influence on the recommended course of treatment, particularly when a serious illness is involved.

Typical responsibilities of pediatric healthcare providers included:

- Identifying and managing diseases, injuries, infections, and dysfunction.
- Make an effort to lower infant and child mortality.
- Promote healthy lifestyles
- Ease the burden of chronic illness on patients' daily lives.
- Determine and deal with behavioral and developmental issues.
- Tracking the development of the body and the mind.
- Delivering vaccinations and screenings according to age.
- Providing parents and patients with guidance and instruction regarding typical developmental challenges.
- Referral of complicated illnesses when necessary and collaborative relationships with other healthcare professionals.

In order to treat complicated illnesses and disorders, general pediatricians frequently work with pediatric subspecialists. They also frequently collaborate with other medical professionals to meet the emotional needs of their patients. The ability to communicate with patients, parents, and educators in an effective manner is essential for providing pediatric care. Pediatric professionals need the consent of parents or legal guardians in order to treat their patients, who are mostly minors.

For the populations they treat, family doctors, internists, gynecologists/obstetricians, and gerontologists are all regarded as primary care providers (PCPs), just as general pediatricians are. When your kids need medical attention, they should go to them first. Physician assistants and pediatric nurse practitioners can also serve as PCPs for annual physicals and the majority of routine, non-emergency medical care. Your pediatrician will refer you to a specialist if they are unable to treat your child. Your PCP will typically supervise care if your child is admitted to the hospital or requires continuous medical attention. PCPs are in charge of providing preventive care to keep their patients healthy. Screenings, immunizations, weight management counseling, and appropriate exercise are all part of preventive care. PCPs provide parents with growth and development advice when caring for younger children.

Pediatric care can include subspecialties that work with young patients in addition to general care. These consist of:

- Adolescent medicine
- Child abuse
- Developmental-behavioral issues
- Hospice and palliative Medicine
- Neonatology
- Cardiology
- Critical care
- Emergency medicine

- Endocrinology
- Hematology
- Oncology
- Infectious diseases
- Nephrology
- Pulmonology
- Rheumatology
- Transplant hepatology
- Sports medicine

As was previously mentioned, infants, kids, and teenagers aren't tiny versions of adults. They require things unique to them. Pediatric medicine offers the best possible healthcare while attending to those needs. Pediatric medical professionals carry out a number of crucial duties that are sometimes invisible. Pediatricians play a vital role in both the overall health of the community and their patients. Pediatricians are personally concerned with all aspects of their patients' development, not just physical growth and illnesses. The public health care system as a whole benefits from comprehensive care aimed at children.

1.1.1. Benefits of Seeing the Same Pediatrician

Studies indicate that kids who see the same pediatrician are generally healthier. A practitioner can provide the best advice and customize care by getting to know a child and their family. The same holds true for young people who suffer from long-term illnesses like diabetes, high blood pressure, asthma, etc.

- **Providing Accurate Medical Information:** Given the deluge of information available online, some parents might find it challenging to verify the accuracy of what they have read. When it comes to safety, nutrition, fitness, development, illness prevention, and treatment options when needed, pediatricians are a reliable source of information.
- **Early Intervention:** Well-child visits are critical for a child's healthy development and the prevention of related issues by serving as a screening and diagnostic tool for conditions like diseases and developmental disorders. Early intervention improves a child's quality of life and supports optimal development so they can become successful adults.
- **Child Advocacy:** Pediatric professionals have a role in advocacy in addition to healthcare. In the absence of pediatricians, some people might make choices that could be harmful to the health of their kids. Ensuring that pediatric needs are legally addressed is another way that presenting a scientific viewpoint before legislative bodies helps address new public health concerns.

1.1.2. Age Limit for Pediatric Patients

Pediatric care can start even before a woman becomes pregnant, and it can go on throughout her pregnancy, delivery, and early adulthood. Pediatric care is defined by the American Academy of Pediatrics (AAP) as patients up to the age of 21, though some pediatricians will treat older college students who have been their long-term patients out of convenience. Subcategories of pediatric care are further separated out as follows:

- Neonates, birth through 28 days
- Infants, 29 days to 2 years

- Children, 2 years to less than 12 years
- Adolescents, 12 years through age 21
- The AAP further categorizes teenagers into three groups: early (ages 11–14), middle (ages 15–18), and late (ages 18–21).

Because many of the young patients they diagnose and treat are unable to express their feelings or are too shy to do so, pediatric professionals need to be skilled communicators. The method used with patients varies according to their age, stage of development, and maturity. When deciding how to approach a patient, it's common practice to first speak with their parents, particularly in the case of younger or developmentally challenged children. In these situations, parents can be very helpful in assisting medical professionals in formulating treatment plans by helping them ask questions. Children who suffer from chronic illnesses often find it difficult to communicate their feelings to medical professionals. When conducting a test or a procedure on these patients, pediatric professionals must reassure them. Treating pediatric patients involves some degree of trust-building. Experts frequently interact with children by asking about their interests and hobbies in order to better treat and help them relax. Just as improving a patient's condition can take time, so too can building trust (Thomas Moshang, 2005; Sandra, 2007; Wetmore, 2007).

1.2. PRIMARY HEALTH CARE

The goal of pediatric primary health care (PPHC) is to provide family-centered care that is continuous, comprehensive, coordinated, accessible, and affordable in order to meet the health needs of infants, children, adolescents, and young adults. Complete care for the whole life cycle—from early childhood to young adulthood—is provided by PPHC. Aspects of PPHC include age-appropriate screening for disease prevention and health promotion, anticipatory guidance and wellness promotion, including mental health and monitoring physical, cognitive, and social growth and development, and health supervision with an emphasis on preventing physical and mental health conditions. Even though 1 in 5 children have a chronic illness or special health care need that has been identified, the prevalence of these conditions is rising and is diverse. Pediatricians who are board-certified or board-eligible face a constant challenge in recognizing and treating serious clinical issues in a population that is generally healthy. As a result, PPHC also includes managing severe and life-threatening illnesses, diagnosing and treating acute and chronic health disorders, and, when necessary, referring patients with more complicated conditions to surgical or medical subspecialty care. In order to attain the best possible health results, PPHC also includes well-planned transitions for all children, particularly those with chronic illnesses, to adult care as well as coordinated management of health issues requiring several professional services. Last but not least, PPHC aspires to be patient- and family-centered, integrating risk and protective factors, sociocultural effectiveness, and community resources and strengths into clinical practice and care delivery strategies.

1.2.1. Different Types of Primary Care Providers

The following are the various categories of primary care physicians.

- **GPs (General Practioner):** Children see their family doctor, or GP, when they are ill. They typically collaborate with nurses, medical assistants, receptionists, and other staff members in a clinic. The pediatrician records the tests, immunizations, and medical history of the child. They offer medical prescriptions, health advice, common ailment treatment, and health assessments. A child's first point of contact before being referred to a pediatrician for more specialized care makes general practitioner visits crucial.

- **Health Visitors:** As part of the Healthy Child Program, a health visitor—a nurse who works with families—will make regular appointments with children ages zero to five. Vaccinations, your child's development, and the parent's opportunity to ask questions regarding their child's health will all be discussed during the appointments. Advice on sleeping, feeding, and teething is available to parents. Health visitors are the individuals who also see children in cases where they suspect maltreatment or failure to attend a crucial referral by parents, in addition to cases involving non-accidental injuries. Children in exceptional situations, such as those with disabilities, asylum seekers, or parents who abuse drugs or alcohol, are given priority.
- **Dentists:** It's crucial for your child to have regular dental examinations, whether they are provided by public or private healthcare, in order to prevent tooth decay and determine whether braces are necessary at a young age.
- **Opticians:** Opticians perform eye exams on children to assess their overall eye health as well as their quality of vision. In addition to prescribing and fitting glasses, they can refer kids who require more care to specialized eye physicians. Children enrolled in the public healthcare system are eligible for free eye exams.

1.2.2. Need for Primary Care

Primary care is usually necessary for children for the following reasons.

- **Prevention of Infectious Diseases:** Primary care physicians make certain that children are vaccinated against serious infectious diseases.
- **Early Detection of Health Problems:** The Child Health Promotion Program offers a structured series of evaluations to monitor a child's growth and well-being and identify any health problems early on.
- **Early Detection of Mental Health Problems:** A diagnosable mental health disorder affects 10% of children between the ages of 5 and 15. A mental health disorder can be identified and early intervention can be provided by routine visits with a primary care provider.
- **Health Promotion for Children:** Primary care physicians encourage healthy eating and lifestyle choices for school-age children, help family members quit smoking, and answer questions from parents regarding their child's growth and health. Additionally, they offer children with special needs additional support.
- **Health Promotion for Teenagers:** Primary care physicians identify unhealthy eating patterns in young people, counsel them on sexual

and contraceptive options, and encourage them to make wise decisions in life (Thomas Moshang, 2005; Sandra, 2007; Wetmore, 2007).

1.2.3. Unique Role of the Pediatrician in Pediatric Primary Care

All facets of pediatric healthcare have been the focus of the extensive education and training that pediatricians have received. Along with this education and training, the individual has a track record of being fully committed to the health care of newborns, kids, teens, and young adults as well as a clear interest in it. The pediatrician is a highly qualified and skilled supervisor of PPHC delivery due to these special qualifications, and they frequently collaborate with other professionals to support team-based care. The only medical specialty where training is solely focused on the needs and special care of newborns, children, adolescents, and young adults is pediatrics. Pediatricians are uniquely positioned to monitor normal growth and development and identify concerns when their patients deviate from their expected developmental path because of the continuity that they typically establish with their patients, often spanning their entire childhood and adolescence. With advantages that last well into adulthood, pediatricians play a unique role in preserving the physical and mental well-being of their patients.

The optimal setting for providing PPHC is a patient- and family-centered medical home that offers continuous, all-inclusive, coordinated, compassionate, and culturally sensitive care that is easily accessible, reasonably priced, and overseen by pediatricians who are board-certified or board-eligible. Collaborating with pediatricians is the most effective way for advanced practice providers, such as nurse practitioners, physician assistants, and other qualified pediatric professionals, to support the medical home.

The incidence of fragmented care, such as that obtained from freestanding or retail-based clinics outside the medical neighborhood, is reduced by team-based care under the supervision of a physician. In fact, the pediatrician is ideally positioned at the center of the medical neighborhood, acting as the "hub" of the entire medical home. In certain cases, the pediatric surgical specialist or pediatric medical subspecialist will lead the child's healthcare team, overseeing the management of complex conditions and coordinating the team's delivery of care. For the care of the patient, family, community, and population to be as efficient, accurate, and effective as possible, cooperation between all PPHC providers working under the direction of the pediatrician is essential.

1.2.4. Evolving Health Care Delivery Models

Pediatricians are particularly well-suited to integrate PPHC into integrated health systems that "allow children to develop and realize their potential" because of their training and holistic approach. Among all medical professionals who focus on treating children, pediatricians have a special responsibility to stay informed about the broader health policy environment and make sure it takes into account the special requirements of children's health. Additionally, pediatricians are often the leaders of larger health organizations, such as accountable care organizations (ACOs), which have been demonstrated to reduce costs and enhance the quality of healthcare. In order to properly integrate this new care pathway into established medical homes, pediatricians' experience and training will be crucial, given the increased use of telehealth platforms as a result of the COVID-19 pandemic. Additionally, pediatricians are in the best position to stay up to date on matters outside of the medical home that may have an impact on children's care. Pediatricians may improve the health of their patients and the viability of child-related public policy by getting involved in the broader health care and policy sphere. This includes interacting with state legislators, agency administrators, and other advocacy organizations (Thomas Moshang, 2005; Sandra, 2007; Wetmore, 2007).

1.2.5. Recommendations for Policymakers

- Acknowledge that the pediatrician is the most qualified specialist to handle the wide range of child health issues that are brought before legislative bodies, executive branches, courts, and health systems. While other medical specialists should share their knowledge, pediatricians' education and experience are essential for guiding policy and figuring out the best ways to advance children's health.
- When making policy decisions, consult the American Academy of Pediatrics (AAP) and any pertinent state chapters. As the leading pediatric organization in the country, the AAP has decades of experience in providing pediatric healthcare, access to pediatricians, pediatric medical subspecialists, pediatric surgical specialists, and policy experts.
- Any policy change should always take into account how it will affect the health and welfare of children. Children are the most vulnerable group in our country, and those who are experiencing health disparities in particular are unable to advocate for themselves; therefore, intelligent policymakers who are able to understand the needs of children and take those needs into consideration when drafting policies are essential to ensuring their well-being.

1.3. MATERNAL AND CHILD HEALTH

The term maternal and child health (MCH) describes the conditions pertaining to mothers, newborns, kids, and teenagers. It also describes a career in public health dedicated to improving the well-being and upcoming difficulties of this susceptible group.

1.3.1. Maternal Health Problems

The health of women during their pregnancies, deliveries, and postpartum periods is referred to as maternal health. To ensure that women and their babies achieve their maximum potential for health and well-being, each stage should be a positive experience. Despite significant advancements over the previous 20 years, 287,000 women lost their lives during or after pregnancy and childbirth in 2020. This figure is simply too high. In addition to indirect causes like anemia, malaria, and heart disease, the most frequent direct causes of maternal injury and death are excessive blood loss, infection, high blood pressure, unsafe abortion, and obstructed labor. The majority of maternal fatalities can be avoided with prompt intervention by a qualified healthcare provider operating in a nurturing setting. The primary priority on the international agenda must continue to be preventing maternal deaths. However, merely making it through pregnancy and delivery cannot serve as a barometer of effective maternal health care. In order to improve health and wellbeing, it is imperative to increase efforts aimed at reducing maternal injury and disability.

Every conception and delivery are distinct. To guarantee that every woman has access to considerate and excellent maternity care, it is imperative to address disparities that impact health outcomes, particularly those related to gender and sexual and reproductive health and rights (Figure 1.1).

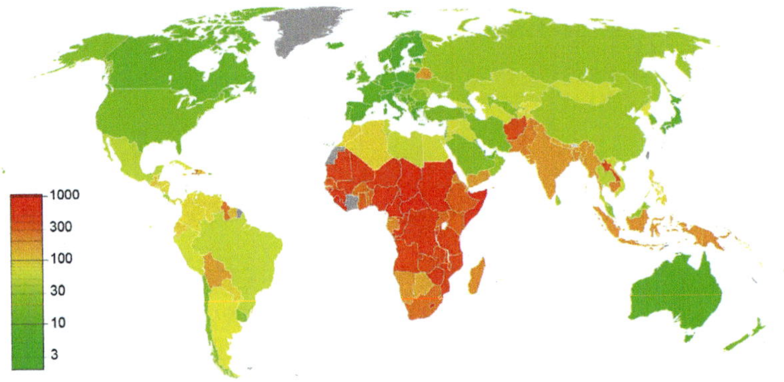

Figure 1.1. *Maternal mortality rate worldwide, as defined by the number of maternal deaths per 100,000 live births from any cause related to or aggravated by pregnancy or its management, excluding accidental or incidental causes.*

Source: By Mikael Häggström – Own work, using Gunnmap, CC0, https://commons.wikimedia.org/w/index.php?curid=20687852.

Every year, about 140 million births occur, and from 58% in 1990 to 81% in 2019, a greater percentage of these are attended by trained medical professionals. This is mostly because more births are occurring at a medical facility. In the past 20 years, there has been a 38% decrease in the number of deaths from complications during pregnancy, childbirth, and the postnatal period; however, this progress has been far too slow, with an average reduction of less than 3% annually. It also conceals enormous disparities both within and between nations.

In vulnerable and humanitarian contexts, over half of all maternal deaths take place. In 2017, 86% of all maternal deaths worldwide occurred in Sub-Saharan Africa and Southern Asia. The international community has a chance to collaborate and advance maternal health for all women, in all nations, and in all situations by working toward the Sustainable Development Goals (SDGs). The SDGs for maternal health include 3.1, which calls for the attainment of universal health coverage, and 3.8, which calls for an average worldwide ratio of fewer than 70 deaths per 100,000 births by 2030. Without universal access to reproductive, maternal, newborn, and child health care, these cannot be fulfilled.

1.3.2. Factors Influencing Maternal Health

1.3.2.1. Poverty and Access to Healthcare

A UNFPA report states that social and economic status, cultural norms and values, and geographic remoteness all contribute to higher rates of maternal mortality. In sub-Saharan Africa, the risk of maternal death (during pregnancy or childbirth) is 175 times higher than in developed countries, and there is also a greater risk of pregnancy-related illnesses and unfavorable outcomes after birth. Maternal health, child outcomes, and poverty are all related. Poverty-stricken women have higher rates of obesity and unhealthy habits like drug and cigarette use, are less likely to receive proper prenatal care or even to participate in it, and are far more likely to experience unfavorable outcomes for both the mother and the unborn child. According to a Kenyan study, hemorrhaging, anemia, hypertension, malaria, placenta retention, premature labor, prolonged/complicated labor, and pre-eclampsia are among the common maternal health issues in areas of extreme poverty.

1.3.2.1.1. Prenatal Care

Pregnancy-related medical attention as well as social, educational, and nutritional services are typically included in adequate prenatal care. For instance, blood pressure checks, uterine measurements to evaluate fetal growth, and serum integrated screening tests for possible chromosomal abnormalities could all be part of prenatal care. In a nationwide study conducted in the United States, 71% of low-income women reported that they had trouble accessing prenatal care even though there are many reasons why women decide not to receive the appropriate care for their unborn child. Furthermore, due to the correlation between education and race, Hispanic and immigrant women are more likely than white or black women to receive little to no prenatal care. In this regard, the level of education is also a risk factor. The likelihood of adolescents receiving any kind of prenatal care is very low. Insufficient funds and lack of transportation were identified by women and adolescents as the most frequent obstacles to getting appropriate prenatal care across multiple studies.

The quality of prenatal care is strongly correlated with income. The availability of prenatal care for women can occasionally be greatly impacted by factors such as transportation accessibility and closeness to medical facilities. According to an analysis of Malian maternal healthcare services, women who resided in rural areas far from medical facilities had a lower likelihood of receiving prenatal care compared to their urban counterparts. Researchers also discovered a much stronger link between prenatal and delivery care and transportation inadequacy. Materia and associates discovered comparable outcomes for proximity and antenatal care in rural Ethiopia, in addition to proximity being a predictor of access to prenatal care. Inadequate and subpar care also plays a role in rising rates of morbidity and mortality among mothers.

1.3.2.2. Pre-Existing Conditions

1.3.2.2.1. Pregestational Diabetes

Preterm birth, preeclampsia, and congenital birth defects are among the known risks associated with pre-existing (pregestational) maternal Type 1 or Type 2 diabetes. According to research from Australia and the United States, pregestational diabetes affects about 1% of pregnancies. Even a well-managed pregnancy can result in hyperglycemia. Mothers who have pregestational diabetes are therefore more likely to experience hyperglycemia.

1.3.2.2.2. HIV/AIDS

Globally, maternal HIV rates range from 1% to 40%; the highest rates are found in Asian and African nations. HIV/AIDS during pregnancy can increase the mother's health risks, even though the child's health is primarily affected by the mother's infection, particularly in nations with high rates of poverty and low levels of education. One major worry for pregnant HIV-positive women is the possibility of getting malaria or tuberculosis in developing nations. Malaria, anemia, HIV/AIDS, and cardiovascular disorders are examples of indirect causes of maternal deaths, accounting for 28% of cases. Indirect causes also include obstructed labor (Thomas Moshang, 2005; Sandra, 2007; Wetmore, 2007).

1.3.2.2.3. Maternal Weight

Women with pre-pregnancy weights ranging from 18.5–24.9 should anticipate gaining 25 to 35 pounds (11 to 16 kg) during their pregnancy. Maternal obesity is associated with higher rates of infections, respiratory problems, diabetes, and hypertension, all of which can negatively impact the course of the pregnancy. One of the biggest risk factors for gestational diabetes is obesity. According to research, mothers who are obese and lose weight (at least 10 pounds or 4.5 kg) in between pregnancies are less likely to develop gestational diabetes during their subsequent pregnancy, while mothers who gain weight are more likely to do so. Pregnant women should try to get in at least 150 minutes of exercise per week, with at least some muscle-building activities. Nonetheless, it is advised that expectant mothers speak with their OB/GYN during the early stages of pregnancy about the types of exercise they can do without risk.

1.3.2.4. Race and Ethnicity

1.3.2.4.1. Statistics

The Centers for Disease Control and Prevention (CDC) analysis of the Pregnancy Mortality Surveillance System shows notable racial and ethnic differences in pregnancy-related deaths. The number of deaths per 100,000 live births due to pregnancy or pregnancy-related causes is known as the pregnancy related mortality ratio, or PRMR. According to a CDC report from 2019, Black and Indigenous women in the US have PRMRs that are three to four times higher than White women's. The PRMR for white women was roughly 13 maternal deaths for every 100,000 live births. In contrast, the PRMRs for Black and Indigenous women were 41 and 30, respectively, per 100,000 live births. The majority of these fatalities were brought on by pregnancy-related illnesses that could have been avoided, like hypertension. Although Black and Indigenous women had a higher death rate from these diseases, the initial prevalence was similar for all racial groups. Asian and Pacific Islander women's PRMR, at 13.5, was marginally higher than that of White women, despite being lower than that of Black and Indigenous women. In recent years, the PRMR for women of Hispanic descent has decreased. State-specific data, however, indicates that Hispanic women continue to experience high rates of maternal morbidity—health issues resulting from pregnancy and childbirth.

1.3.2.4.2. Contributing Factors

The racial disparity in maternal mortality has several causes, according to the CDC. It is said that three to four contributing factors come together to cause the majority of pregnancy-related deaths. Several factors contribute to this, such as lower rates of prenatal care, lower rates of insurance coverage, and higher rates of chronic conditions in minor communities. Minority communities also have higher rates of teen pregnancies, which increases the risk of pregnancy or birth complications. Healthcare professionals may harbor racial bias against Black and Indigenous women, which could compromise the standard of care provided to treat or prevent a deadly illness. For instance, according to an NIH study, Black women have a two to three times higher risk of dying from embolisms or hemorrhages during pregnancy or the postpartum period. The racial disparity in maternal mortality can be caused by structural factors other than interactions between patients and providers. This covers the disparity in primary and preventive care access as well as other social determinants of health like community support and education.

1.3.2.5. Religion

The availability of resources and maternal health are influenced by a variety of factors. Religion is one of these elements that recent research has brought to light. For instance, one such study claimed that immigrant Muslim women in Canada received inadequate health information and care as a result of the physicians' insensitivity and ignorance.

The medical care they received from doctors did not address their cultural or religious customs, nor did it offer much in the way of emotional support or cultural adaptations. It has been established that Muslim women require greater support in order to connect with the immigrant community and receive health-related information, as well as a more secure and comfortable environment. One factor affecting the maternal health care that women from different backgrounds receive is discrimination based on religion. Studies showing the difficulties women face with regard to their religion and childrearing are not often discussed. In the context of religion, stigmatizing specific maternal and reproductive practices is not uncommon.

For instance, during a one-hour interview, a participant in a study that focused on speaking with women who had abortions used the word guilt 16 times. She stated that her upbringing as a Catholic was the reason behind her guilt. Overall, the data indicated a strong correlation between self-stigma and religion. 65% of the women who self-identified as practicing Christians made claims that demonstrated the negative impacts of self-stigma. Religious stigma and conventions are pervasive and put women at risk when seeking medical care. It has been demonstrated that certain religious customs and practices have a detrimental effect on mother health.

1.3.3. Effects on Child Health and Development

1.3.3.1. Prenatal Health

An essential component of basic maternal health care is prenatal care. It is advised that expectant mothers have at least four prenatal checkups, during which a medical professional can monitor the fetus's health and status and look for any indications of illness, such as underweight, anemia, or infection. Women receive nutrition and hygiene advice during these visits in order to maximize their health both before and after delivery. Any pre-existing medical conditions the woman may have had before getting pregnant, such as diabetes, hypertension, or renal disease, can also be maintained during these visits. The patient can work with her healthcare provider to create a birth plan that details what to do in case of an emergency and how to get help.

A relatively recent addition to prenatal healthcare, the Centering Pregnancy model (group prenatal care) has been shown to improve patient and provider satisfaction as well as birth outcomes. In particular, a randomized controlled trial (n=995) revealed a 33%decrease in preterm birth, with the reduction being even more noticeable for participants who identified as Black or African American. Pregnant women with similar due dates are given physical examinations, education, and peer support by Centering Pregnancy. There hasn't been enough research done on race concordant group prenatal care, like the EMBRACE group at UCSF, to suggest better results yet. However, it has been demonstrated that racial concordant care enhances patient satisfaction and communication between patients and providers. Additionally, racial concordance between the newborn and the physician was strongly linked to reductions in infant mortality among Black babies.

Poverty, malnutrition, and substance use can lead to cognitive, motor, and behavioral issues in children. When a mother is not healthy during pregnancy and the fetus is exposed to harmful substances, the child may experience health problems or developmental delays. The environment in which the mother supports the fetus is crucial for its well-being both during and after birth. A teratogen is any substance that can cause birth defects or impact cognitive and behavioral development. The amount, genetic factors, and timing of exposure all play a role in how severely a teratogen may affect an embryo or fetus.

Both over-the-counter medications like diet pills and prescription medications like streptomycin, tetracycline, some antidepressants, progestin, synthetic estrogen, and Accutane can have teratogenic effects on the developing embryo or fetus. Furthermore, while low-dose aspirin is typically safe, high dosages have been linked to bleeding in both mothers and fetuses.

Babies whose moms use heroin during pregnancy frequently show signs of withdrawal at birth and are more likely to experience health problems and attention deficit disorders as they get older. Stimulants like cocaine and methamphetamine used during pregnancy have been related to a host of issues for the fetus, including small head circumference and low birth weight, delays in motor and cognitive development, and behavioral issues throughout childhood. Six-year-olds whose mothers had smoked during pregnancy performed worse on an intelligence test than kids whose mothers had not, according to research published in the American Academy of Child and Adolescent Psychiatry.

There are several harmful consequences that smoking cigarettes during pregnancy can have on the development and health of the fetus. Preterm births, low birth weights, fetal and neonatal deaths, respiratory issues, sudden infant death syndrome (SIDS), and an increased risk of cognitive impairment, attention deficit hyperactivity disorder (ADHD), and other behavioral issues are common outcomes of smoking during pregnancy. Furthermore, a study in the International Journal of Cancer found that children whose mothers smoked while they were pregnant had a 22% higher risk of non-Hodgkin lymphoma.

The US Surgeon General recommends against drinking alcohol at all while pregnant, despite the fact that moderate alcohol consumption (one to two servings a few days a week) is not generally known to cause fetal alcohol spectrum disorder (FASD). Overindulgence in alcohol during pregnancy can result in Fetal Alcohol Syndrome (FASD), which is characterized by abnormalities in the child's body and mind, including learning difficulties, intellectual disability (ID), facial deformities, and defects of the heart, limbs, and face.

While there are other times when HIV/AIDS can be passed from mother to child, pregnancy is the most common period when this happens. The virus can enter the embryo or fetus during the perinatal stage by way of the placenta. There is a direct correlation between obesity in offspring through adolescence and gestational diabetes. Moreover, Type II diabetes is more likely to strike children whose moms had the disease. Pregnant women with gestational diabetes are more likely to give birth to babies that weigh 10 pounds (4.5% kg) or more. This is the reason behind macrosomia. Compared to babies of mothers without diabetes, neonates with macrosomia have noticeably higher rates of hypoglycemia. This is because high blood sugar levels during pregnancy cause macrosomic newborns to naturally have high insulin levels. When the neonates' gestational source of blood sugar is suddenly cut off at birth, their blood sugar drastically drops.

The nutrition of the embryo or fetus depends on the mother's protein, vitamin, mineral, and total calorie intake; therefore, babies born to malnourished moms are more likely to have deformities. Furthermore, there are direct and indirect effects that maternal stress can have on the fetus. Stress causes physiological changes in a mother's body that may be harmful to the growing fetus. Furthermore, the mother is more likely to participate in activities like alcohol consumption, drug use, and tobacco smoking that may have a harmful impact on the fetus.

1.3.3.2. Childbirth and Sexually Transmitted Infections

During delivery, the baby may contract enteroviruses, rubella, cytomegalovirus, varicella, parvovirus B19, and genital herpes. 25% of babies delivered through an infected birth canal suffer brain damage, and 1/3 of those babies die, in pregnancies in which the mother carries the virus. HIV/AIDS can also be passed from mother to fetus through the placenta or through contact with the mother's bodily fluids during childbirth. To lessen the chance of the virus spreading through the birth canal, mothers in developed nations frequently choose to have a cesarean section performed; however, this option is not always available in developing nations.

1.3.3.3. Postpartum Period

Out of the 136 million women who give birth worldwide each year, over eight million experience heavy bleeding after giving birth. This illness, known medically as postpartum hemorrhage (PPH), is the leading cause of maternal deaths worldwide, responsible for one in every four fatalities that occur each year. Women in developing nations are disproportionately affected by postpartum hemorrhage deaths.

An estimated 20 to 30 women experience significant complications for every woman who passes away from pregnancy-related causes. A potentially fatal condition complicates at least 15% of all births. If a woman survives such complications, she may have long-term physical, psychological, social, and financial repercussions as well as prolonged recovery times. Nearly all of these complications are treatable, despite the fact that many are unpredictable. According to results from a systematic review of the literature published in 2023, there is a connection between postpartum health outcomes and health insurance coverage. This suggests that women who have little to no coverage are more likely to experience poor postpartum health outcomes.

Many moms breastfeed their babies in the postpartum period. Breastfeeding-related HIV/AIDS transmission is a major problem in developing nations, particularly in African nations. Even though antiretroviral therapy (during pregnancy, delivery, and breastfeeding) reduces the risk of HIV transmission by more than 90%, the majority of infants who get the virus from breast milk do so within the first six weeks of life. Nonetheless, breastfeeding has several advantages for healthy moms' babies. The American Academy of Pediatrics and the American Academy of Family Physicians advise mothers to breastfeed their children for at least the first six months of their lives and for as long as is mutually desired, in contrast to the World Health Organization's recommendation that mothers breastfeed their children for the first two years of their lives. Breastfeeding babies of healthy mothers (not HIV/AIDS positive) reduces the risk of gastrointestinal and lower respiratory tract infections, otitis media, group B streptococci, hemophilus influenza, *Streptococcus pneunoniae*, Vibrio cholerae, *Escherichia coli*, *Giardia lamblia*, rotavirus, respiratory syncytial virus, and herpes simplex virus-1. Not only do breastfed babies have lower incidence of SIDS, but they also have lower rates of infant mortality. Children who are breastfed also have lower rates of obesity and conditions like childhood cancers, asthma, atopic dermatitis, Type I diabetes, and childhood metabolic disease.

In order to monitor maternal health, it is essential to follow up with women who have given birth. It is simple to put women on a follow-up and make sure they are doing well as the baby grows because healthcare facilities have records of the women who have given birth. These records are used when the women are followed to monitor the health and progress of their babies. Nutritional guidance is given along with follow-up to make sure the mother and her child are in good health. This keeps them healthy and avoids illnesses that could harm them both. Furthermore, mental health screening and support must be part of the longitudinal follow-up, since approximately 15% of women will experience postpartum depression, commonly referred to as the "baby blues," within the first year of giving birth, though the symptoms usually appear 1–3 weeks after delivery.

1.3.4. Recommended Maternal Health Practices

Prenatal health is the foundation for both maternal and fetal health care. A balanced diet that consists of an assortment of fruits, vegetables, nuts, whole grains, fish, meat, and beans is recommended by the World Health Organization as the first step towards good health. Pregnant women should also take folic acid and iron supplements on a daily basis. The US Surgeon General advises taking these supplements to help moms and babies avoid birth complications like low birth weight, anemia, hypertension, and premature birth. Folic acid should be advised as soon as possible because it can help a fetus's neural tube formation, which occurs early in gestation. Supplements containing calcium and vitamin A are also advised when these nutrients are either scarce in the natural diet or only present in low amounts; however, supplements containing vitamins D, E, C, and B6 are not advised. The World Health Organization also recommends low-impact exercise and limiting caffeine consumption to under 330 mg per day as ways to lower the risk of neonatal morbidity. Pregnant women should continue with light exercise, as it has been shown to mitigate the negative health effects, side effects, and birth complications associated with obesity. If any of the potential pregnancy side effects—which include heartburn, nausea, vomiting, leg cramps, lower back pain, and constipation—occur, the World Health Organization advises low-intensity exercise, a balanced diet, or natural herb supplements to help lessen the effects. Throughout the course of a pregnancy, the US Surgeon General advises against consuming alcohol or nicotine in any form, as well as against using it to lessen some of the previously mentioned pregnancy side effects.

Moms should receive ongoing medical care from a doctor during and after pregnancy, either in-person or through telehealth if necessary, to track the development and condition of the fetus. In order to help anticipate any potential growth abnormalities and avoid further gestational concerns, maternal health organizations recommend that pregnant women should, at the very least, undergo one ultrasound at week 24. It also states that women who are expecting should get any immunizations that they may have missed as soon as possible, such as the influenza and tetanus shots. It is possible to prevent preeclampsia in pregnant women who are at risk by taking a low-dose aspirin dietary supplement prior to 20 weeks of gestation. Because blood sugar monitoring can detect the possible onset of gestational diabetes, pregnant women should also keep an eye on their blood sugar levels. Additional tests for prenatal screening consist of nuchal translucency ultrasounds, serum integrated protein tests, and blood tests using cell free

DNA to check for chromosomal abnormalities. Mothers can also have more invasive diagnostic procedures, like an amniocentesis or chorionic villous sampling, if their medical system can offer them, in order to more accurately identify anomalies.

It is usually advised that mothers and babies stay at the hospital for 24 hours following a successful vaginal birth before leaving. It is advised to give yourself enough time to evaluate the mother and child for any potential issues, like bleeding or more contractions. The World Health Organization advises that infants should see a doctor on days 3, 7, 14, and 6 weeks following delivery. It is important to take the mother's emotional health into account during these follow-up visits. The WHO also recommends paying close attention to the possibility of postpartum depression, which affects 10–15% of mothers in 40 countries. Mothers can also get advice from a doctor regarding beginning the breastfeeding process during these check-ins.

1.3.5. Long-term Effects for the Mother

Complications from childbirth that do not result in death are among the issues related to maternal health. Approximately 20 women experience an infection, harm, or disability for every woman who passes away during childbirth. If they had access to healthcare interventions and pregnancy prevention, about 75% of women who die during childbirth would still be alive today. Pregnant black women are more likely to die from pregnancy-related causes and to receive subpar medical care.

Prior to becoming pregnant, women with chronic hypertension are more likely to experience complications like early birth, low birthweight, or stillbirth. Compared to women with normal blood pressure who experienced no pregnancy complications, those with high blood pressure who experienced complications during their pregnancy have a threefold increased risk of developing cardiovascular disease. Blood pressure monitoring during pregnancy can aid in preventing problems and subsequent cardiovascular illnesses.

In developing nations, about half of all births still occur without a medically trained attendant present to assist the mother; in South Asia, this percentage is considerably higher. The majority of women in Sub-Saharan Africa rely on traditional birth attendants (TBAs), who may or may not have received formal training in healthcare. To increase the likelihood that moms and babies will have better health outcomes, some nations and non-governmental organizations are working to train TBAs in maternal health-related subjects.

Women who breastfeed reap a number of long-term advantages. Breastfeeding women have improved blood pressure, glucose and lipid metabolism, and they lose pregnancy weight more quickly than non-breastfeeding women. In addition, type 2 diabetes, ovarian cancer, and breast cancer are less common in breastfed women. It is crucial to remember, though, that breastfeeding offers significant advantages to women who are HIV-negative. HIV/AIDS is a major cause of maternal death in nations with high rates of infection, like South Africa and Kenya, particularly in cases where breastfeeding mothers are affected. One issue is that a lot of moms who are HIV positive cannot afford formula, which means they are unable to protect their own health or prevent HIV from being passed on to the child through breast milk. In situations such as these, mothers are forced to breastfeed their children even though they are aware of the risks.

1.3.6. MCH Programs

Over the years, a wide range of public health initiatives have been developed with the goals of enhancing the health of underprivileged moms, babies, and kids and minimizing gaps in health and access to care. Some of the most important programs are mentioned below.

- **MCH Block Grant Program:** The Social Security Act of 1935's Title V permitted the use of public funds for MCH initiatives. When seven MCH programs were combined into one MCH block grant in 1981, the Title V program underwent its largest modification. State governments now oversee MCH programs, which facilitate the direct provision of MCH services in public health settings. Federal and state governments split the associated costs.
- **Medicaid:** Medicaid was established in 1965 by Title XIX of the Social Security Act with the goal of assisting low-income Americans in receiving health care. The program is jointly administered and its costs are shared by the federal and state governments. Medicaid is not so much a service delivery program as it is a financing program. States are required to provide coverage for all children up to age 19 in families with incomes below the federal poverty line, as well as for pregnant women and children six years of age and under who are living at up to 133% of that level. Medicaid, which funds EPSDT, maternity and obstetric care, and health services for kids with special needs, is by far the biggest MCH program. Women and children make up three out of every four Medicaid recipients, but they only account for one-fourth of all Medicaid spending.
- **Community and Migrant Health Center Program:** Established in 1965, the Community and Migrant Health Center Program offers primary care services to underserved populations, predominantly in rural areas. It is run locally with funding provided by the federal government. Improving the health of moms and children and lowering infant mortality are top priorities for these centers. Children under the age of 15 make up one-third of the program's clientele, and women who are capable of bearing children make up one in four.
- **The Special Supplemental Food Program for Women, Infants, and Children (WIC):** Established in 1972, WIC offers low-income expectant mothers, nursing moms, and children identified as nutritionally vulnerable additional food and education. It is funded by the federal government and administered by the U.S. Department of Agriculture. Although WIC is not technically a health care program, assessments have shown that it is beneficial in lowering infant mortality, low birth weight, anemia, and other issues.
- **Head Start, Early Head Start, and Healthy Start:** In order to guarantee that preschoolers from low-income families have a similar foundation when they enter school as their peers who are more affluent, Project Head Start was established in 1965 with the goal of fostering social and behavioral competence in these kids. Preventive health services are among the many health services offered by the program. A portion of 10% of enrolled Head Start students are designated as disabled children. Assessments have demonstrated a decrease in juvenile delinquency and an increase in

school completion rates among kids participating in the Head Start initiative. Congress created the Early Head Start program in 1994 to assist low-income families with young children. The Department of Health and Human Services' Head Start Bureau is in charge of overseeing both initiatives. Established in 1991, the Healthy Start Initiative aims to address the root causes of low birthweight and infant mortality in nearly 100 American communities by implementing a wide range of community-based interventions. The Maternal and Child Health Bureau is in charge of overseeing the Healthy Start Initiative.

- **Temporary Assistance for Needy Families (TANF) Program:** 1996 saw the U.S. The Personal Responsibility and Work Opportunity Reconciliation Act, a historic welfare reform bill passed by Congress, replaced the Aid to Families with Dependent Children (AFDC) Program with the TANF Program. The goal of TANF was to provide states with fresh chances to design and execute original and inventive plans and methods for breaking the cycle of family dependency on public assistance and enabling them to find gainful employment. Although opinions regarding TANF's effects on women's and children's health have been divided, the program has brought in more funding for mental health services. For instance, Los Angeles County used its TANF funds to establish the Long-Term Family Self-Sufficiency Plan. Programs to assist expectant mothers in accessing prenatal care as well as extra support services like parenting skills training are part of the plan.
- **State Children's Health Insurance Program (SCHIP):** In order to offer insurance to children from families whose incomes were too high for them to be eligible for Medicaid but too low for them to afford private health insurance, SCHIP was created in 1997. Just 3 million of the more than 10 million children in the US without health insurance in 1997 qualified for Medicaid before the introduction of SCHIP. SCHIP has enrolled more than 3 million children in its first three years of operation. Despite the initial slow enrollment, states have responded by coming up with creative ways to connect with children and families who don't have insurance in an effort to boost enrollment. The Health Care Financing Administration (HCFA) oversees the administration of SCHIP.
- **State Programs:** Numerous state and local governments have created their own MCH programs in addition to the ones mentioned above. Proposition 10, also known as the California Children and Families First Initiative, is one prominent example. The initiative, which was passed in 1998, raises about $700 million a year from a tobacco surtax to support early childhood development programs for kids up to age five. The funds will go toward child care programs, parental education and support services, and health care services for kids and families. It is sufficiently flexible to accommodate various approaches that transcend the conventional boundaries of MCH, a flexibility that is frequently prohibited under categorical funding and grant making, thanks to the independence of its governance structure and its broadly defined goals. There is a chance that Proposition 10 will serve as a template for other states in the country.

1.3.7. Future Challenges

As we enter the 21st century, MCH still faces numerous obstacles. Below is a description of some of the most significant areas of concern.

- **Maternal Mortality and Morbidity:** Since 1982, the decrease in maternal mortality in the US has reached a plateau. A third to half of the deaths that still happen are most likely avoidable, so this does not imply that it has reached an irreducible minimum. But maternal deaths are just the tip of the iceberg: one in four pregnant women have problems, many of which can be avoided. There needs to be a greater effort made to evaluate and guarantee the standard of care provided to expectant mothers. Similarly, more needs to be learned about the relationship between women's health and maternal health. Maternal and child health are likely to be improved most when women's health is improved throughout their lives, not just during pregnancy.
- **Infant Mortality and Morbidity:** About 3% of all live births are affected by birth defects, which are the primary cause of infant mortality. Preconceptional and early prenatal care is the best way to prevent birth defects because they are most common during the first three months of pregnancy. Most birth defects have unknown causes, necessitating more research. The majority of infant deaths and congenital neurological disabilities unrelated to birth defects are caused by low birthweight and prematurity. Additionally, they are the main reason why African Americans lose infants. Preventing low birthweight and prematurity during pregnancy has not proven to be effective in the majority of cases to date.
- **Prenatal and Preconceptional Care:** Though generally acknowledged, there is insufficient evidence to prove that prenatal care improves pregnancy outcomes, specifically in preventing low birthweight and prematurity. This may indicate that prenatal care is not given appropriately, and some researchers have started to doubt the suitability of the information included in prenatal care. It may also indicate methodological problems in the research on prenatal care. Others have maintained that the cumulative effect of lifetime exposures and habits on pregnancy outcomes cannot be undone with fewer than nine months of prenatal care. The majority of women do not seek preconceptional care prior to becoming pregnant, and a large number of medical professionals either do not know how to offer preconceptional care or only do so for those who are actively trying to become pregnant. As a result, chances to improve the outcomes of unplanned pregnancies are lost.
- **Breast-Feeding:** Breastfeeding has been shown to have numerous health benefits for both moms and babies, including increased immunity to infections, better cognitive development, and a stronger bond between the mother and child. Notwithstanding these

advantages, breastfeeding rates in the US are still low, especially for underprivileged women. Hospital campaigns promoting the WHO/UNICEF 10 Steps to Successful Breastfeeding have not been very successful. It also takes adjustments to social policy, employment practices, and cultural norms to support breastfeeding among American women.

- **Immunization:** Even though the country's childhood immunization rate has been gradually rising, it still falls short of the 90% target by the age of two, especially for children from low-income families. Experts in public health cannot agree on a plan to raise this to the point where children who are not vaccinated would be protected by herd immunity.
- **Child Care:** Over half of U.S. mothers with children under six work outside the home, and 60% of these children receive care outside their homes. Children cared for in daycare centers may receive less support for their cognitive and social development than children cared for at home, in addition to having a higher risk of infections and injuries. Support is scarce for parents who require child care, especially for families with low incomes.
- **Family Violence:** A U.S. woman's lifetime chances of experiencing physical abuse are one in five. The incidence of physical abuse by an intimate partner during pregnancy is estimated to be between 4 and 8 percent, but it could potentially reach 20%. The majority of communities lack the resources necessary to support abused women. Many medical professionals fail to screen for domestic violence or are unable to recognize it. Along with a lack of coordination between the health care, social service, and legal systems, shortages of shelter beds, social workers, and other essential services are common in communities. In half of the families where women are abused, there are also children. Although there is a lack of knowledge and action regarding primary prevention of family violence, it is evident that addressing the social and economic factors that jeopardize children and families is essential to ending family violence.
- **Unintentional and Intentional Injury:** For children and teenagers, injuries are the main cause of death, with motor vehicle accidents accounting for the majority of these cases. Drowning and fires/burns are two more causes. Of teenage injury-related deaths, homicides and suicides account for one-fourth of the cases. Little progress has been made in preventing deaths related to homicides and suicides, despite advancements in the prevention of motor vehicle injury deaths, which are mostly attributable to a decline in alcohol-related fatalities.
- **Tobacco, Alcohol, and Other Drugs:** Approximately one-third of teenagers smoke at the moment, and half have consumed alcohol in the previous month. 5% have used

cocaine, and nearly one-third have used marijuana. Teenagers who use alcohol and other drugs are more likely to sustain unintentional or intentional injuries, such as car accidents, homicides, suicides, unplanned pregnancies, STDs, and a variety of other health and social issues. The efficacy of neighborhood- and community-level interventions has not yet been proven, and the success of clinical interventions at the individual level is limited.

- **Sexual Behavior and Unintended Pregnancy:** By the time they are in the ninth grade, one-third of girls and almost half of boys in the US have engaged in sexual activity, and 20% of all adolescents in grades nine through 12 report having had four or more sexual partners. Although these figures are comparable to those in Europe, the rates of STDs and unwanted pregnancies are significantly higher among U.S. teenagers. By the time they are 20 years old, one in four sexually active teenagers will have contracted an STD. In the US, approximately one million teenage girls fall pregnant each year, and half of these pregnancies end in live births. Teenage moms are more likely to be dependent on welfare, have lower educational attainment, and earn less money in the future. Of these teenage pregnancies, two thirds happen outside of marriage.

Outside of public health, maternal and child health has advanced significantly. MCH has benefited greatly from and will continue to benefit greatly from advancements in public policy, gender and race relations, education, health care, and many other social fields. Promoting change outside of MCH's traditional bounds in order to enhance the health of moms, newborns, kids, and teenagers is a significant challenge for the field of MCH (Thomas Moshang, 2005; Sandra, 2007; Wetmore, 2007).

A Closer Look

Abortion

The removal of a fetus from the uterus before it reaches the viable stage (typically around the 20th week of gestation in humans) is known as an abortion. Abortions can happen naturally, in which case they are also referred to as miscarriages, or they can be intentionally caused, in which case they are commonly referred to as induced abortions. Miscarriages, also known as spontaneous abortions, can happen for a variety of reasons, such as illness, trauma, genetic defects, or the mother's and the fetus's incompatibility. Sometimes a fetus passes away inside the uterus without being expelled; this is known as a missed abortion.

Four general categories exist for the use of induced abortions: protecting the mother's life or her physical or mental health; stopping the continuation of a pregnancy that resulted from rape or incest; preventing the birth of a child who has a serious deformity, mental illness, or genetic abnormality; and preventing a birth for social or economic reasons (like the pregnant woman's extreme youth or the family's severely stretched resources). According to certain definitions, therapeutic, or justified, abortions are those carried out to protect the woman's health or in situations of rape or incest. There are several medical methods available for carrying out abortions. The contents of the uterus may be extracted using endometrial aspiration, suction, or curettage during the first trimester (up to roughly 12 weeks after conception). In endometrial aspiration, the endometrium—the lining of the uterus—is suctioned out using an electric pump after a thin, flexible tube is inserted up the cervical canal, or the neck of the womb.

There are several medical procedures available for performing abortions, especially during the first trimester (within the first 12 weeks of conception). Techniques such as endometrial aspiration, suction, or curettage are commonly used to remove the contents of the uterus. Endometrial aspiration involves inserting a thin flexible tube through the cervical canal and utilizing an electric pump to suction out the lining of the uterus (endometrium).

In order to induce uterine contractions, a saline solution injection can be used between weeks 12 and 19. Alternatively, prostaglandins can be administered by injection, suppository, or other means, but these drugs have the potential to have serious side effects. During the second trimester or beyond, a hysterotomy—the surgical removal of the uterine contents—may be performed. Generally speaking, a woman is more likely to die after an abortion or experience major complications the further along the pregnancy is.

A novel approach to inducing abortion was identified in the latter part of the 20th century, employing the synthetic steroid medication RU-486 (mifepristone), which bears close resemblance to the contraceptive hormone norethnidrone. The way that RU-486 functions is by inhibiting progesterone, a hormone that is essential for the growth of a fertilized egg. RU-486 efficiently starts the menstrual cycle and flushes the fertilized egg out of the uterus when taken within weeks of conception. Usually, RU-486 is taken with misoprostol, a medication that relaxes the cervix and causes contractions in the uterus. By 2020, more than half of all abortions performed in the US were performed using the two-drug combination, also known as a "medication abortion" or the "abortion pill."

The question of whether and to what degree induced abortions should be socially acceptable, promoted, or strictly prohibited has long caused disagreement among theologians, philosophers, and lawmakers. In the Greco-Roman world, abortion seems to have been a common and socially acceptable way to limit one's family. Even though Christian theologians strongly opposed abortion from the beginning, it wasn't until the 19th century that harsh criminal penalties were frequently used to discourage the practice. Throughout the 20th century, several nations altered these sanctions in one way or another: the Soviet Union in 1920, the Scandinavian nations in the 1930s, Japan and a number of eastern European nations in the 1950s. The lack of access to birth control methods contributed to the acceptance of abortion in some nations. China employed widespread abortion as a population control measure in the late 20th century. Despite strong opposition from the church, some jurisdictions decriminalized abortion in the early 21st century, like Portugal and Mexico City, while other jurisdictions, like Nicaragua, tightened restrictions on the procedure.

Throughout the 1960s, a widespread social movement advocating for the easing or abolition of laws restricting the practice of abortion led to the passage of more permissive laws in United States. In the US, in 1973, the Supreme Court decided in the case of Roe v. Wade that states' unduly restrictive restrictions on abortion were unconstitutional. This effectively allowed women to have abortions for any reason during the first three months of pregnancy. Soon after, a countermovement emerged calling for the return of tight restrictions on the conditions under which abortions might be legalized, and the matter became entangled in political and social unrest. Though it was unwilling to overturn Roe v. Wade itself, a more conservative Supreme Court maintained the legitimacy of new state restrictions on abortion in decisions in 1989 (Webster v. Reproductive Health Services) and 1992 (Planned Parenthood v. Casey). The federal prohibition on intact dilation and evacuation, a procedure for abortion that is rarely used, was also upheld by the Court in 2007. The Court reversed both Roe and Casey in a subsequent decision, Jackson Women's Health Organization v. Johnson (2022), concluding that there is no constitutional right to an abortion.

The federal Food and Drug Administration's (FDA) 2,000 approval of RU-486 was essentially nullified by an order issued by a federal district court judge in Texas in April 2023. A federal district court judge in Washington state issued an order roughly at the same time that forbade the FDA from further restricting access to RU-486 in 17 states as well as the District of Columbia. Shortly after the two rulings, the U.S. Court of Appeals for the Fifth Circuit temporarily blocked the Texas judge's finding that RU-486 had been improperly approved but declined to reverse his separate stays of measures that the FDA had taken since 2016 to make RU-486 accessible to more patients, including extending the period during which the drug could be used from 7 to 10 weeks of pregnancy and permitting the drug to be mailed to patients rather than administered at an in-person visit with a doctor. These actions included allowing the drug to be mailed to patients instead of being given at a doctor's appointment and extending the drug's use window from 7 to 10 weeks of pregnancy. The administration of Pres. The FDA approved RU-486 and has been taking steps to make the medication more widely available since 2016. Joe Biden then filed an emergency appeal with the Supreme Court, requesting that the court temporarily maintain these actions. The Supreme Court approved the administration's request a week later. December 2023 saw the Supreme Court agree to review the case Food and Drug Administration v. after the Fifth Circuit's August ruling upholding the district court's invalidation of the FDA's accessibility measures since 2016. Alliance for Hippocratic Medicine, the first significant case pertaining to abortion on its caseload since Dobbs v. The Jackson Women's Health Organization. Oral arguments in the case were heard by the Court in March 2024, and a decision was anticipated by the end of June.

The public discussion surrounding the abortion issue has brought to light the significant challenges political institutions face in addressing the nuanced and confusing ethical issues this topic raises. Abortion opponents contend that there is no logical basis for differentiating between a fetus and a newborn baby because both are completely dependent on their mothers, have the potential to become members of society, and share some human characteristics. They also oppose abortion for any reason other than saving the mother's life. Proponents of less restrictive laws on abortion contend that only a woman has the right to control her pregnancy, not the government, and that abortion is dangerous, if not lethal, when it is not legal and must be performed under medical supervision.

Summary

- The practice of pediatrics is different from that for adults as children are more than miniature versions of grownup males and females.
- Pediatric care can begin even before a woman conceives and continue through gestation and birth and into young adulthood.
- Pediatric primary health care (PPHC) always aspires to be continuous, comprehensive, and coordinated care that is accessible and affordable to meet the health needs of the infant, child, adolescent, and young adult by providing family-centered care.
- Pediatricians have received comprehensive education and training devoted to all aspects of pediatric health care. This education and training is coupled with a demonstrated interest in and total professional commitment to the health care of infants, children, adolescents, and young adults. Because of these unique qualifications, the pediatrician is a highly skilled and qualified supervisor of PPHC delivery, often partnering with other professionals to support team-based care.
- Maternal health refers to the health of women during pregnancy, childbirth and the postnatal period. Each stage should be a positive experience, ensuring women and their babies reach their full potential for health and well-being.
- Prenatal care is an important part of basic maternal health care. It is recommended expectant mothers receive at least four antenatal healthcare visits, in which a health worker can check for signs of illness - such as underweight, anemia or infection - and monitor the health and status of the fetus.
- Genital herpes, rubella, cytomegalovirus, varicella, parvovirus B19, and enteroviruses can be passed to the baby through the birth canal during delivery. In pregnancies where the mother is infected with the virus, 25% of babies delivered through an infected birth canal become brain damaged, and 1/3 die.
- Globally, more than eight million of the 136 million women giving birth each year have excessive bleeding after childbirth. This condition—medically referred to as postpartum hemorrhage (PPH)—causes one out of every four maternal deaths that occur annually and accounts for more maternal deaths than any other individual cause.
- Maternal health care and care of the fetus starts with prenatal health. The World Health Organization suggests that the first step towards health is a balanced diet which includes a mix of vegetables, meat, fish, nuts, whole grains, fruits and beans. Additionally, iron supplements and folic acid are recommended to be taken by pregnant women daily.

References

1. Ackerman, N. D., Brown, K. M., et al. (2015). Patient- and family-centered care of children in the emergency department. *Pediatrics, 135*(1), e255–e272. https://doi.org/10.1542/peds.2014-2666.
2. Akinbami, L. J., Moorman, J. E., Simon, A. E., et al. (2014). Trends in racial disparities for asthma outcomes among children 0–17 years, 2001–2010. *Journal of Allergy and Clinical Immunology, 134*(3), 547–553. https://doi.org/10.1016/j.jaci.2014.07.023.
3. Alakeson, V., & Frank, T. (2010). Health care reform and mental health care delivery. *Psychiatric Services, 61*(11), 1063. https://doi.org/10.1176/ps.2010.61.11.1063.
4. Alakeson, V., Pande, N., & Ludwig, M. (2010). A plan to reduce emergency room "boarding" of psychiatric patients. *Health Affairs (Millwood), 29*(9), 1637–1642. https://doi.org/10.1377/hlthaff.2010.0572.
5. Basch, E. (2014). New frontiers in patient-reported outcomes: Adverse event reporting, comparative effectiveness, and quality assessment. *Annual Review of Medicine, 65*, 307–317. https://doi.org/10.1146/annurev-med-010713-141500.
6. Bethell, C. (2013). Engaging families (and ourselves) in quality improvement: An optimistic and developmental perspective. *Academic Pediatrics, 13*(6 Suppl), S9–S11. https://doi.org/10.1016/j.acap.2013.08.001.
7. Cassedy, A., Fairbrother, G., & Newacheck, P. (2008). The impact of insurance instability on children's access, utilization, and satisfaction with health care. *Ambulatory Pediatrics, 8*(5), 321–328. https://doi.org/10.1016/j.ambp.2008.07.005.
8. Donnelly, L. F. (2002). *Pediatrics: Top 100 Diagnoses*. Amirsys.
9. Guevara, J., Moon, J., Hines, E., et al. (2014). Continuity of public insurance coverage: A systematic review of the literature. *Medical Care Research and Review, 71*(2), 115–137. https://doi.org/10.1177/1077558713509913.
10. Iedema, R., & Angell, B. (2015). What are patients' care experience priorities? *BMJ Quality & Safety, 24*(6), 356–359. https://doi.org/10.1136/bmjqs-2014-003391.
11. Kenney, G., & Pelletier, J. (2011). Monitoring duration of coverage in Medicaid and CHIP to assess program performance and quality. *Academic Pediatrics, 11*(3 Suppl), S34–S41. https://doi.org/10.1016/j.acap.2011.03.008.
12. Kim, S. I. (2007). *Pediatrics* (4th ed.). Lippincott Williams & Wilkins.
13. Kirk, T., Di Leo, P., Rehmer, P., et al. (2013). A case and care management program to reduce use of acute care by clients with substance use disorders. *Psychiatric Services, 64*(5), 491–493. https://doi.org/10.1176/appi.ps.201200258.
14. Kroger, A. T., Sumaya, C. V., Pickering, L. K., et al. (2011). General recommendations on immunization: Recommendations of the Advisory Committee on Immunization Practices. *MMWR Recommendations and Reports, 60*(RR-2). https://www.cdc.gov/mmwr/preview/mmwrhtml/rr6002a1.htm (accessed on 11 September 2024).
15. Markowitz, L. E., Dunne, E. F., Saraiya, M., et al. (2007). Quadrivalent human papillomavirus vaccine: Recommendations of the Advisory Committee on Immunization Practices (ACIP).

MMWR Recommendations and Reports, 56(RR-2). https://www.cdc.gov/mmwr/preview/mmwrhtml/rr5602a1.htm (accessed on 11 September 2024).

16. Neuspiel, D., & Taylor, M. (2013). Reducing the risk of harm from medication errors in children. *Health Services Insights, 6*, 47–59. https://doi.org/10.4137/HSI.S11965.
17. Okelo, S., Butz, A. M., Sharma, R., et al. (2013). Interventions to modify health care provider adherence to asthma guidelines: A systematic review. *Pediatrics, 132*(3), 517–534. https://doi.org/10.1542/peds.2013-0886.
18. Olmstead, T., Cohen, J., & Petry, N. (2012). Health-care service utilization in substance abusers receiving contingency management and standard care treatments. *Addiction, 107*(8), 1462–1470. https://doi.org/10.1111/j.1360-0443.2012.03794.x.
19. Panitch, H. B. (2005). *Pediatric Pulmonology: The Requisites in Pediatrics*. Elsevier Mosby.
20. Phillips-Salimi, C., Haase, J., & Kooken, W. (2012). Connectedness in the context of patient-provider relationships: A concept analysis. *Journal of Advanced Nursing, 68*(1), 230–245. https://doi.org/10.1111/j.1365-2648.2011.05716.x.
21. Ramphul, M., Kennelly, M. M., Burke, G., et al. (2015). Risk factors and morbidity associated with suboptimal instrument placement at instrumental delivery: Observational study nested within the Instrumental Delivery & Ultrasound randomized controlled trial ISRCTN 72230496. *BJOG: An International Journal of Obstetrics & Gynecology, 122*(4), 558–563. https://doi.org/10.1111/1471-0528.13186.
22. Sarzynski, E. M., Luz, C. C., Rios-Bedoya, C. F., et al. (2014). Considerations for using the "brown bag" strategy to reconcile medications during routine outpatient office visits. *Quality in Primary Care, 22*(4), 177–187. https://doi.org/10.1016/j.qc.2014.05.003.
23. Simon, A. E., Pastor, P. N., Reuben, C. A., et al. (2015). Use of mental health services by children ages six to 11 with emotional or behavioral difficulties. *Psychiatric Services*. Advance online publication. https://doi.org/10.1176/appi.ps.201400342.
24. Thomas, M. (2005). *Pediatric Endocrinology: The Requisites in Pediatrics*. Mosby.
25. Wetmore, R. F. (2007). *Pediatric Otolaryngology: The Requisites in Pediatrics*. Mosby/Elsevier.

Chapter

HISTORY ELICITATION AND PHYSICAL EXAMINATION

2

Contents

INTRODUCTION

The core of pediatrics is working with kids and their families. Although it might seem scary at first, consultations can be very rewarding on both a professional and personal level, and they can even be enjoyable when done well!

There are a few significant variations between adult consultations and the comparisons you may find useful.

- In general, children are less able to communicate their symptoms to you.
- Children are frequently terrified or depressed, in part due to their presenting complaint but also because the clinical setting can be very daunting.
- Communication styles need to be adjusted based on these factors because the pediatric population spans the antenatal and late teenage years.

Children typically come in with their parents or other legal guardians, and it's important to take into account how the presenting complaint will affect the entire family as well as the patient (Coulehan, 2001; DeMyer, 2009. Bickley and Lynn, 2013).

Orientation and Directional Terms

Term	Definition	Illustration
Pulse	A pulse represents the tactile arterial palpation of the cardiac cycle by trained fingertips.	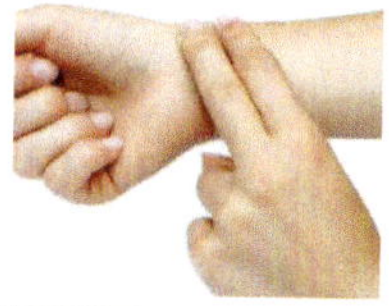
Temperature	Temperature is a physical quantity that quantitatively expresses the attribute of hotness or coldness.	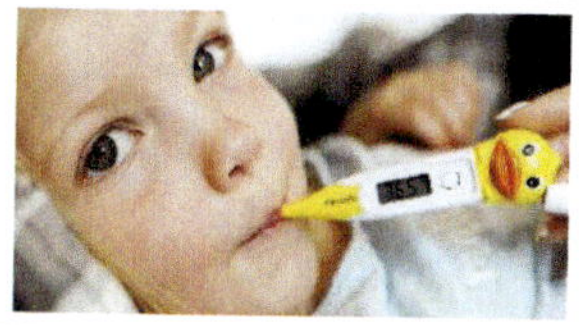
Blood pressure	Blood pressure is a measure of how forcefully your blood goes through your arteries.	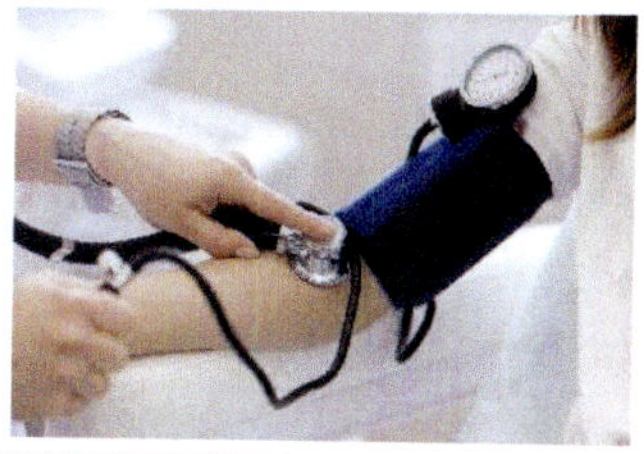
Heart	The heart is a muscular organ that is situated in the front of the chest. It pumps blood all through the body in a process called circulation.	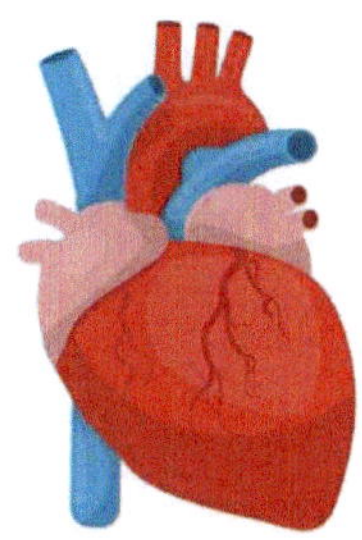
Abdomen	The abdomen is the part of the body that is between the chest and the thigh.	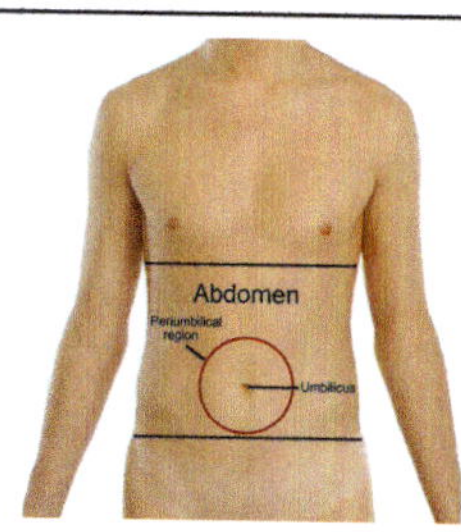

2.1. HISTORY ELICITATION IN PEDIATRICS

Studying children, particularly those who are young, calls for a unique methodology, familiarity with specific pediatric practice methods, and expertise in behavior and treatment. This applies not only to patients but also to parents who are worried about their child's health and experiencing anxiety. The Centers for Disease Control and Prevention (CDC) advises wellness visits for kids at 1, 2, 4, 6, 9, 12, 15, 18 months, 2 years, 2.5 years, and 3 years, and then every year until they turn 21.

One of the most important aspects of providing young patients with quality healthcare is gathering accurate medical histories. It serves as the cornerstone upon which medical professionals build their comprehension of the symptoms, medical history, and general health of a child. We will look at key methods and best practices in this section to help medical practitioners provide the best possible care for pediatric patients. This will guarantee thorough and efficient care.

2.1.1. Conditions for a High-quality Examination

Your reputation matters. A clean robe and tucked hair under a cap are appropriate attire for doctors. It's important to use cosmetics sparingly. Before examining any child, hands should be washed, warm, and free of short, clipped nails.

2.1.1.2. Building Trust

Establishing a relationship with the child and their parent or caregiver is the first step in gathering a pediatric history. To elicit accurate information, it is essential to establish trust and foster open communication. To help the child and their family feel at ease, establish a cozy atmosphere, speak in a language that is appropriate for their age, and practice active listening. To the extent that the child's condition permits, communication with him must occur before the examination. Elderly kids ought to get to know one another better by learning each other's names, and showing interest in their interests, habits, and hobbies.

For younger children, speak in plain English; for older children, progressively introduce more sophisticated vocabulary. Inquire in a non-aggressive way to promote truthful answers.

The doctor should:

- have an even, calm mood
- show patience, self-control
- Never lose your patience with the child, his mother, or other family members.

2.1.1.3. Involving Parents and Caregivers

To provide vital medical and developmental information about the child, parents and other caregivers are essential. To ensure that they understand the significance of their input into the diagnostic process, ask them for insights and encourage their active participation.

2.1.1.4. Prioritizing the Chief Concerns

Early on in the process of gathering a history, identify the main concerns. After the child or caregiver has expressed their primary concerns, get information about those concerns. This keeps the evaluation on target and ensures that no important information is missed.

2.1.1.5. Conditions for the Premises

You should keep the following in mind as you examine the child physically:

- To examine the patient under bright lighting, ideally during the day, with the child closer to the source of light.

- The child should be naked before the age of three, and as the study goes on, school-age children—especially girls going through puberty—should be gradually undressed. But, due to the possibility of hypothermia, the child shouldn't be left unclothed for an extended period of time;
- The room should be warm, 71–77°F (22–25°C).

2.1.2. The Process of Pediatric History-Taking

In pediatric practice, anamnesis is obtained from family members, usually the mother. However, it's crucial to question the young person directly, particularly if they are older.

The child's study begins with questioning, which goes in 5 main directions:

- Clarification of passport data (name, date of birth).
- Signs of the disease (presenting complaints).
- the earlier course of the illness's onset.
- The social history of the patient, including their living circumstances, birth history, and inheritance.
- Drug history and epidemiology (details regarding interactions with infected patients).

The initial symptom is where the collection of diseases known as amnesia starts. You should list each sign's specific characteristics along with how it changes when the other appears, all in chronological order. This section ought to encompass the outcomes of all earlier investigations, therapeutic approaches, and their efficacy. The process of gathering disease anamnesis is methodical and is enhanced with new data as the patient is observed.

These are some lists of essential questions to ask when examining children.

- Taking the Medical History of a Small Child (up to age 3):
    - How did the pregnancy of this child proceed?
    - Prenatal regime and nutrition. Was maternity leave used and how?
    - How did the birth proceed (duration, complications, mode of delivery)?
    - Did the child cry out immediately after birth?
    - Birth weight and height.
    - Characteristics of the newborn period: evaluation on the Apgar scale one and five minutes following delivery, feeding methods (free, hourly, at night, etc.), vaccinations administered in maternity hospitals.
    - Infants with borderline conditions (jaundice, uric acid infarction, natural weight loss and recovery period, etc.).
    - Illnesses that affect newborns, such as rheumatoid arthritis, birth trauma, rashes, septic illnesses, wheezing, gastrointestinal disorders, etc.).
    - The child's development dynamics include head holding, sitting, walking, and mental growth.

- Sleep, its features and duration.
- Kind of feeding (natural, artificial, mixed).

- An older Child's History Taking:
  - How did he develop at an early age?
  - The way the child acts at home and in a group, how well the child performs in school, and which subjects she/he likes to study.
  - Previous health issues and surgical procedures.
  - Preventive vaccinations.
  - Results of tuberculin tests when they are performed.
  - Sexual development of the child.
- Family History:
  - Surname, first name, and occupation if the parents.
  - The physical condition of the mother's and father's immediate relatives as well as their parents.
  - Three generations of the family tree's status, from a sick child to the grandparents, i.e., both horizontally, up to siblings, and vertically.
  - The number of children in the family and their overall health.
- Social and Living Conditions:
  - What is the occupation, total income, number of family members, and place of employment of parents?
  - Features of the living environment (heating, cooling, light, ventilation, humidity, etc.), the quantity of adults and children that are alive.
  - The caliber of child care (does the child have a separate bed, how often does he wash, is he given linen, does he have toys, a children's library, clothes appropriate for the season, does he follow the daily schedule, the diet, how long do walks and sleep for, etc.)
- Epidemiological History:
  - Find out if there have been any interactions with sick adults or kids in the neighborhood or family where you live, or get more information from the district physician.

Anamnesis of life, particularly family history, should be meticulously gathered in order to determine a child's susceptibility and risk factors for a given illness. Even in adults, this is frequently realized in later stages of ontogenesis.

Let's examine a case study of a pediatric patient's history being taken for abdominal pain (Coulehan, 2001; DeMyer, 2009. Bickley and Lynn, 2013).

2.1.3. Example of History Taking for Abdominal Pain

- Patient Information
  - Name: Sarah
  - Age: 8 years
  - Gender: Female
  - Date of Visit: July 20, 2024
- Chief Complaint

Sarah has presented with abdominal pain for the past 2 days.

- History of the Present Illness
  - When did the pain start? (2 days ago)
  - **Onset:** Was the pain sudden or gradual? (Gradual)
  - **Location:** Sarah gestures to her lower right side of her abdomen, asking where the pain is.
  - **Character:** Could you explain the nature of the pain? Sarah's mother says it's a dull, continuous ache.
  - **Intensity:** How bad is the pain, according to you, on a scale of 1 to 10? Sarah gives it a 6.
  - **Aggravating Factors:** Does anything exacerbate the pain? Sarah's mother reports that eating and moving around seem to exacerbate the pain.
  - **Alleviating Factors:** Is there anything that relieves the pain? (Sarah finds that resting and lying down help).
  - **Timing:** Does the pain always exist or does it only occasionally occur?
  - **Associated Symptoms:** Does Sarah's mother mention any other symptoms in addition to the pain? She mentions a slight nausea but no vomiting or diarrhea.
- Past Medical History
  - Has there ever been a history of gastrointestinal problems or abdominal pain? (No)
  - Has Sarah ever had surgery or been admitted to the hospital before? (No)
  - Are there any known food, supplement, or medication allergies? (No)
- Family History
  - Does the patient have a family history of digestive disorders or other pertinent medical conditions? (No).
- Social History
  - Is Sarah a regular student? (Yes, she attends the third grade).
  - Are there any noteworthy occurrences or pressures in your life lately? (No)
- Systems Review
  - Has Sarah's appetite or eating habits changed recently? Sarah's mother claims that her pain is causing her to eat less.
  - Urinary patterns or changes in bowel movements? (No unusual bowel movements or changes in urination).
  - Has there been any recent travel or contact with sick people? (No travel history or known contact with sick people).
- Developmental Milestones
  - Is Sarah reaching developmental milestones that are appropriate for her age? (Yes, she is meeting expected developmental milestones).
- **Conclusion:** Sarah, an 8-year-old girl, has lower right abdominal pain that is localized, according to the history she has provided. The pain is consistent, dull, and rated at a six out of ten. It began gradually two days ago, and eating and moving

make it worse. When Sarah lies down, she feels relieved. The only noticeable side effects are a slight nausea. Her family history and medical history are not noteworthy. It will take more investigation and a physical examination to identify the source of her stomach ache and suggest the best course of action.

Taking an accurate pediatric medical history is the first step toward providing young patients with comprehensive, individualized care. Children, in contrast to adults, frequently struggle to express their symptoms and worries intelligibly. This makes making an accurate physical examination diagnosis difficult. Healthcare providers can obtain vital information about a child's medical history, developmental milestones, family history, and any recent changes in their health status through a well-conducted history-taking session. It directs medical professionals toward the proper investigations and interventions by helping them recognize potential warning signs, early indicators of health problems, and potential risk factors (Coulehan, 2001; DeMyer, 2009. Bickley and Lynn, 2013).

2.2. GENERAL APPROACHES TO PHYSICAL ASSESSMENT

Advanced medical technology has shown to be extremely helpful in the diagnosis process, but the clinician's most crucial instruments are still a thorough history and physical examination. They are the greatest set of diagnostic tests available and are highly regarded components of the medical arts. All patients should receive a fairly thorough physical examination, regardless of the reason for the visit. Many anecdotes in medicine describe situations where an examination produced results that were unexpected and unrelated to the patient's primary complaint and concerns. Sometimes a small or insufficient examination can miss a large lesion, serious ailment, or potentially fatal condition.

2.2.1. General Principles

2.2.1.1. The Approach

The clinician should check the patient's file and verify the patient's and everyone else's identities before entering the room. By doing this, you might avoid calling the patient, parent, or caregiver by the incorrect name. The examiner should always gently open the door after knocking and waiting for a response before going inside. Little ones on the other side run the risk of being hurt by the door's impact when it is being opened or by the handle. Whether the caregiver and the clinician have met before or not, it is appropriate to greet each other politely and keep a professional yet approachable manner. In particular, if the clinician is unsure of the relationship between the caregiver(s) and the child, they should introduce (or reintroduce) themselves, as well as any colleagues or students watching or participating in the visit. They should also ask those present to introduce themselves.

Holding their caregiver makes babies over six months old and nervous toddlers who are wary of strangers much more comfortable. A soothing smile, a calm demeanor, and a toy or bright object as a distraction can help the clinician win the child over and prevent the beginning of an adversarial relationship. It is important to keep a suitable distance during the history-taking phase. When the actual physical examination is about to commence, the clinician should proceed with caution and in a non-threatening manner. Children older than 30 to 36 months who are accustomed to the examining clinician and/or have a trusting demeanor, as well as infants younger than six months who do not experience stranger anxiety, typically cooperate during the examination without being restrained. Children aged 5 to 12 make good subjects for physical examinations because they are generally cooperative and not overly fearful.

2.2.1.2. General Appearance

When visiting the patient's room, the examiner may learn a great deal about crucial social and family dynamics just by observation alone. The following terms are used to characterize a patient's overall appearance:

- Degree of comfort (calm, nervous, shy)
- State of well-being (normal, ill-appearing, distressed)
- activity level (sedate, alert, active, fidgety)
- Physical appearance (neat, disheveled, unkempt)
- Behavior and attitude (happy, sad, irritable, combative)
- Body habitus (overweight, underweight, short, tall)
- Nutritional status (malnourished, normal, corpulent)

The doctor may develop a theory based on preliminary observations that is then confirmed by physical examination results. As illustrations:

- Neglect is one possibility if there is no eye contact between the patient and caregiver, or if the patient is uninterested and does not smile socially. Psychosocial support might be necessary.
- When a child seems sick, the doctor should take note of the patient's favored posture.
- An acute abdomen may be present in a child who lies motionless on the examination table, responds verbally, but winces conspicuously when they are moved.
- When a dyspneic patient sits up straight, leans forward slightly, and puts their hands on their knees, they may be going through an asthma attack or another respiratory distressing event.
- When a baby cries, pay attention to the tone and volume of the cry.
- A loud, resilient cry is comforting.
- A feeble and listless cry could be a sign of a very sick baby.
- An intense, high-pitched cry could be a sign of a strangulated inguinal hernia, elevated intracranial pressure, a reaction to a painful injury, a toxic reaction, or other serious conditions.

Observe the breathing pattern of the patient. Primary pulmonary disease or respiratory compensation for metabolic acidosis may be the underlying cause of rapid, shallow breathing in a patient who does not appear to be in acute distress. Before making any physical contact with the child, even when taking a history, the examiner should assess the child's developmental state. The patient's response to sounds, speech pattern, motor function, and interactions with people and objects in the environment all provide indicators of whether or not the patient is developing normally and doesn't require a more thorough developmental evaluation.

2.2.1.3. History

When it comes to patients in the neonatal through early childhood age range, historical information is almost entirely dependent on the caregiver. Although patient comments are frequently relevant, the clinician still has to rely primarily on the caregiver to obtain pertinent information regarding a 5- to 12-year-old child. Adolescent patients should, when possible, spend some time alone with the clinician without the presence of caregivers. This will allow for a more candid discussion of important medical history, preventive care concerns, and guidance ahead of time.

Creating a friendly, caring environment and asking questions in a calm, non-aggressive way are important components of taking a history. The examiner's vocabulary and style should be suitable for the patient's and caregiver's level of health literacy. Maintaining eye contact and a feeling of complete focus is important. The doctor should take a comfortable seat across from the patient and/or caregiver, away from any big furniture like desks or tables. The amount of time that the medical staff and phone calls interrupt outside patients should be minimized. Clinicians should disclose that they might occasionally need to consult the written or electronic medical record to review imaging reports, laboratory results, or other relevant information before starting the history. A concerted effort should be made to keep the conversation flowing, take minimal notes, and try not to turn away from the patient or caregiver to review the medical record.

2.2.1.4. Physical Examination

It is recommended that examiners thoroughly wash their hands both before starting and following the examination. When it's appropriate, protective gloves should be worn. Competent medical professionals use a variety of strategies to win over pediatric patients. When examining young children, infants, and toddlers, the use of toys, distracting objects, and pictures can be helpful. Often, telling stories to a two- to four-year-old or having a conversation about imaginary animals works well as a diversion. Depending on the examination stage, food can be used as a pacifier in the form of liquid refreshments or chewable snacks.

When a child over four years old who is normally well-behaved refuses to cooperate during an examination—even when a familiar caregiver is present—it could be a sign of a traumatic past encounter between the patient and another examiner or a sign that the current examiner needs to try a different approach. If a child is over four and very uncooperative or combative, there may be an underlying psychosocial issue or behavior disorder to take into account. The examiner should explain what will be done during the examination to patients who are old enough to understand but who seem nervous. They should also be allowed to view and handle any instruments that will be used. It is important to alert elderly patients ahead of time to possible pain or discomfort.

A parent or guardian should be present when an infant, toddler, or child is being examined; if the parent or guardian's presence could interfere with the examination (for example, if there is a suspicion of child abuse), a chaperone should be present. When examining the anorectal and genital regions, as well as the breasts, of adolescents, both male and female, a chaperone should be used. The doctor should give a brief explanation of the purpose of the examination as well as its methodology. When it comes to the patient's comfort and wishes, the chaperone's gender should be chosen (if possible). A staff member would be preferable to a family member as the chaperone. The medical record should specify the chaperone's role and identity.

The examination should be completed last if the patient presents with a complaint, sign, or symptom that seems to involve a specific anatomical area. For instance, if a patient reports right lower quadrant abdominal pain that is suspected to be caused by appendicitis, the clinician may be able to distract the patient from the affected area and rule out other potential causes of the pain by not first examining that part of the body.

Respecting patient privacy is important. Allow the patient to stay clothed until a particular area of the anatomy needs to be examined if they object to being undressed or to wearing an examination gown. The patient should be asked to take off or remove any clothing that is obstructing their ability to see, feel, or hear sounds in the affected area. The sequence in which the physical examination is performed is frequently determined by the examiner's preference and is age-specific. A clinician may choose to start with an examination of the eyes in an infant or younger child, noting the red-light reflex, extraocular eye muscle movements, and visual tracking. Then, the clinician may proceed to other parts of the body or organ systems before performing the often delicate ear examination. The examination may start at the head and work its way down the body, finishing with the neurologic examination for the older, more cooperative child. Typically, the pediatric examination starts with the parts that need the patient's cooperation the most: taking their blood pressure, auscultating their heart and lungs, and doing an eye and neurologic examination. The more uncomfortable parts of the examination, which include the measurement of head circumference and examinations of the abdomen and ears, come after these.

2.2.1.5. Primary Assessment

Every shift should begin with a primary assessment, which should also be done whenever clinically indicated or if the patient's condition changes. This evaluation is recorded in flowsheets; additional evaluations or modifications are recorded in progress notes. Using clinical judgment, one should determine the necessary scope of the assessment (Allan and Max, 2003; Lissauer and Carroll, 2018; Guidelines for Protecting Children: 2020).

Information from the primary assessment comprises, but is not restricted to (Table 2.1):

Table 2.1. American (AAN) and European (EAU) DoC Practice Guideline Recommendations Addressing Neurobehavioral Assessment

Recommendations to improve diagnostic accuracy	• Use standardized serial assessment deemed reliable by American Congress of Rehabilitation Medicine.
	• Reassessment intervals dependent upon patient presentation (AAN)
	• Optimize patient arousal prior to assessment, especially when observed to be diminished (AAN)
	• Use of mirror to diagnose visual pursuit (EAN).
	• Observe for spontaneous motor behaviors to diagnose signs of consciousness (EAN).
	• Use of FOUR consciousness assessment in ICU (EAN).
	• Use of CRS-R for consciousness assessment in subacute and ICU (EAU).

Recommendations to mitigate diagnostic confounds	• Use multi-modal assessment tools when bedside assessment results are unclear (AAN).:
	• Utilize serial assessment results to identify and address complications (AAN).
	• Use of PET, FMRI, EEG to identify covert consciousness and differentiate between UWS/MCS (EAN).
Recommendations related to prognosis	• Utilize serial standardized assessment inform prognosis (AAN).
	• Use CRS-R to inform prognosis with non-traumatic vegetative state presentation (AAN).
	• EAU does not provide Guidelines addressing prognosis.

Adapted from Giacino et al. (2018), Kondziella et al. (2020).

Source: Murtaugh B and Shapiro Rosenbaum A (2023) Clinical application of recommendations for neurobehavioral assessment in disorders of consciousness: an interdisciplinary approach. Front. Hum. Neurosci. 17:1129466. doi: 10.3389/fnhum.2023.1129466.

2.2.2. Examination by System

Depending on many variables, the examination's focus will change (indications, age of the child, etc.). The following is a list of some crucial elements of the pediatric examination in the primary systems.

2.2.2.1. Cardiovascular System

If the child is calm and cooperative, it might be a good idea to begin the examination at this point. Allowing the child to stay sitting or held in a caregiver's lap will comfort them:

- Start by taking notes on the character, strength, rhythm, and pulse rate.
- Make sure the capillary refill time is less than two seconds by checking for central perfusion.
- Feel and rape the front of the chest wall to determine the size of the heart and the location and rhythm of the peak beat.
- Find out if there are any thrills as well.
- The first heart sound, the second heart sound, the sounds in between these, and any murmurs in between heart sounds should all be heard.
- Observe the occurrence, nature, volume, location, and dispersion of any murmurs.
- Verify whether the neck is being affected by this.
- Take a blood pressure reading if you suspect heart or kidney disease.

2.2.2.2. Respiratory System

Observe the respiratory rate and the diaphragm and chest wall's movement when breathing quietly and when exerting more force on your respiration (as required by an older child or when a baby is crying). Examine the breathing effort: are accessory muscles being used, or are there intercostal or subcostal recessions?

To find out if the lung is overinflated, tap the top edge of the liver.

In the very young, breath sounds and other noises can be challenging to interpret. Depending on the location, kind, and narrowness of the aperture, noises can range from fine, high-pitched to low, coarse.

- When a baby appears normal, careful auscultation may reveal crepitations, which are tiny crackling noises made during inspiration. When a distressed toddler exhibits persistent, bilateral crepitations, it usually indicates bronchiolitis or, less frequently, left heart failure.
- Rales, which are irregular noises made during inspiration and expiration, typically signify liquid debris in the larger airways and can be emitted from the throat's back.
- Children are less likely to experience rhonchi, which are harsh noises that are added to breathing sounds and indicate a more persistent obstruction.
- The main airway is typically the source of bronchial breathing, which is characterized by continuous noises over the baby's upper back that harden and extend the breath sounds.
- A stridor is a harsh sound that comes from the upper respiratory tract, as in croup cases. Usually, inspiration is when it happens.
- Wheezing is a condition in which the airways narrow in the middle. It can be unilateral due to airway obstruction, such as that caused by a foreign body, or bilateral due to asthma or viral wheeze. Usually, it's expiratory.

2.2.2.3. Ear, Nose and Throat Examination

Probably the most often studied system is this one.

- A young child should ideally be sat sideways on the parent's lap with one hand holding the child's hands and the other holding the child's head, with one ear pressed against the parent's shoulder while the other ear is examined.
- A tongue depressor can be used to see into the throat of a stubborn toddler by being inserted between the clamped teeth and cheek. For a moment, the teeth might open, enabling you to skillfully insert the tongue depressor. Usually, it is best to save this until the very end of the test.

2.2.2.4. Gastrointestinal System

Initially, examine the abdomen, searching for any swellings or motions.

- Ask if there is any tenderness, and while you palpate the abdomen, try to keep an eye on the child's face. Ask the child to swell up their stomach ('like a balloon') before you palpate if the child is experiencing systemic illness and there is tenderness. Without physically touching the child and inadvertently harming them, this could cause rebound.

- To systematically ascertain the location and dimensions of the liver, spleen, kidneys, and bladder, palpate the four quadrants.
- Take note of any enlarged organ's location, dimensions, surface, texture, and, if present, the nature of its edge and tenderness.
- Examine whether a digital rectal examination is necessary, then inform the parent or parents.
- Check the child's fluid intake, especially if they have experienced vomiting or diarrhea in the past. In early babies, the fontanelle may be depressed, the skin turgor may be diminished, and the eyes and lips may appear dry and sunken if dehydration progresses.

2.2.2.5. Musculoskeletal System

- Keep an eye out for any unusual curvature or spinal deformities, especially on the lower end.
- Pay close attention to the sacrum of small babies and keep an eye out for any hairy naevi or sinuses.
- Recognize typical variations in gait, such as "in-toeing," femoral anteversion, genu valgus, genu varus, and so forth.
- Precise inspections of the feet and hips.

2.2.2.6. Central Nervous System

Examine the child's motor skills, speech and language, and social interaction during the consultation to determine if they are developing normally. Take note of any particular worries that the parent or parents may have expressed.

In newborns and infants, the anterior fontanelle should always be palpated. Make note of any pulsation and whether it is typical.

- By the midpoint of the second year, the fontanelle ought to close. It must be either flat or full.
- Take note of the child's ability to hear, see, move their head and eyes freely in all directions, move all of their limbs, and determine whether or not these movements are full and normal.
- Check to see if each limb's shape and location are normal and have adequate strength. As you handle the child, pay attention to the limb's tone of movement and any limitations.
- If the joints are excessively flexible and lax, take note. Move the limbs while keeping an eye on the child's face.

Using the percussion finger instead of a hammer, you might be able to elicit reflexes, though this is rarely helpful (Allan and Max, 2003; Lissauer and Carroll, 2018; Guidelines for Protecting Children: 2020).

2.2.3. Examination at Different Ages

The examination will be broken down by age group. These are not meant to be comprehensive checklists; rather, they are meant to draw attention to key components of the examination in these particular age groups, especially in cases where there are significant variations from adult examinations. The specific objectives and purposes of the examination mentioned above will dictate the focus and specifics of any examination.

All children undergo only the newborn and six-week checkups.

- Newborn babies.
- 6-week-old babies.
- 7- to 9-month-old babies.
- Toddlers or children aged under 2 years.
- Pre-school children.
- School-age children.
- Adolescents.

2.2.3.1. Newborn Babies

It is frequently necessary to perform a precise and thorough set of checks, observations, and measurements on newborns and neonates (those younger than four weeks old), in addition to getting a thorough medical history from the parents. At six to eight weeks of age as well as upon birth, babies undergo routine examinations and checks.

2.2.3.2. 6-Week-Old Babies

- Important Elements of the Analysis:
  - The assessment is comparable to that of a newborn.
  - Talking about feeding progress is necessary.
  - Ask the parent(s) for their thoughts and address any concerns they may have.
- Growth:
  - Plotting should be done for weight, length, and head circumference.
  - Disturbances from centiles ought to be examined and investigated further.
- Development:
  - Every baby should have their milestones reviewed in brief.
- General Examination:
  - The guidelines and procedures are the same as those described for infants and young children.
  - Hips could be checked once more.

2.2.3.3. 7- to 9-Month-Old Babies

- Important Aspects of the Examination:
  - Doctors see this age group regularly.
  - From approximately three months of age, viral infections are prevalent.
  - It's a time of tremendous development and expansion.
  - In this age group, routine examinations are no longer typically carried out.
  - Growth and development assessments are typically made opportunistically.
- Growth:
  - Growth is extremely quick, doubling the birth weight on average in just five months.
  - Plotting length and weight and comparing the results to earlier readings is necessary.
  - In this age group, getting an accurate measurement can be very challenging.
- Development:
  - When there are worries about their child's developmental

progress, parents frequently come with their kids.

- This is a time of fast developmental advancement.
- It is best to review developmental milestones when the opportunity arises. For instance:

- It should have been socially smiling by eight weeks.
- Eight months is when children should be able to sit unassisted.
- By eight months old, children should be babbling.
- General examination:
  - Common skin conditions like eczema and viral infections can both cause rashes.
  - Important rashes (like the purpuric rashes of meningococcal septicemia, idiopathic thrombocytopenic purpura, and Henoch-Schönlein purpura) should be known to doctors.
- Cardiovascular examination:
  - Heart rate variations primarily control cardiac output (as with newborn and younger babies). Tachycardia is a significant symptom that requires clarification.
- Respiratory examination:
  - This is a common practice for people in this age range.
  - Again, observation is crucial.
  - Differentiating between stridor and wheeze is crucial.
- Gastrointestinal examination:
  - Once more, observation is crucial. For instance, a child with peritonitis will lie motionless, flexing their knees and breathing shallowly.
  - If necessary, examine the anogenital region. As kids get older, this examination gets harder and harder and needs to be handled carefully.
  - A sick child's abdomen cannot be palpated; instead, warm hands and assurance are required.
- An analysis of development and neurology
  - A formal examination is quite challenging. Many times, improvisation is necessary.
  - The examination of cranial nerves involves observation, such as facial and behavioral movements. In this age range, there are various abnormalities of the cranium nerve:

- Bell's palsy.
- impairment of the eighth cranial nerve (sensorineural deafness).
- Convergent squint, a sixth cranial nerve deficit, accompanied by elevated intracranial pressure.

2.2.3.4. Toddlers

Important aspects of the examination:

- Toddlers are babies who are under two years old but have typically been walking for more than a year.
- Once more, this group confers frequently.
- Attendance will probably be dispersed among various locations (e.g., hospitals, primary care, clinics, walk-in centers).

- Effective communication is crucial between these various agencies.
- Rapid development and growth occur.
- Monitoring growth and development will frequently need to be done on an as-needed basis.
- In this age group, genu varus is physiological.
- Growth:
  - Beginning at the end of the first year, growth slows.
  - As the brain grows through myelination in cortical areas, the head grows quickly.
- Development:
  - Important milestones should be identified. Briefly:
- During the first year, hand dexterity and visual acuity both increase from palmar to pincer grip. It is possible to build a six-brick tower by the second year.
- At 18 months, speech progresses from babbling to six or more words, and in the second year, it reaches short phrases.
- About a year can follow basic instructions due to comprehension.
- By the time they are one year old, they have gone from crawling to cruising to walking (before 18 months).
- General examination:
  - Examining infants on a parent's lap and building a comfortable relationship is usually the best approach.
  - Play will help to make the examination easier.
  - It might be essential to be extremely picky and look at significant or pertinent systems first.
  - Save the more invasive or uncomfortable tests (such as throat exams) for last.
- Cardiovascular examination:
  - Refer to normal values.
  - Identify innocent murmurs (often heard).
- Respiratory examination:
  - Note and recognize the typical breathing pattern, rate, and sounds.

The gastrointestinal examination, neurological and developmental analysis are as previously mentioned.

2.2.3.5. Pre-School Children (Age 2 to 5 Years)

- Important aspects of the examination:
  - Additionally, this age group comes in a lot for advice and medical care.
  - Attendance will be required due to illness and, more often, accidents.
  - Once more, for an easier examination, rapport and confidence need to be built

and maintained. Future exams can be prepared for by developing trust.

- This genu valgum of this age group is physiological.

- Growth:
  - At this point, growth is slowing.
  - Centile charts ought to be utilized and examined.
- Development:
  - The areas with the biggest improvements are language usage and communication abilities.
  - Every child should have their language skills briefly assessed.
- General examination:
  - Once more, usually accomplished by sitting on a parent's lap or by being near the parent.
  - As procedures are carried out, provide explanations and commentary. Respond to inquiries; at this age, they are typically quite observant.
- Cardiovascular examination:
  - In this age range, exams are simpler.
  - Once more, quiet whispers are typical.
  - Slower heart rates make it easier to identify heart sounds.
- Respiratory examination:
  - Once again, observation is crucial.
  - Before the age of five, peak flow measurement is not very accurate.
- Gastrointestinal examination:
  - Examining while kneeling next to the patient is usually the most effective.
  - Youngsters might prefer to have their hands palpated beneath the examiner's.
- Hip and knee examination:
  - At this age, irritable hip and other hip conditions can develop and need to be evaluated.
  - At this age, reassurance is frequently needed for normal genu varus (physiological in toddlers) and valgus (physiological in preschoolers).
- Neurological and developmental examination:
  - This is getting closer to what is achievable in adulthood.
  - By matching letters or shapes, a three-year-old's vision can be evaluated.
  - The replication time of a circle is 3 years, a cross is 4 years, a square is 4+5 years, and a triangle is roughly 5 years.

2.2.3.6. School-Age Children (From 5 to 10 Plus Years)

- Key elements of the assessment:

- Doctors examine people in this age group less frequently.
- Problem presentation starts to involve more and more psychological elements.

• Growth:
- The pubertal growth spurt will precede steady growth.
- Expressions of concern regarding development and growth in connection to puberty may start.

• Development:
- The behavioral and social dimensions of development gain significance.
- Aspects of development that are closer to adulthood exist.

• Examination:
- Nowadays, the examination differs little from that of an adult.

2.2.3.7. Adolescents (From the Onset of Puberty) (Table 2.2)

• Important aspects of the examination:
- Adolescents seldom come for medical advice.
- Building rapport and effective communication can be challenging.
- Psychological aspects are probably going to be crucial.
- Adolescents tend to be highly self-conscious, which can make an adequate examination difficult.
- The presence of a chaperone is advised.
- Consent and confidentiality take on greater significance.

• Growth:
- Growth picks up speed during puberty.
- Recognizing normal and abnormal puberty is important.

• Examination:

The examination is extremely similar to what adults do (Sharma and Cockerill, 2014).

Table 2.2. The Most Often Used Pain Scales in Pediatrics

Acronym	Age Range
CHIPPS	Under 5 years
CHEOPS	1–7 years
FLACC	2 months–7 years
OPS and MOPS	8 months–13 years
Poker Chip Tool	From 3 years
Oucher Scale	3–12 years
Wong-Baker FACES® Pain Rating Scale	From 3 years
FPS-R	From 4 years
VAS	From 5 years
NRS	From 8 years

Abbreviations: CHIPPS (Children and Infants Postoperative Pain Scale); CHEOPS (Children's Hospital of Eastern Ontario Pain Scale); FLACC (Face, Legs, Activity, Cry and Consolability); OPS/MOPS (Objective Pain Scale/Modified Objective Pain Scale); FPS-R (Faces Pain Scale—Revised); VAS (Visual Analog Scale); and NRS (Numeric Rating Scale).

Source: Sansone L, Gentile C, Grasso EA, Di Ludovico A, La Bella S, Chiarelli F, Breda L. Pain Evaluation and Treatment in Children: A Practical Approach. Children. 2023; 10(7):1212. https://doi.org/10.3390/children10071212.

A Closer Look

First Aid for Fracture Medication Administration

Giving children oral medicine can be a difficult task in and of itself. Oral liquids can be administered to infants mixed with a small amount of milk or formula through a bottle nipple after measurement with the proper equipment, or to older children mixed with a small amount of edible food or drink before administration. Oral liquids can also be simply spit into the cheek, which has no taste buds, and then followed by a drink of something edible. Rinsing the mouth after using iron liquid is crucial (if the medication has been diluted in a liquid, use a straw as well). Iron liquid can stain teeth. Keep in mind that while these safety measures are not necessary for newborns without teeth, they are crucial for those who have permanent teeth.

Oral medication administration is made easier when a child can swallow oral solid dosage forms, which typically happens around age 5 or 6. Children who have trouble swallowing pills can practice by using candies that get bigger (e.g., begin with sprinkles and gradually increase the size of the candies until they reach the desired tablet size). Most medications can be adequately sized by using small jelly beans. To help with this, children can drink a large amount of liquid, tilt their heads back, and place the medication or candy on the back of their tongue. In rare circumstances, infants and young children who receive the proper guidance from licensed professionals may be able to swallow small oral dosage forms. Levothyroxine is one medication where part-tablets are the recommended dosage form and crushed tablets and suspensions might not offer the required accuracy.

Prescription drugs to be given through feeding tubes e.g., palatability issues; however, the intestinal site of the medication administration should be taken into consideration in the context of the intestinal administration site (e.g., nasogastric tubes, gastrojejunal tubes) to make sure the drug can be absorbed if given into the jejunum), and the tubes should be cleaned with water afterward to guarantee that the entire dosage has been delivered.

Summary

- The study of children, especially at an early age, requires a special approach, knowledge of certain techniques used in pediatric practice, and skills in behavior and treatment.
- Pediatric history-taking begins with building a rapport with both the child and their parent or caregiver. Establishing trust and open communication is crucial to eliciting accurate information.
- Pediatric practice collects anamnesis from relatives, most often from the mother. Nevertheless, it is important to question the child himself, especially if the child is older.
- A relatively complete physical examination should be performed on each patient, regardless of the reason for the visit. Numerous medical anecdotes relate instances in which the examination revealed findings unrelated to and unexpected from the patient's chief complaint and major concerns.
- Before entering the room, the clinician should review the patient's record and confirm the identity of the patient and others in the room. This may avoid greeting the patient, parent, or caregiver by the wrong name.
- The examiner should evaluate the developmental status before touching the child, including during history taking. The patient's motor function, interaction with surrounding objects and people, response to sounds, and speech pattern give clues about whether the patient is developing typically or is in need of a more comprehensive developmental assessment.
- Primary assessments should be completed at the start of every shift and then as clinically indicated or if the patient's condition changes. This assessment is documented in flowsheets, further assessments, or changes to be documented in the progress notes. Clinical judgment should be used to decide on the extent of assessment required.
- The emphasis of the examination will vary depending on various factors (indications, age of the child, etc.).
- The examination will be outlined in different age groups. These are not intended to be exhaustive checklists but aim to highlight important aspects of the examination in the selected age groups, particularly where there are notable differences to adult examination.

References

1. Allan, M. A. (2003). *History and Examination* (2nd ed.). Mosby.
2. Bickley, L. S. (2013). *Bates' Guide to Physical Examination and History-Taking.* Wolters Kluwer Health/Lippincott Williams & Wilkins.
3. Coulehan, J. L. (2001). *The Medical Interview: Mastering Skills for Clinical Practice* (4th ed.). F.A. Davis Co.
4. DeMyer, W. (2009). *Taking the Clinical History: Eliciting Symptoms, Knowing the Patient, Ethical Foundations.* Oxford University Press.
5. Department of Health. (2019). *National Action Plan for the Health of Children and Young People: 2020–2030.* Government of Western Australia.

6. Department of Health: Child and Adolescent Health Services. (2020). *Guidelines for Protecting Children: 2020*. Government of Western Australia.
7. Duderstadt, K. (2019). *Pediatric Physical Examination: An Illustrated Handbook* (3rd ed.). Elsevier Health Sciences.
8. Feigelman, S. (2018). Developmental and behavioral theories. In *Nelson's Textbook of Pediatrics* (21st ed., pp. 117–123). Elsevier.
9. Fishman, J. M. (2005). *History Taking in Medicine and Surgery*. PasTest.
10. Frank, A. L. (2001). *Taking an Exposure History*. U.S. Dept. of Health & Human Services, Public Health Service, Agency for Toxic Substances and Disease Registry.
11. Hagan, J., Shaw, J., & Duncan, P. (2020). *Bright Futures: Guidelines for Health Supervision of Infants, Children and Adolescents* (4th ed.). [eBook]. https://doi.org/aappublications.org/bright-futures-guidelines.
12. John, B. (2008). *History and Examination* (3rd ed.). Mosby.
13. Lissauer, T., & Carroll, W. (2018). *Illustrated Textbook of Paediatrics* (5th ed.). Elsevier.
14. Sharma, A., & Cockerill, H. (2014). *From Birth to Five Years: Practical Developmental Examination*. Taylor & Francis.
15. Sharma, A., & Cockerill, H. (2014). *From Birth to Five Years: Children's Developmental Progress* (4th ed.). Routledge.

Chapter 3

NEWBORN CARE

Contents

INTRODUCTION

A baby's first four weeks of life are referred to as the neonatal period. During this time, the infant interacts with various stimuli and undergoes numerous complex physiologic changes. Efficacious and ongoing care should be provided during this time. The provision of prophylactic medication and vaccinations, assessment of the need for resuscitation, a thorough physical examination, appropriate feedings, secure sleep, newborn hygiene, and other critical areas for baby wellness comprise newborn care.

Orientation and Directional Terms

Term	Definition	Illustration
Neonatal jaundice	Neonatal jaundice is yellow discoloration found on a newborn baby's skin and eyes. It occurs due to an excess of bilirubin —a yellow pigment of red blood cells— in the baby's bloodstream. It is a common condition, particularly in premature babies and some breast-fed babies, which usually occurs when a baby's liver is not developed enough to get rid of the excess bilirubin in the blood.	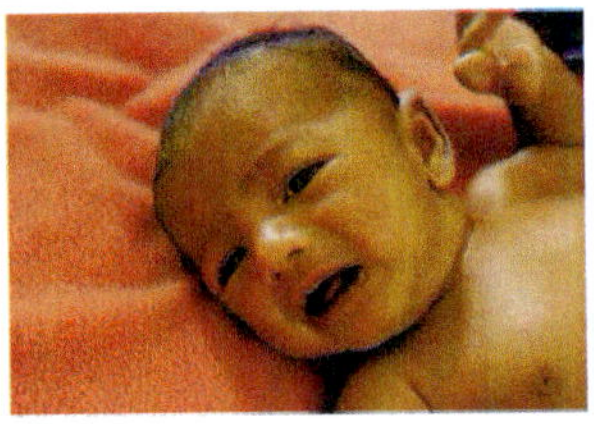
Sepsis	Neonatal sepsis is a blood infection that occurs in infants younger than 90 days old. Early-onset sepsis is diagnosed in the first week of life, usually within 24 to 48 hours of birth, while late-onset sepsis occurs after 1 week until 3 months of age.	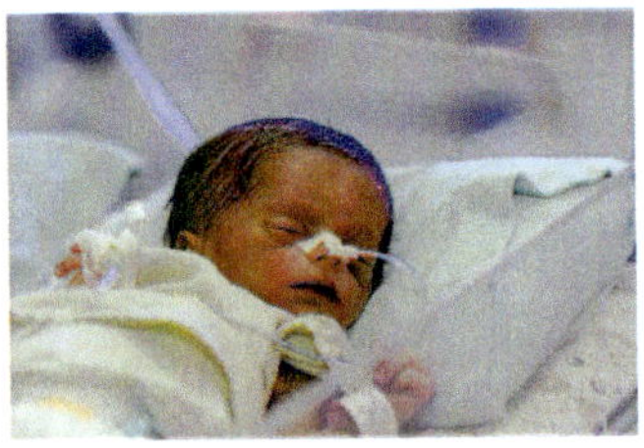
Congenital hypothyroidism	Congenital hypothyroidism (CH) is defined as thyroid hormone deficiency present at birth. CH must be diagnosed promptly because delay in treatment can lead to irreversible neurological deficits.	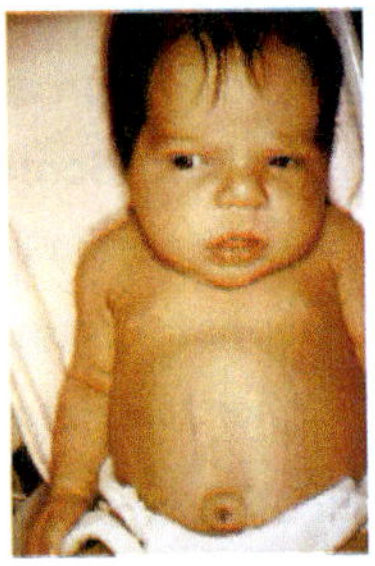
Down's syndrome	Down syndrome is a genetic condition where a person is born with an extra copy of chromosome 21.	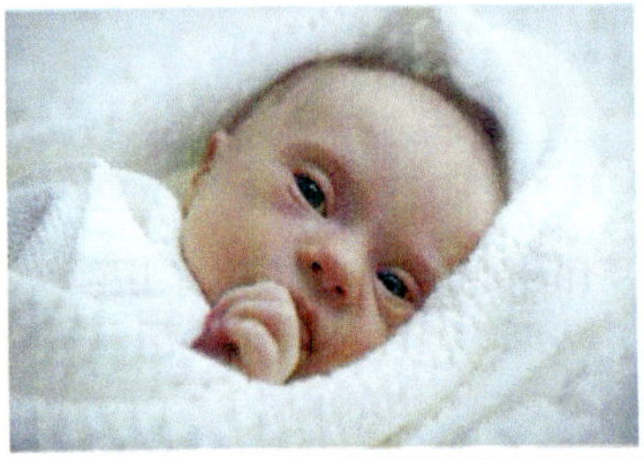

3.1. PERINATAL-NEONATAL NOMENCLATURE

In the neonatal unit, a lot of new vocabulary will be used. Many of these terms and words may be entirely unfamiliar to you. Many new terms that you might not be familiar with will be used (Table 3.1).

Table 3.1. Alberta's Newborn Screening Panel

Classification	Disorders	Screening Initiated	Assay and Instrumentation
Metabolic Disorders—Organic Acid	GA1	2007	PerkinElmer NeoBase™ Non-derivatized MSMS kit PerkinElmer NeoBase™ Succinylacetone Assay Solution Waters™ ACQUITY UPLC™ with XEVO™ TQD
	HMG deficiency	2007	
	IVA	2007	
	MMA	2007	
	PA	2007	
Metabolic Disorders—Fatty Acid Oxidation	CUD	2007	
	LCHAD deficiency	2007	
	MCAD deficiency	2007	
	TFP deficiency	2007	
	VLCAD deficiency	2007	
Metabolic Disorders—Amino Acid	CIT	2007	
	MSUD	2007	
	PKU	1967	
	TYR1	2019	
Metabolic Disorders—Other	BIOT	1990	PerkinElmer Neonatal Biotinidase kit PerkinElmer VICTOR2 ™D Instrument
	GALT	2019	PerkinElmer GSP® Neonatal GALT kit PerkinElmer GSP® Neonatal Total Galactose kit PerkinElmer GSP® Instrument
Endocrine Disorders	CAH	2007	PerkinElmer AutoDELFIA® Neonatal 17α-OH-progesterone kit PerkinElmer AutoDELFIA® Instrument
	CH	1977	PerkinElmer AutoDELFIA® Neonatal hTSH kit PerkinElmer AutoDELFIA® Instrument

Other Disorders	CF	2007	PerkinElmer AutoDELFIA® Neonatal IRT kit PerkinElmer AutoDELFIA® Instrument Luminex® xTAG® CF39v2 Kit Luminex® 200™
	SCID	2019	Laboratory developed test Applied Biosystems™ QuantStudio™ 12K Flex Real-Time PCR System
	SCD	2019	Bio-Rad VARIANT™ Sickle Cell Program kit Bio-Rad VARIANT™ nbs Newborn Screening System

Source: De Souza A, Wolan V, Battochio A, Christian S, Hume S, Johner G, Lilley M, Ridsdale R, Schnabl K, Tran C, et al. Newborn screening: Current status in Alberta, Canada. International Journal of Neonatal Screening. 2019; 5(4):37. https://doi.org/10.3390/ijns5040037.

3.1.1. Standard Terminology for Fetal, Infant, and Perinatal Deaths

Understanding the scope and causes of these significant events requires first accurately defining and reporting perinatal deaths, also known as fetal and infant deaths. Neonatologists and pediatricians, in addition to obstetric healthcare professionals, should have simple access to up-to-date, easily obtainable materials that define and specify US standards for live births, fetal deaths, and infant deaths. Accurately identifying these crucial occurrences will enhance data at the local, state, and federal levels, enabling more effective prevention and management of these fatalities.

3.1.1.1. Live Birth

A live birth occurs when a human conception product is fully expelled or extracted from the mother, regardless of the length of pregnancy. Following this expulsion or extraction, the child breathes or exhibits any other signs of life, such as heartbeat, umbilical cord pulsation, or distinct voluntary muscle movement, regardless of whether the placenta is attached or not. It is important to distinguish between heartbeats and brief cardiac contractions, as well as between respirations and gasps.

3.1.1.2. Fetal Death

Eight weeks after conception to term while still inside the uterus is when a fetus is defined. Fetal death is defined as any death, regardless of the length of pregnancy, that occurs before the full extraction or expulsion of a human conception product from the mother and is not an induced pregnancy termination. The fact that the fetus does not breathe or exhibit any other signs of life—such as a beating heart, pulsing umbilical cord, or distinct voluntary muscle movement—after such expulsion or extraction indicates that it has died. It is important to distinguish between heartbeats and brief cardiac contractions, as well as between respirations and gasps.

Fetal deaths are further classified as "early" (20–27 weeks gestation) or "late" (≥28 weeks gestation) for statistical purposes. Fetal deaths that occur at 20 weeks or more of gestation are also referred to as "stillbirths." Although stillbirth is not clearly classified as occurring at early or late gestation, the World Health Organization defines it as occurring at or after 28 weeks of gestation for international comparisons. Miscarriages are the specific term used to describe fetuses that pass away in utero before 20 weeks of gestation.

3.1.1.3. Infant Death

An infant dies when a live birth ends in death within the first year (less than 365 days). Neonatal (less than 28 days) infant deaths are classified into three categories: early neonatal (less than 7 days), late neonatal (between 7 and 27 days), and postneonatal (between 28 and 364 days).

3.1.1.4. Perinatal Death

Fetal deaths and live births with only a brief survival period (days or weeks) are combined to form the term "perinatal deaths," which is based on the idea that similar factors are linked to these losses. Although used for statistics, neonatal death is not a vital event that needs to be reported in and of itself. There are three accepted definitions of perinatal deaths:

- Definition I comprises deaths of infants under 7 days of age and deaths of fetuses with a stated or assumed gestational period of 28 weeks or longer.
- Definition II comprises deaths of infants under 28 days of age and deaths of fetuses with a stated or assumed gestational period of 20 weeks or longer.
- Definition III comprises deaths of infants under 7 days of age and deaths of fetuses with a stated or assumed gestation of 20 weeks or longer.

Perinatal deaths have significant implications for public health and clinical interventions on a national and global scale. Different interpretations of these deaths exist worldwide due to cultural perspectives, clinical definitions of viability, and data availability. The National Center for Health Statistics currently categorizes perinatal deaths using two definitions. Definition I, used by the National Center for Health Statistics and World Health Organization, allows for international comparisons by including deaths between 20 and 27 weeks' gestation. Definition II is more comprehensive and suitable for monitoring perinatal deaths throughout gestation, as most fetal deaths occur before 28 weeks' gestation.

3.2. NEONATAL RESUSCITATION

Because of the physiological shift from fetal to neonatal life, resuscitation at the time of birth differs from all other forms of resuscitation. Most newborns will successfully navigate this transition without the need for major medical interventions. Resuscitation guidelines, however, place a strong emphasis on priorities that take into account these particular physiological circumstances for those newborns who do require assistance at birth. Table 3.2 provides a summary of current key recommendations for neonatal resuscitation. The guidelines also stress the importance of effective communication, preparedness and teamwork.

Table 3.2. Comparison of Apparently Stillborn Neonate Resuscitation Algorithms with International Guidelines (NRP, 2015) and Chinese Neonatal Resuscitation Guidelines (CNR, 2016)

	NRP algorithm	**CNR algorithm**	**Apparent stillbirth algorithm**	**Illustration**
Team	Three people	Three people	Four people	(1) Resuscitation of apparently stillborn neonates often requires intubation, heart compressions, and umbilical venous catheter (UVC) placement simultaneously; therefore, multiple people are needed.
Assessment	Term, tone, breathing, or crying	Term, clean amniotic fluid, tone, breathing, or crying	Any breathing, tone or HR > 10 bpm?	(1) Apparently stillborn neonates are mostly in asystolia or approaching it (HR < 10 bpm). (2) Infants may die from complications of MAS [such as pneumothorax and persistent pulmonary hypertension (PPHN)] in low-resource areas of China. Therefore, to prevent subsequent complications, the CNR still recommends suctioning the airway in fluid-contaminated newborns with low vitality*.
Drying and stimulation	Yes	Yes	No	Apparently stillborn neonates are at the terminal stage of secondary apnoea, and stimulation does not help. In addition, apparently stillborn infants often need therapeutic hypothermia later to prevent brain injury; warming and drying are less important than aeration in this case.
Intubation	Initiate after 1 min (if needed)	Initiate after 1 min (if needed)	Preferably finish within 30 s	(1) Intubation facilitates the recovery of heart beat and cerebral perfusion. (2) Heart compression is mostly needed in resuscitation of apparent stillbirth and NRP guidelines recommend to intubate before heart compression. (3) Only experienced neonatologists are allowed to perform the resuscitation of apparent stillbirths in most level III centers in China, which ensures intubation to be accomplished within 20 s and less intubation-related injury.

Initiate FiO_2%	>35 weeks 21%, <35 weeks 21–30%	21, 40, and 100%**	100%	Evidences about the injury of 100% oxygen are slightly conflicting. According to our experience, restoring cerebral perfusion is the top priority in these infants and recommend using pure oxygen to initiate ventilation; however, we are always aware of potential hyperoxia injury.
Frequency of ventilation	40–60 times/min	40–60 times/min	>60 times/min	Facilitate aeration and restore oxygenation in cerebral blood.
First assessment of heart rate	100 bpm	100 bpm	10 bpm	Apparently stillborn neonates are mostly in asystolia or approaching to it.
Initiation of chest compressions	After 1–2 min if needed	After 1–2 min if needed	After 30 s	Timely chest compressions facilitate perfusion of well-oxygenated blood throughout the body, preventing organ injury caused by hypoxia.
Frequency of heart compression	90 times/min	90 times/min	>120 times/min	Facilitate perfusion of the well-oxygenated blood throughout the body.
Chest compression to ventilation ratio	3:1	3:1	Not restricted to 3:1	Evidence from piglets shows sustained inflations (SIs) combined with chest compressions significantly shortened the time needed to induce spontaneous circulation compared to the standard 3:1 compression: ventilation ratio.
UVC	After ~2 min	After ~2 min	After 30 s, initiate at the same time as chest compressions	Epinephrine is often needed in the resuscitation of apparently stillborn neonates. Therefore, the UVC can be placed concurrently with chest compressions.
First dose of epinephrine	After ~4 min	After ~4 min	After 1.5 min, if needed.	Since the UVC is established early, epinephrine can be administered early if needed.

The key to resuscitation of apparently stillborn neonates is to deliver oxygenated blood to the body. Therefore, never start chest compressions before the establishment of effective ventilation.

*Low vitality refers to one of the following symptoms: low tone, no breathing or gasping, HR < 100 bpm.

**In rural areas of China, self-inflating bags are the most common devices for resuscitation. Air-oxygen mixers and blenders are not available. The CNR is aware of the toxicity of 100% oxygen and therefore suggests removing the corrugated tube from the self-inflating bag to generate a concentration of 40% oxygen after mixing ambient air with 100% oxygen.

Source: Chen X, Li H, Song J, Sun P, Lin B, Zhao J and Yang C (2020) The resuscitation of apparently stillborn neonates: A peek into the practice in China. Front. Pediatr., 8, 231. doi: 10.3389/fped.2020.00231.

One of the most dreaded situations for an anesthetist who is actively caring for a mother is having to lead her struggling neonate's resuscitation at the same time. Neonatal resuscitation should not be performed by an anesthetist caring for a mother, according to numerous national and international practice guidelines. Survey results show that anesthetists are frequently asked to assist with or oversee the resuscitation of the newborn despite this recommendation. Naturally, depending on the practice setting, anesthetists' involvement in neonatal resuscitation varies greatly, with a higher probability of involvement in hospitals with fewer deliveries.

If an anesthetist is asked to care for a mother and her newborn at the same time, the mother is the anesthetist's primary concern, and calling for assistance should always be the first course of action. If the mother is stable and a second anesthesia provider is not available, it might be reasonable to think about helping to resuscitate the baby while another medical professional (e.g., a midwife or an operating room nurse) keeps an eye out for any changes in the mother's clinical condition or vital signs.

Given that their participation in neonatal resuscitation is frequently spontaneous and irregular, anesthetists who provide obstetric care ought to stay up to date on the most recent advancements in this field. Neonatals are not "tiny adults," as the saying goes, and adult or pediatric life support does not take into account the physiological factors that are relevant to the change from fetal to neonatal life (Cheng, 2020; Wyckoff et al, 2020).

3.2.1. Preparation

Neonatals are typically delivered with enough notice for a team of medical professionals to get ready for a resuscitation if needed. Risk factors that are known before delivery can be used to estimate the possibility that resuscitation will be required. To let the neonatal resuscitation team know how high the risk is for resuscitation, there must be clear communication between the anesthesia and obstetric teams. Teams dedicated to neonatal resuscitation ought to be structured and equipped with a strategy for handling different degrees of resuscitation needs. Identifying which team members will be present and what tasks they should be prepared to complete is part of this plan. When the team is called in to assist with the birth of a baby who might require resuscitation, everyone on the team should be clearly informed about all possible risk factors, their roles should be clearly defined, and their equipment should be ready. To start preparing the parents for what's going to happen, the neonatal resuscitation team may also get in touch with them. As things develop, the anesthetist can frequently help with communication with the mother (Table 3.3).

Table 3.3. Summary of Selected Narrative and Systematic Reviews and Observational Studies Evaluating Volume Replacement During Neonatal Resuscitation

Study	Topic	Number of Articles Included	Findings and Recommendations
Finn et al. (2017); Holmes (2013), narrative review	Volume resuscitation in the delivery room	none	No current clinical tools allow differentiation of an asphyxiated infant who will benefit from volume replacement from a normovolemic asphyxiated infant who may deteriorate with volume replacement. Consider volume expansion in the setting of presumed blood loss, with fresh blood if available, or with crystalloid.
Keir et al. (2016); Visscher, Adam, Brink, & Odio, (2015), systematic review	Late preterm and term neonates with hemodynamic compromise, excluding acute hemorrhage	Two studies	No robust evidence to support fluid bolus for infants with hemodynamic compromise without acute blood loss. Complications of fluid boluses include volume overload (affecting end-organ function), dilutional coagulopathy, electrolyte imbalance with hyperchloremic metabolic acidosis after normal saline and adverse effects from blood transfusions. Routine use of fluid boluses is to be avoided in absence of acute hemorrhage.
Shalish et al. (2017); Wyckoff et al. (2015), systematic review	Albumin use as volume expander in various settings including the delivery room.	none	Albumin appears to be equally effective as crystalloids in improving hemodynamics such as blood pressure but is associated with higher mortality. In asphyxiated infants, albumin may increase oncotic pressure and cause transudation of fluid in interstitial space. Crystalloids (normal saline) are preferred for fluid resuscitation over albumin.
Keir et al. (2019); Warren, & Phillipi, (2012), cross-sectional survey	International multicenter observational study in 41 neonatal units—fluid bolus for suspected hemodynamic compromise		5/163 infants received a fluid bolus for neonatal resuscitation. No further details provided.

Source: Sankaran D, Lane ECA, Valdez R, Lesneski AL, Lakshminrusimha S. Role of volume replacement during neonatal resuscitation in the delivery room. Children. 2022; 9(10), 1484. https://doi.org/10.3390/children9101484.

Equipment for neonatal resuscitation needs to be easily accessible at all times. To keep the baby warm, open their airway, watch over them, ventilate them, place a backup airway, and support their circulation, equipment will be required. Making sure the right sizes of all the equipment are on hand is essential. Additionally, equipment needs to be examined to make sure it operates properly and is primed for use (i.e., full power was applied to the radiant warmer, and the gas flow and suction were activated and ready for use). The team members should think about having the emergency supplies ready to go rather than just having them on hand for high-risk scenarios like an emergency Caesarean section. In these cases, opening, prepping, and flushing an umbilical catheter could save vital minutes during a life-saving resuscitation (Table 3.4).

Table 3.4. The Steps of MRSOPA (modified from the Textbook of Neonatal Resuscitation)

MRSOPA	Action
M:	adjust **M**ask
R:	**R**eposition mask
S:	**S**uction mouth and nose
O:	**O**pen mouth
P:	increase **P**ressure
A:	**A**lternate airway

Source: Eckels M, Zeilinger T, Lee HC, Bergin J, Halamek LP, Yamada N, Fuerch J, Chitkara R, Quinn J. A Neonatal intensive care unit's experience with implementing an in-situ simulation and debriefing patient safety program in the setting of a quality improvement collaborative. Children. 2020; 7(11), 202. https://doi.org/10.3390/children7110202.

Maintaining strong resuscitation skills appears to require regular, small-scale resuscitation training. Teamwork is enhanced by regular practice through interdisciplinary simulation, which makes it possible for members of the resuscitation team to function comfortably in all roles and collaborate in an organized and effective way. This kind of simulated training is best carried out in situ, or the location where resuscitations typically take place, during the working day to allow teams to become as familiar as possible with their surroundings and teammates. When these abilities are required, a cohesive team is likely to carry out resuscitation in a highly effective way (Figures 3.1 and 3.2).

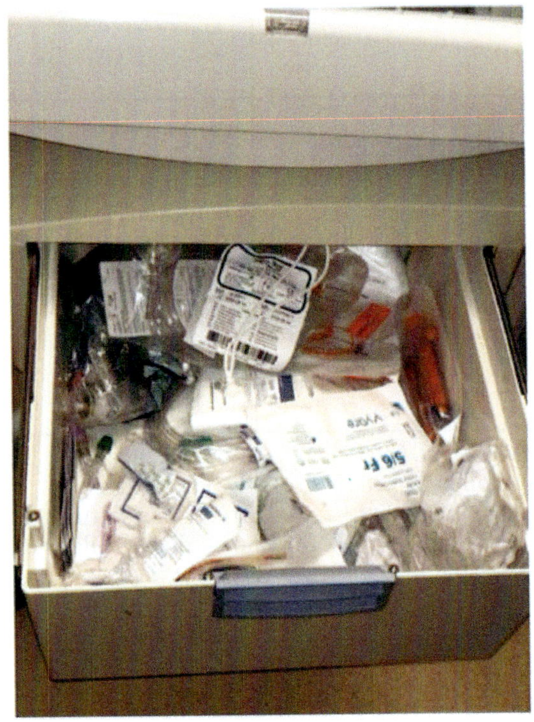

Figure 3.1. *The equipment should be ready.*

Source: Eckels M, Zeilinger T, Lee HC, Bergin J, Halamek LP, Yamada N, Fuerch J, Chitkara R, Quinn J. A neonatal intensive care unit's experience with implementing an in-situ simulation and debriefing patient safety program in the setting of a quality improvement collaborative. Children. 2020; 7(11):202. https://doi.org/10.3390/children7110202.

5SW NURSERY INFANT WARMER SUPPLY LIST

MONTH

DATE														
	7A	7P	7A	7P	7A	7P	7A	7P	7A	7P	7A	7P	7A	7P
ON WARMER: (checked & connected)														
T-piece														
Suction tubing														
TOP SHELF:														
Skin temp probe														
Pulse ox probe														
Suction catheters 8 & 10 FR.														
INSIDE DRAWER:														
LAB COLLECTION SUPPLIES														
2 heel warmers														
Lancets (Gentlefeet) 2 newborn & 2 preemie														
5 spot bandaids														
5 sterile 2 x 2's														
10 alcohol pads														
1 plastic tape														
Miscellaneous Supplies														
2 urine collection bags														
5 cotton balls														
2 pulse ox probes														
2 temp probes														
1 cord clamp														
3 saline bullets														
2 tape measures														
3 KY jelly														
Anesthesia bag & mask														
Airway supply bag (content label on bag)														
TIME:														
INITIALS:														

Figure 3.2. *A sample checklist.*

Source: Eckels M, Zeilinger T, Lee HC, Bergin J, Halamek LP, Yamada N, Fuerch J, Chitkara R, Quinn J. (2020). A Neonatal intensive care unit's experience with implementing an in-situ simulation and debriefing patient safety program in the setting of a quality improvement collaborative. Children, 7(11):202. https://doi.org/10.3390/children7110202.

3.2.2. Cord Management

In the past few years, the practice of clamping the umbilical cord after birth has received a lot of attention. In an attempt to stop postpartum hemorrhage, the obstetric practice of immediately clamping the umbilical cord was introduced as part of the active management of the third stage of labor. Nevertheless, lower neonatal blood volumes are the outcome of clamping the cord as soon as possible after birth as opposed to waiting a longer time (referred to as "delayed or deferred" cord clamping). If the umbilical cord is clamped right away, a sizable amount of the volume of feto-placental blood will stay in the placenta rather than transfer into the newborn. The amount of blood that is given to the newborn depends on how long the umbilical cord remains intact after delivery. The placenta transfers a greater volume of blood to a newborn who starts breathing on its own before the cord clamps than to a newborn who does not start breathing on its own. This is because the respiratory status of the infant influences the placenta's ability to transfer blood to the newborn.

Improved iron stores in infancy may benefit neurological development in term infants due to the effect of increased blood volume transferred from the placenta to the newborn in response to later cord clamping. Preterm babies experience better hemodynamic stability during the shift from fetal to neonatal life, which is evident more quickly in the newborn stage. A meta-analysis of the available clinical trials also showed a decrease in the incidence of intraventricular hemorrhage, fewer blood transfusions, and lower mortality rates in infants treated with delayed cord clamping.

Many ongoing studies are assessing the practice of providing respiratory support before the cord is clamped in infants who do not breathe spontaneously after birth. This approach is based on physiological observations in animal models that show a more stable hemodynamic transition from fetal to newborn life when ventilation begins before the cord is clamped. Previous research has assessed the practice of "milking" or "stripping" the cord, wherein an obstetrician tries to speed up the transfer of blood from the placenta to a neonate that is not breathing on its own. Regrettably, more preterm babies who are susceptible to intraventricular hemorrhage may suffer harm as a result of this practice.

Currently, the Royal College of Obstetricians and Gynecologists advises waiting at least two minutes after delivery to perform cord clamping whenever possible. The European Resuscitation Council (ERC) advises against performing cord clamping on infants who do not require immediate resuscitation until the infant has been alive for at least one minute. To provide the right care, there must be sufficient communication regarding the plan for managing the cord between the anesthetist, pediatrician, and obstetrician. Although not thoroughly investigated, the administration of uterotonic medications in connection with cord clamping does not seem to have an impact on the outcomes of mothers or newborns.

3.2.3. Initial Assessment

A brief assessment of the newborn in the initial moments following birth will assist in deciding the course of action. The newborn may remain with the mother and receive skin-to-skin care if they are healthy, crying, breathing, and at term. If any of those conditions are not met, the infant needs to be evaluated more thoroughly. The infant should be placed in a neutral position and placed near a radiant warmer once the umbilical cord has been clamped. When a newborn reaches 32 weeks gestation, it should be dried right away. To maintain a suitable temperature, newborns under 32 weeks gestation should be wrapped in plastic without drying, except for their faces. For infants born before 28 weeks of pregnancy, the ERC advises keeping the delivery room (DR) temperature between 23°C and 25°C, and higher than 25°C. Thermal mattresses are another useful tool for preserving normothermia in preterm infants. Gentle stimulation, such as drying the baby, should be tried to encourage the newborn to breathe regularly and adequately if during the first assessment, the baby is not breathing well.

While suctioning the Oro- and nasopharynx was once advised for all newborns, it is now only advised in cases of obviously excessive secretions, particularly if the airway appears to be blocked. When positive-pressure ventilation (PPV) is indicated, suctioning should also be tried if face mask-assisted PPV fails to produce adequate ventilation as evidenced by a rise in the chest.

Notably, unless resuscitation is unsuccessful due to airway obstruction, suctioning the trachea through a tracheal tube (TT) is no longer advised in newborns born through meconium-stained amniotic fluid. The lack of evidence supporting the benefits of universal tracheal suctioning and the possible risks associated with postponing resuscitation and performing needless laryngoscopy are the reasons behind this change in practice.

3.2.4. Monitoring

A crucial component of neonatal resuscitation, the assessment of heart rate (HR) and oxygen saturation (SpO_2) directs clinical care. The most crucial vital sign to consider when assessing the success of resuscitation efforts is heart rate. During neonatal resuscitation, the following techniques are acceptable for measuring HR: ECG, cardiac auscultation, pulse oximetry monitoring, and umbilical cord palpation. But in the early newborn stage, palpation of pulses—including those of the umbilical cord—becomes less accurate. Continuous monitoring of the newborn can be facilitated by the same ideal tools that are used to assist the neonatal resuscitation team in measuring vital signs in the DR. The benefit of pulse oximetry is that it can measure both HR and SpO_2 at the same time. To measure the oxygenation of cerebral blood flow, or pre-ductal SpO_2, a newborn's right wrist or hand should be the site of the pulse oximeter sensor application. During the first 10 minutes of life, there is a typical pre-to post-ductal difference of 10–15%. Erroneous or delayed readings may be caused by motion artifacts, acrocyanosis, skin edema, or low-volume conditions. This can be lessened by warming and drying the baby as well as by using sensors made specifically for neonatal resuscitation, which have a short average time and maximum sensitivity.

ECG is currently the gold standard for assessing the newborn's heart rate during advanced neonatal resuscitations requiring advanced airway for ventilation or additional interventions due to its efficiency and reliability. Crucially, using the ECG enables the team to continuously see the baby's heart rate on a monitor while the resuscitation is underway. While ECG is a reliable and effective tool, it shouldn't be the only way to measure a newborn's heart rate during resuscitation because, despite being uncommon, pulseless electrical activity can happen. If the leads do not stick firmly to the baby's chest due to amniotic fluid, vernix, or meconium, additional ECG problems may occur. The main obstacle to using ECG for neonatal resuscitation in many institutions is that it's not always available in the neonatal intensive care unit.

It has also been demonstrated that controlling temperature is crucial to neonatal resuscitation, especially in cases of preterm newborns. Neonatals who are admitted with hypothermia are more likely to experience morbidity and mortality. The optimal temperature range to aim for is between 36.5°C and 37.5°C. A newborn can be kept at the minimum target temperature to maintain normothermia without developing hyperthermia by setting a temperature target on the radiant warmer and using a skin temperature probe.

3.2.5. Positive Pressure Ventilation

Reevaluating the infant after the first stages of resuscitation are finished will aid in deciding what to do next. After a short period of drying and stimulation, PPV should be started if the newborn is gasping, apneic, or has a <100 beats min^{-1}. A mask that fits the newborn well and covers their mouth and nose while minimizing mask leakage without putting too much pressure on their eyes should be selected. Flow-inflating bags, self-inflating bags, or neonatal T-piece resuscitators can all be used to provide ventilation. Devices known as neonatal T-piece resuscitators produce controlled assisted inflations employing a continuous flow of mixed air and oxygen.

Assisting the neonate in moving from the fetal state of fluid-filled lungs to the neonatal state of air-filled lungs is the aim of assisted ventilation during resuscitation. Through this change, the fetus can develop a functional residual capacity (FRC), which keeps the lungs inflated. Peak inspiratory pressure (PIP) or PEEP levels that are best for initiating resuscitation are unknown, but according to current ERC guidelines, a PIP of 30 cm H_2O should be used for term newborns and 20–25 cm H_2O for preterm newborns.

To aid in lung opening, the ERC advises holding the first five inflations for two to three seconds each. The team should watch for visible chest rise and an increase in HR, which are indicators of efficient and sufficient ventilation, once PPV has started. As an alternative, ventilation with color change can be demonstrated using a CO_2 detector.

Particularly in very preterm infants, giving ventilation with an excessive tidal volume for more than a few inflations can result in lung damage. Consistent PIP delivery provided by the T-piece may help prevent the delivery of excessive tidal volumes. Providing a recruitment maneuver, such as sustained inflation (holding the PIP at a constant level for more than 5 s), has been another strategy to minimize PIP delivery. It has not been demonstrated that this method is safe, and it is not advised at this time.

According to physiological parameters, a newborn's SpO_2 is roughly 60% at one minute of life and rises to 85% at five minutes. The use of oxygen during the resuscitation of newborns has been thoroughly researched. Short-term mortality in term newborns is reduced when a lower FiO_2 (0.21–0.30) is used during neonatal resuscitation as opposed to a higher FiO_2 (0.6–1.0). The ideal starting Fio2 in preterm infants is still unknown, but the majority will need some extra oxygen during the first stages of stabilization. The starting Fio_2 is therefore set at 0.21 for term newborns and 0.21–0.30 for preterm newborns. Fio_2 should be raised if the newborn's HR does not rise with PPV and 0.21. At any point during resuscitation, if an infant needs chest compressions, the Fio_2 should be raised to 1.0 right away.

If corrective measures are taken to optimize mask ventilation but the heart rate does not improve, placement of an advanced airway (TT or supraglottic airway [SGA]) is indicated. Based on the newborn's size, the team should select the TT and laryngoscope or SGA that are the proper sizes. While it's important to have a spare SGA on hand in case of challenging intubation, size restrictions may prevent preterm or growth-restricted neonates from using an SGA.

When a newborn is breathing on their own but exhibits symptoms of respiratory distress, like grunting or the use of auxiliary muscles, CPAP may be a viable option to help stabilize the baby. The use of continuous positive airway pressure (CPAP) can help prevent the need for mechanical ventilation in preterm newborns and improve long-term outcomes, like death or bronchopulmonary dysplasia.

3.2.6. Chest Compressions

When ventilated properly, the great majority of newborns respond to resuscitation. As a result, the establishment of efficient ventilation, which includes creating an advanced airway before initiating chest compressions, is supported by neonatal resuscitation guidelines. Chest compressions are recommended if a newborn has severe bradycardia with HR <60 beats min^{-1} despite receiving effective ventilation for 30 seconds.

Breaths and chest compressions should be timed in a 3:1 ratio. Using the two-thumb technique, compress the newborn's chest to one-third of the anterior-posterior diameter at the lower third of the sternum is the optimal way to perform chest compressions. In manikin studies, it has been demonstrated that the two-thumb technique consistently produces compressions of the right depth when compared to the two-finger technique. The two-thumb method of placing the hands is demonstrated in Figure 3.3. Using either method, the healthcare professional applying chest compressions must always maintain contact with the newborn's chest with their thumbs or fingers.

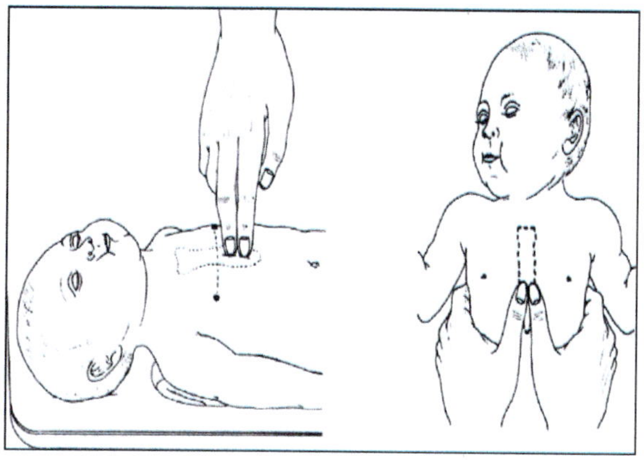

Figure 3.3. *Two methods of chest compression.*

Source: Chadha IA. Neonatal resuscitation: Current issues. Indian J Anaesth. 2010 Sep;54(5):428–38. doi: 10.4103/0019-5049.71042. PMID: 21189881; PMCID: PMC2991653.

ECG and pulse oximetry can give the entire resuscitation team continuous HR monitoring while performing chest compressions. The person doing the ventilation should stand to the side to provide inflations once an advanced airway has been established. This will allow the person doing the chest compressions to stand at the head of the bed and perform the most efficient chest compressions. To aid in the coordination of ventilation and chest compressions, the healthcare provider should count aloud while executing the technique. Assessing heart rate is necessary following 60 seconds of chest compressions. Chest compressions should cease during the HR assessment. With successful resuscitation, a newborn's heart rate—which is a sensitive indicator of their clinical status—will rise.

3.2.7. Medications

Adrenaline (epinephrine) may be helpful for critically ill newborns who maintain bradycardia with a heart rate >60 beats per min^{-1} despite receiving chest compressions and adequate ventilation. It is advised to standardize the adrenaline concentration to 0.1 mg ml^{-1} during neonatal resuscitation. The i.v. route is the most effective. Adrenaline can also be given *via* an i.o. catheter or through a TT if no other route is available. The i.v. or i.o. dose is 10–30 mcg kg^{-1} (0.1–0.3 ml kg^{-1}), whereas the intratracheal dose of adrenaline is 50–100 mcg kg^{-1} (0.5–1 ml kg^{-1}).

One of the key competencies in neonatal resuscitation is the prompt placement of an umbilical venous catheter when necessary. An umbilical venous catheter needs to be easily accessible and flushed with saline to be inserted during resuscitation quickly. Povidone iodine should be used to clean the umbilical cord, it should be tied to stop bleeding, and it should be cut to make room for the vessels. In contrast to the two arteries with thicker walls, the vein is recognized by the clinician as a single vessel with a larger lumen and a thinner wall. After blood return is verified, the medical professional moves the umbilical catheter to a location slightly past the cord. Then, volume and medications can be administered quickly.

Some babies are born hypovolemic and respond to fluid infusion, though this is uncommon. For infants whose medical history suggests that they may be hypovolemic (e.g., from blood loss), 10 ml kg^{-1} boluses of saline or O-negative blood can be given as infusions. For newborns with suspected severe blood loss, an emergency blood transfusion is preferred to restore lost volume and treat any resulting anemia; however, preparation time may be longer.

Other causes of newborn compromise should be taken into consideration for any newborn that is not responding to resuscitation efforts. Successful resuscitation may be impeded by pneumothorax or undetected anomalies, such as congenital diaphragmatic hernia. When deciding whether resuscitation has failed in an infant who is still bradycardic, these factors should be taken into account. It may be decided to stop resuscitation for newborns who are born with no detectable heart rate and who have not responded to efficient resuscitation efforts for longer than 20 minutes. Maintaining communication with the family is essential, as is giving them time to see and cuddle their child as needed.

The majority of newborns can be stabilized at birth with little assistance. If sufficient ventilation is available, resuscitation efforts are typically successful when required. The circumstances surrounding a child's birth can have a significant long-term impact on their health and neurological development. All healthcare professionals who might assist in resuscitation at birth should be knowledgeable about the most recent guidelines as well as the special requirements of the newborn leaving the womb. Maintaining resuscitation skills requires regular training and improvement techniques (Cheng, 2020; Wyckoff et al, 2020).

3.3. EXAMINATION OF A NEWBORN

Every newborn is closely examined for indications of complications or issues at the time of birth. Every bodily system will be examined thoroughly by the medical professional. Doctors, nurses, and other medical professionals keep a close eye on the baby's health during the hospital stay. They are keeping an eye out for indications of issues or disease. Evaluations might cover the following.

3.3.1. Apgar Scoring

Finding breathing difficulties and other health problems is aided by the Apgar score. It is a component of the particular care given to a newborn in the initial moments of life. The baby's heart and breathing rates, muscular tone, reflexes, and color are assessed one and 5 minutes after birth. Throughout those first 5 to 10 minutes, a baby who requires assistance with any of these problems is receiving continuous care. In this instance, the real Apgar score is provided after the pressing problems have been resolved.

A maximum of 10 points can be scored in any area, with scores ranging from 0 to 1. The majority of babies receive a score of 8 or 9, with 1 or 2 points deducted for having blue hands and feet due to immature circulation. A baby's Apgar score will drop if they have a difficult time giving birth and require additional assistance after. Apgar ratings of six or lower typically indicate that a newborn requires medical attention right away (Table 3.5).

Table 3.5. Apgar Score

APGAR Evaluation of newborn infants

SIGN	0	1	2
Heart rate	Absent	Below 100	Over 100
Respiratory effort	Absent	Slow, irregular	Good, crying
Muscle tone	Limp	Some flexion	Active motion
Reflex*	No response	Grimace	Cough or sneeze
Color	Blue, Pale	Body pink Extremities blue	Completely pink

➤7 to 10 is normal ➤ 4 to 6 is moderately depressed ➤ 0 to 3 needs immediate resuscitation

Source: https://upload.wikimedia.org/wikipedia/commons/b/ba/APGAR_score.jpg.

3.3.2. Birth Weight

The weight of a newborn is a crucial indicator of health. In between 37 and 41 weeks of pregnancy, full-term babies are born. A full-term baby typically weighs around 7 pounds (3.02 kg). Large babies and very small babies are generally more likely to have issues. In the nursery, babies are weighed daily to monitor their growth as well as their dietary and hydration needs. Typically, newborns lose between 5% and 7% of their birth weight. This implies that a newborn weighing seven pounds, three ounces may lose up to eight ounces in the first few days of life. Usually, within the first two weeks of life, babies regain this weight. Babies that are premature or unwell might not gain weight right away.

The majority of hospitals weigh newborns using the metric system. Using this chart, you can convert grams to pounds.

Grams to pounds and ounces conversion (Figure 3.4):

1 lb. = 453.59237 grams; 1 oz. = 28.349523 grams; 1,000 grams = 1 Kg.

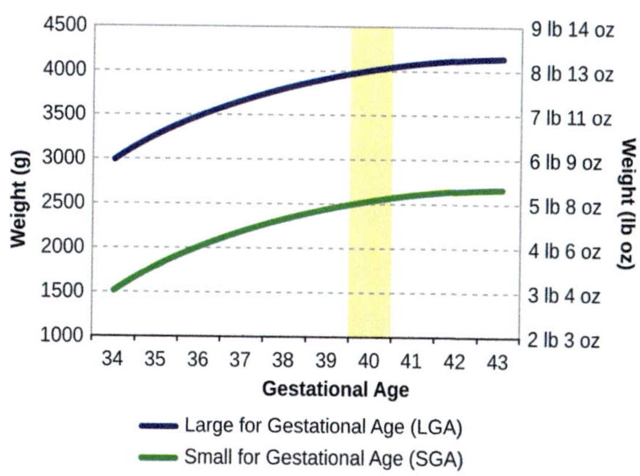

Figure 3.4. *Birthweight conversion chart.*

Source: https://en.m.wikipedia.org/wiki/File:Birth_weight_chart_2.svg.

3.3.3. Measurements

For every baby, the hospital staff measures them again. These consist of:

- **Head Circumference:** The circumference of the infant's head.
- **Abdominal Circumference:** The circumference of the abdomen.
- **Length:** The distance between the top of the head and the heel.

These vital signs are also checked by the staff:

- **Temperature:** This verifies that the infant can maintain a consistent body temperature in a typical room.
- **Pulse:** A newborn's heartbeat typically ranges from 120 to 160 beats per minute.
- **Breathing Rate:** A newborn typically breathes between 40 to 60 times per minute.

3.3.4. Physical Exam

An essential component of newborn care is a thorough physical examination. The medical professional closely examines each body system to ensure that it is healthy and operating normally. The doctor also searches for any indications of disease or birth abnormalities. A newborn's physical examination frequently entails:

3.3.4.1. Cardiorespiratory System

When the baby is quiet, the heart and lungs are assessed. To rule out dextrocardia, the physician should determine the location of the loudest heartbeats. Checks are made on heart rate and rhythm (normal: 100 to 160 beats per minute). Although an irregular rhythm due to premature atrial or ventricular contractions is not unusual, the rhythm should be regular. The most common cause of a murmur detected within the first 24 hours is a patent ductus arteriosus. A daily cardiac exam verifies that this murmur has disappeared, usually in three days.

Brachial and femoral pulses are compared and checked. An aortic coarctation or other obstruction of the left ventricular outflow tract is indicated by a weak or delayed femoral pulse. Central cyanosis is indicative of sepsis, pulmonary illness, or congenital cardiac disease. Because newborns breathe irregularly—40 to 60 breaths per minute is the normal rate—the respiratory system is assessed by counting respirations over the course of a full minute. Lung sounds should be consistent throughout, and the chest wall should be inspected for symmetry. Respiratory distress manifests as retractions, nasal flaring, and grunting.

3.3.4.2. Head and Neck

During a vertex delivery, the head is often shaped with some swelling and scalp ecchymosis (caput succedaneum) along with the cranial bones overriding at the sutures. When a baby is born breech, the head experiences less molding, and the presenting part— (i.e., buttocks, genitals, or feet)— experiences swelling and ecchymosis. The fontanelles range in diameter from a few millimeters to the width of a fingertip. Hypothyroidism may be indicated by a large anterior fontanelle and anything greater than the width of a fingertip in the posterior fontanelle.

Blood builds up between the periosteum and the bone, resulting in a swelling that does not cross suture lines, which is a common finding in cephalohematomas. It sometimes occurs over the occiput and over one or both parietal bones. Cephalohematomas typically take months to manifest; they usually go undetected until soft-tissue edema goes down. Congenital hydrocephalus is detected by examining the size and shape of the head. Craniofacial abnormalities are caused by a variety of genetic syndromes. The mandible, palate, pinnae, and external auditory canals are among the features of the face that are examined for symmetry and normal development.

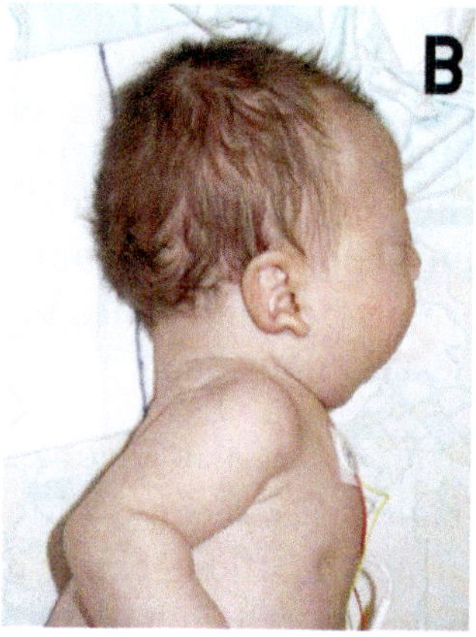

Figure 3.5. *Low-set ears in an infant with Noonan syndrome.*

Source: By Gregor Nosan, Sara Bertok, Samo Vesel, Helger G. Yntema, and Darja Paro-Panjan – https://www.ncbi.nlm.nih.gov/pmc/articles/PMC3893993/, CC BY 4.0, https://commons.wikimedia.org/w/index.php?curid=75310051.

Due to swelling around the eyelids from the birth process, it might be simpler to examine the eyes the day after delivery. The red reflex should be checked in the eyes; if it is absent, glaucoma, cataracts, or retinoblastoma may be the cause. Forces used during delivery are the common cause of subconjunctival hemorrhages. Low-set ears can be a sign of genetic disorders such as Down syndrome's trisomy 18 and 21. Numerous genetic syndromes may involve malformed ears, external auditory canals, or both. Physicians should search for external ear pits or tags, as these can occasionally be linked to renal abnormalities and hearing loss (Figure 3.5).

To check for soft or hard palate defects, the clinician should examine and palpate the palate. One of the most prevalent congenital conditions is orofacial clefts. A benign gum hamartoma known as an epulis, which can obstruct the airway and cause feeding difficulties in certain newborns, is a birth defect. These are non-recurrent lesions that can be removed. Some newborns have natal teeth, also known as primary teeth. Since natal teeth lack roots, it might be necessary to extract them to stop them from falling out and becoming aspirated. The roof of the mouth may develop Epstein pearls, which are inclusion cysts.

The doctor must lift the chin when performing a neck examination to check for anomalies like goiters, cystic hygromas, and remnants of the branchial arch. Birth trauma can result in a sternocleidomastoid hematoma, which can cause torticulosis.

3.3.4.3. Abdomen and Pelvis

The abdomen ought to be symmetrical and round. A diaphragmatic hernia, which allows the intestine to migrate through it to the chest cavity in utero, may be indicated by a scaphoid abdomen. Pulmonary hypoplasia and postnatal respiratory distress may ensue. An abdominal mass is suggested by an asymmetric abdomen. About 30% of newborns have a palpable splenic edge. If the splenic edge is palpable more than two centimeters below the left costal margin, it may indicate hemolytic anemia or a congenital infection. Deep palpation may reveal the kidneys; the left kidney is easier to reach than the right. Large kidneys could be a sign of cystic illness, tumor, or obstruction. Normally, one can feel the liver one to two centimeters below the costal margin. Because of a weakness in the muscles surrounding the umbilical ring, umbilical hernias are common but infrequently serious. It is important to confirm if a normally positioned, patent anus is present. It is important to check the penis of boys for hypo- or epispadias. The testes should be in the scrotum in term boys. Swollen scrotum can indicate hydrocele, inguinal hernia, or, less frequently, torsion of the testicles. The scrotum transilluminates when hydrocele occurs. Torsion is a surgical emergency that results in firmness and ecchymosis. Term girls have noticeable labia. Pseudomenses, or mucoid vaginal and serosanguineous secretions, are normal and arise from the mother's hormone exposure during pregnancy and withdrawal after delivery. Sometimes there is a tiny tag of hymenal tissue at the posterior fourchette; this tag disappears over a few weeks and is thought to be caused by hormonal stimulation from the mother. Intersex, also known as ambiguous genitals, can be a sign of several rare conditions, (e.g., congenital adrenal hyperplasia; 5-alpha-reductase deficiency; Klinefelter syndrome, Turner syndrome, or Swyer syndrome). It is recommended to discuss the advantages and disadvantages of immediate versus delayed sex assignment with the family and to refer the patient to an endocrinologist for evaluation.

3.3.4.4. Musculoskeletal System

The extremities are checked for maldevelopment, contractures, amputations (partially or completely missing limbs), and deformities. Birth trauma-related brachial nerve palsy can sometimes cause pronation of the forearm, internal rotation of the shoulder, and limited or absent spontaneous arm movement on the affected side. A meningomyelocele, or exposure of the spinal cord or meninges, is one of the symptoms of spina bifida that is looked for when examining the spine.

The goal of an orthopedic examination is to find hip dysplasia, but it also involves palpating the long bones for birth trauma, especially clavicle fractures. Female sex, breech position in utero, twin gestation, and family history are risk factors for dysplasia. One way to check for dysplasia is to perform the Barlow and Ortolani maneuvers. Neonates need to be quiet during these maneuvers. Both babies begin in the same way: on their backs, with their hips and knees bent to a 90° angle (the feet will not be on the bed), their feet facing the healthcare professional, who places a thumb on the lesser trochanter and an index finger on the greater trochanter.

When performing the Barlow maneuver, the medical professional pushes the thigh posteriorly while adducting the hip, or drawing the knee across the body. The femur head has moved out of the acetabulum when there is a felt but unheard clunk; the Ortolani maneuver moves the head and validates the diagnosis. To perform the Osteolani maneuver, the hip must first be brought back to its initial position. Next, the hip under test must be gently pulled anteriorly and abducted, which involves moving the knee away from the midline and toward the examination table in a frog-leg position. A test result for hip dysplasia is positive if there is a palpable clunk of the femoral head with abduction, which indicates movement of an already dislocated femoral head into the acetabulum.

Due to tighter hip muscles and ligaments, the maneuvers may be mistakenly negative in infants older than three months. Hip ultrasonography should be performed at 4 to 6 weeks if the examination is unclear or the infant is at high risk (such as girls who were breech). Some experts advise screening ultrasonography at 4 to 6 weeks for all infants with risk factors (Figure 3.6).

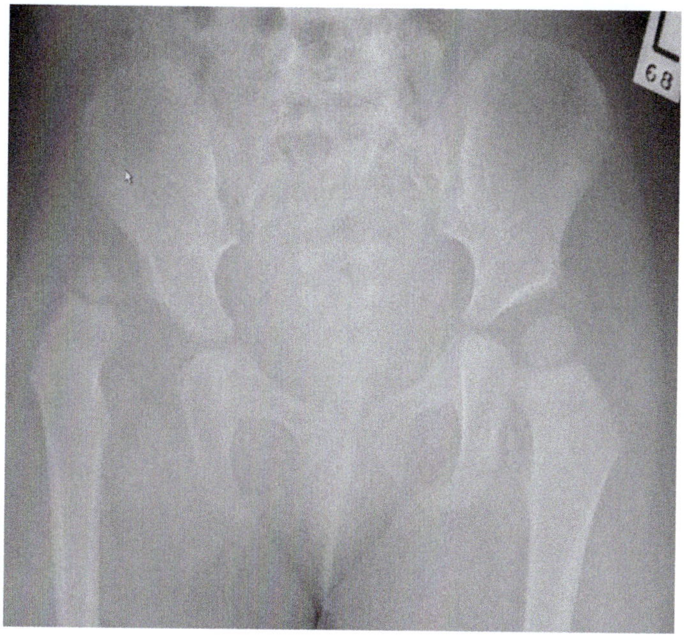

Figure 3.6. *Hip dysplasia.*

Source: By Heather (The original uploader was Glitzy queen00 at English Wikipedia.) – Own work (Transferred by hellerhoff), Public Domain, https://commons.wikimedia.org/w/index.php?curid=14631661.

3.3.4.5. Neurologic System

Evaluations are made of the neonate's tone, degree of alertness, extremity movement, and reflexes. Neonatal reflexes, such as the suck, rooting, and Moro reflexes, are typically elicited as follows:

- **Moro Reflex:** A newborn will pull their arms just a little bit off the bed and then release them abruptly in response to being startled. The newborn cries and flexes their hips in response, extending their arms with fingers outstretched.
- **Rooting Reflex:** A newborn will turn their head toward contact and open their mouth when their cheek or lateral lip is stroked.
- **Suck Reflex:** To trigger this reflex, a gloved finger or pacifier is used.

These reflexes are indicators of a healthy peripheral nervous system and persist for several months following birth.

3.3.4.6. Skin

Neonatals typically have ruddy skin, and during the first few hours of life, cyanosis of the fingers and toes is common. Vernix caseosa affects the majority of neonates born after 24 weeks. Peeling and dryness, especially at the creases of the wrists and ankles, frequently appear within days. When the face is the affected area, such as after delivery, petechiae may appear there. Nevertheless, newborns with diffuse petechiae need to have their thrombocytopenia assessed. Erythema toxicum, a benign rash with an erythematous base and a white or yellow papule, affects a lot of newborns.

This rash can last up to two weeks and typically shows up 24 hours after birth. It is scattered over the body.

3.3.5. Gestational Assessment

The baby's maturity will be assessed by the healthcare professional. This is a crucial aspect of medical care. When a pregnancy's dates are unclear, this check helps determine the best course of action for the unborn child. A very small baby, for instance, might be more mature than their size would suggest and require different care than a premature baby. A test known as the Dubowitz/ Ballard Examination for Gestational Age is frequently used by medical professionals. A baby's gestational age can be accurately estimated with this exam. The examination examines the skin, other anatomical features, movement, and reflexes of the infant. Within the first two hours of life, the physical maturity portion of the exam is completed. Within 24 hours of birth, the movement and reflexes portion of the examination is completed. The results of this exam are frequently used by the provider to assist with additional maturity estimates.

3.3.6. Physical Maturity

The Dubowitz/Ballard exam's physical maturity section examines physical characteristics that change in appearance depending on a baby's gestational age. Physically mature babies typically score higher than premature babies. For every assessment area, there are points awarded. A baby is extremely immature if the low is -1 or -2. A 4 or 5 indicates that the infant is postmature, or extremely mature. The following areas were examined:

- Skin textures. Is the skin peeling, smooth, or sticky?
- The baby's body has soft, downy hair (lanugo). Babies who are not yet mature do not have this hair. In a mature infant, it manifests itself, but in a postmature infant, it disappears.
- Plantar creases. These are furrows found on the foot soles. They may be completely absent or extend to cover the entire foot.
- Breast. The physician examines the size, thickness, and darker area (areola) surrounding each nipple.
- Eyes and ears. The medical professional observes whether the eyes are open or fused. Additionally, he or she assesses the ears' stiffness and cartilage content.
- Genitals, male. The provider examines the appearance of the scrotum and the testes. It could be wrinkly or smooth.
- Genitals, female. The provider measures the clitoris and labia and examines their appearance.

3.3.7. Maturity of Nerves and Muscles

The infant's muscles and nerves are examined six times by the medical professional. Each area examined is assigned a score. The higher the score, the more mature the baby is on average. These areas have been verified:

- Posture. This examines the baby's arm and leg holding technique.
- "Square window." This examines the range of motion of the infant's hands in relation to the wrist.
- Arm recoil. This examines the extent to which the baby's arms rebound to a flexed position.
- Popliteal angle. This examines the baby's knee length.
- "Scarf sign." This examines the range of motion of the infant's elbows across its chest.
- Heel to ear. This examines the proximity of the baby's feet to their ears.

The healthcare provider can estimate the baby's gestational age by adding the scores for the nerves and muscles and the physical assessment. Mature and postmature babies receive very high scores, while immature babies receive very low scores. These examinations are all crucial means of finding out about the health of your unborn child. Your baby's doctor can plan the best possible care by identifying any issues (Baily et al, 2009; Levine et al, 2019; Jasani et al, 2021).

3.4. NEWBORN SCREENING

A public health initiative known as newborn screening (NBS) examines infants for treatable conditions that are not clinically evident in the newborn period. The objective is to identify infants who are at risk for these conditions at an early age so that the diagnosis can be confirmed and treatment can be started to change the disease's clinical course and prevent or lessen its clinical manifestations. The discovery that dietary modifications could be used to treat the amino acid disorder phenylketonuria (PKU) and that early intervention was necessary for the best result led to the founding of NBS. PKU babies seem normal at birth, but they have irreversible intellectual disability because they cannot metabolize the essential amino acid phenylalanine. Robert Guthrie created a directtechnique in the 1960s that used a bacterial inhibition assay to find high phenylalanine levels in blood soon after a baby was born. Guthrie also invented the practice of collecting blood on transportable filter paper because he realized that a direct system was required for large-scale screening. Filter paper similar to this is still used for newborn screening worldwide. NBS was first implemented as a public health initiative in the United States in the early 1960s, and it has since spread to other nations.

The purpose of screening programs, which are frequently conducted by national or state regulatory bodies, is to check for a specific panel of treatable disorders in all newborns born within the jurisdiction. Each jurisdiction determines how many diseases are screened for, and the number can vary widely. Measurements of metabolites or enzyme activity in whole blood samples collected on filter paper are used for the majority of NBS tests. Certain NBS programs include bedside tests for congenital heart defects using pulse oximetry and hearing loss using automated auditory brainstem response. When an infant tests positive, more testing is done to see if the result was a false positive or if the infant is actually afflicted with a disease. Follow-up testing is usually coordinated by the infant's primary care physician or pediatrician and geneticists.

3.4.1. Inclusion of Disorders

Initially, newborn screening programs used screening standards that were mostly derived from JMG Wilson and F. Jungner in the year 1968. Their publication, Principles and Practice of Screening for Disease, suggested 10 requirements that screening programs should fulfill before being used as a public health measure, even though it did not directly address newborn population screening programs. Every jurisdiction administers newborn screening programs, and a panel of experts usually reviews additions to and removals from the panel. The four criteria from the publication that were relied upon when making decisions for early newborn screening programs were:

- having a workable treatment plan in place that improves the prognosis for individuals with the illness who are diagnosed early.
- knowledge of the condition's progression over time
- a comprehension of who will receive medical treatment
- a public-acceptable screening test that is dependable for patients with and without the condition.

Discussions about how screening programs should change have arisen as diagnostic techniques have advanced. Even in cases where a patient does not meet all other screening criteria, the number of diseases that may potentially be detected has significantly increased thanks to tandem mass spectrometry. In many countries across the world, Duchenne muscular dystrophy has been included in screening programs, even though there isn't enough data to say whether or not a patient's clinical outcome is improved by early detection.

3.4.2. Targeted Disorders

The goal of newborn screening is to detect infants with curable conditions before they exhibit clinical symptoms or sustain irreversible harm. It is meant to be a public health initiative. The first condition for which newborn screening was intended was phenylketonuria (PKU), which was first introduced in a few hospitals before swiftly spreading throughout the United States and the rest of the world. Guthrie and colleagues searched for other disorders that could be detected and treated in infants after the success of newborn screening for PKU (39 infants were identified and treated in the first two years of screening, with no false negative results). Eventually, they developed bacterial inhibition assays to identify classic galactosemia and maple syrup urine disease. Since the 1960s, newborn screening has increased, though national guidelines can differ significantly. PKU testing was first used in this regard. While France and Hong Kong only screened for one condition (PKU and congenital hypothyroidism, respectively), the United States screened for 54 conditions in 2011, Germany for 12, and the United Kingdom for two (PKU and medium-chain acyl-CoA dehydrogenase deficiency, or MCADD). Globally, newborn screening programs cover a wide range of conditions, depending on factors such as legal requirements, population prevalence of specific diseases, political pressure, and the availability of resources for testing and patient follow-up.

3.4.2.1. Congenital Disorders of Amino Acid Metabolism

The practice of newborn screening began with the identification of phenylketonuria (PKU), an amino acid disorder that can lead to severe intellectual disability if left untreated. Robert Guthrie developed the screening test for PKU in the early 1960s, allowing for early detection and intervention before symptoms appear. This led to the widespread adoption of newborn screening programs globally. Ireland was the first country to implement a nationwide screening program in February 1966, followed by Austria and England in subsequent years. Other amino acid disorders tested for include Tyrosinemia and Maple Syrup Urine Disorder.

3.4.2.2. Fatty Acid Oxidation Disorders

To include several fatty acid oxidation disorders

in newborn screening programs, tandem mass spectrometry was developed as a screening tool. One of the first conditions to be considered for inclusion was medium chain acyl-CoA dehydrogenase deficiency (MCADD), which has been linked to multiple cases of sudden infant death syndrome. When the United Kingdom expanded its screening program from PKU only, MCADD was the first condition added. According to population-based studies conducted in Australia, Germany, and the US, the combined incidence of fatty acid oxidation disorders in Caucasians is 1:9300. While other nations screen for a subset of these, the United States screens for all known fatty acid oxidation disorders, either as primary or secondary targets.

It has been demonstrated that the introduction of screening for fatty acid oxidation disorders has decreased the morbidity and mortality linked to the conditions, especially MCADD. According to an Australian study, compared to individuals who presented clinically before screening, those identified by newborn screening as having MCADD experienced a 74% reduction in episodes of severe metabolic decompensation or death. Infants identified before clinical presentation resulted in better outcomes at a lower cost, according to studies conducted in the UK and the Netherlands.

Programs for newborn screening have also increased the amount of information available about certain uncommon conditions. Short-chain acyl-CoA dehydrogenase deficiency (SCADD) was considered a life-threatening condition before it was included in newborn screening. The majority of individuals diagnosed with this enzyme deficiency through newborn screening were asymptomatic, to the point where SCADD was taken off screening panels in several areas. This clinical phenotype most likely would not have been discovered in the absence of the cohort of patients found through newborn screening.

3.4.2.3. Endocrinopathies

The two endocrine system conditions that are most frequently mentioned are congenital adrenal hyperplasia (CAH) and hypothyroidism (CH). The standard newborn screening card can be used to collect blood samples for testing for both disorders. Measurements of thyroxin (T4), thyrotropin (TSH), or a mix of the two analytes are used to screen for CH. The main marker used to screen for CAH is elevated 17α-hydroxyprogesterone (17α-OHP). This is most commonly achieved using enzyme-linked immunosorbent assays, although many programs also use a second tier tandem mass spectrometry test to lower the number of false positive results. Examining screening results carefully for CAH may also reveal cases of congenital adrenal hypoplasia, which manifests as abnormally low 17α-OHP levels. The immunoassay method shows a high rate of false positive results when used as a screening technique to measure 17α-OHP in dried blood spots. According to the Endocrine Society's 2018 clinical practice guideline, using LC-MS/MS to measure adrenal steroid hormones (like androstenedione and 21-deoxycortisol) and 17α-OHP is advised as an additional screening method to improve the accuracy of positive predictions.

In the 1970s, CH was incorporated into numerous newborn screening programs as the second condition following PKU. The main cause of CH is thyroid gland dysgenesis. Despite years of screening, the global incidence of CH was estimated at 1:3600 births without significant differences among ethnic groups. However, recent data from certain areas, such as New York, have shown a higher incidence of 1:1700 births. The reasons for this apparent increase have been investigated, but no clear explanation has been identified.

The condition known as classic CAH, which is the focus of newborn screening programs, is brought on by a lack of the steroid 21-hydroxylase enzyme and manifests itself in two ways: a simple virilizing form and a salt-wasting form. Between populations, the incidence of CAH can differ significantly. The Yupic Eskimos of Alaska (1:280) and the French island of Réunion (1:2100) have the highest recorded incidence rates.

3.4.2.4. Hemoglobinopathies

Any condition that leads to the abnormal production of hemoglobin falls under the category of hemoglobinopathies. It is believed that 7% of the global population may carry a hemoglobinopathy that has clinical significance. The most well-known disorder within this group is sickle cell disease. Newborn screening for numerous hemoglobinopathies is conducted by identifying abnormal patterns using isoelectric focusing, which can detect various types of abnormal hemoglobins. In the United States, newborn screening for sickle cell disease was recommended for all infants in 1987, but it was not fully implemented across all 50 states until 2006 (Figure 3.7).

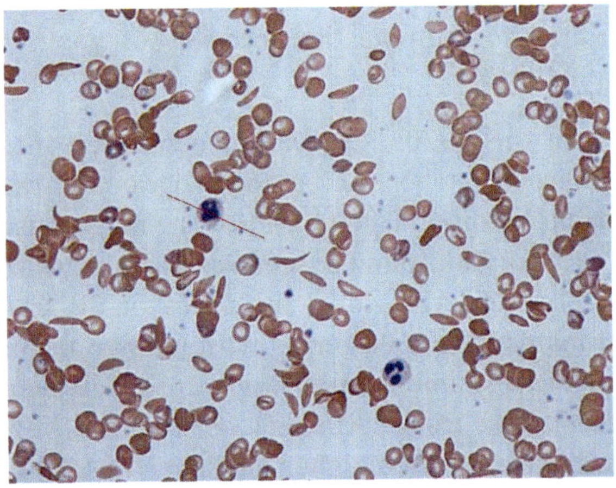

Figure 3.7. *Sickle cells in human blood: both normal red blood cells and sickle-shaped cells are present.*

Source: By Dr Graham Beards – Own work, CC BY-SA 3.0, https://commons.wikimedia.org/w/index.php?curid=18421017. Treatment for hemoglobinopathies, including sickle cell disease, can be started on time when patients are identified early. Blood transfusions are administered to patients diagnosed with severe thalassemia, and penicillin has been used in children with sickle cell disease.

3.4.2.5. Organic Acidemias

0The majority of states did not begin screening for any of the organic acidemias before tandem mass spectrometry considerably increasing the range of conditions that could be identified through newborn screening. Since 1971, Quebec has operated a voluntary second-tier screening program that uses thin layer chromatography to screen urine samples taken at three weeks of age for an expanded list of organic acidemias. Several organic acidemias, such as propionic acidemia, methylmalonic acidemia, and isovaleric acidemia, can be identified through newborn screening with tandem mass spectrometry.

3.4.2.6. Cystic Fibrosis

In 1981, newborn screening programs in New Zealand and some Australian regions included the diagnosis of cystic fibrosis (CF) based on the measurement of immunoreactive trypsinogen (IRT) in dried blood spots. Australia implemented a two-tier testing program following the discovery of the CTR gene to lower the quantity of false positive results. Samples that showed an increased IRT value were subsequently sent back to parents and medical professionals after being subjected to molecular analysis to determine whether any disease-causing mutations were present. All 50 states have recommended that CF be included in the core panel of conditions. Texas was the last to start a CF screening program in 2010. In 2007, Alberta became the pioneer province in Canada to introduce CF screening. CF is not included in the screening programs in Prince Edward Island, New Brunswick, Nova Scotia,

Newfoundland, or Quebec. Both the United States and many European Union nations screen for cystic fibrosis (CF). One of the most recent nations to include CF in its newborn screening options is Switzerland, which did so in January 2011.

3.4.2.7. Urea Cycle Disorders

In many jurisdictions, newborn screening programs include disorders of the distal urea cycle, such as citrullinemia, argininosuccinic aciduria, and argininemia, which are identified using tandem mass spectrometry to identify essential amino acids. Because they cannot be reliably detected with current technology and because severely affected infants will present with clinical symptoms before newborn screening results are available, proximal urea cycle defects, such as ornithine transcarbamylase deficiency and carbamoyl phosphate synthetase deficiency, are not included in newborn screening panels. The identification of elevated ornithine levels in the newborn screening dried blood spot is the basis for some regions' claims to screen for HHH syndrome (hyperammonemia, hyperornithinemia, homocitrullinuria). However, other sources have demonstrated that affected individuals do not have elevated ornithine at birth.

3.4.2.8. Lysosomal Storage Disorders

Programs for frequent newborn screening do not cover lysosomal storage disorders. They are heterogeneous in general, with only about 40 disorders having been identified for which screening is practical. The benefits of early treatment (when available), avoiding a diagnostic maze for families, and giving couples with an affected child information on family planning are the main justifications for their inclusion in newborn screening programs. The challenges of accurately identifying those who will be impacted by a severe form of the disorder, the relatively unproven nature of the treatment approaches, and the high risk/high cost of some treatment options are the main points of contention against including these disorders, either collectively or individually.

Due in large part to Jim Kelly's efforts, whose son Hunter had the disease, New York State launched a pilot study in 2006 to screen for Krabbe disease. In Austria, a pilot screening program using anonymized dried blood spots for four lysosomal storage diseases—Gaucher disease, Pompe disease, Fabry disease, and Niemann-Pick disease—was finished in 2010. Their data revealed several late-onset diseases, which are not usually the focus of newborn screening programs, as well as an increased incidence compared to what was expected in the population.

3.4.2.9. Hearing Loss

Undiagnosed hearing loss in children can have detrimental effects on language, social interactions, emotions, cognitive function, academic performance, and vocational skills, among other developmental domains. These effects can all have an adverse effect on a child's quality of life. Screening programs aimed at identifying infants with hearing loss as early as possible have been motivated by the high incidence of the condition (estimated at 1–3 per 1,000 live births, and as high as 4 percent for patients in neonatal intensive care units) and the serious consequences of a delayed diagnosis. These patients and their families can get the resources they need to maximize their developmental outcomes thanks to early identification.

Transiently evoked otoacoustic emissions, automated auditory brainstem responses, or a combination of the two are used for bedside newborn hearing testing. Depending on the technology employed, hearing screening programs have found that the initial testing can cost anywhere from $10.20 to $23.37 per baby. There may be false positive results because these are merely screening tests. A fussy baby, environmental noise in the testing room, user error, or fluid or congestion in the baby's outer or middle ear could all be the cause of false positive results. The initial referral rates (screen positive results) for hearing screening programs ranged from 0.6% to 16.7%, according to an analysis of the programs. 0.517% was the highest overall incidence of hearing loss detection. In all screening programs, a sizable fraction of screen-positive infants were lost to follow-up before a diagnosis could be confirmed or ruled out.

3.4.2.10. Congenital Heart Defects

Prenatal ultrasound and postnatal physical examination may fail to detect critical congenital heart defects (CCHD) in certain cases. Recently, bedside screening for congestive heart failure (CCHD) at 24 to 48 hours postpartum has included pulse oximetry. This approach, which solely looks at blood oxygen levels, can't, however, identify every cardiac issue. If a baby's test results are positive, an immediate follow-up examination—such as an echocardiography—is performed to identify the reason for the low oxygen levels. After a diagnosis of CCHD, babies are examined by cardiologists.

3.4.2.11. Severe Combined Immunodeficiency

T-cell deficiency-induced severe combined immunodeficiency (SCID) is a disease that has recently been included in newborn screening programs in some United States. In 2008, Wisconsin became the first state to require the inclusion of SCID in its screening panels, and in 2010, it was suggested that panels in every state should follow suit. As of December 2018, SCID screening is conducted in every United states. In January 2018, Norway became the first nation in Europe to implement nationwide SCID screening. Using real-time polymerase chain reaction (qPCR), T-cell receptor excision circles (TRECs) are detected in infants with sickle cell disease (SCID). The TRECs in infants with SCID are reduced.

There are several reasons why SCID has not been widely included in newborn screening. Since PCR is not used for any other assays included in screening programs, it requires technology that is not currently used in the majority of newborn screening labs. Affected infants must also receive follow-up and treatment from qualified immunologists, who may not be available in every area. Stem cell transplants, the main treatment for SCID, are not available in all centers.

3.4.2.12. Other Conditions

An X-linked condition called Duchenne muscular dystrophy (DMD) is brought on by a malfunction in dystrophin synthesis. Numerous countries have either tested for or attempted to screen for DMD by measuring the elevated levels of creatine kinase in dried blood spots. The lack of universal newborn screening for DMD has resulted in a significant delay in diagnosis for affected individuals. Interest in including a newborn screening test rises as DMD treatment options become more and more successful. Since 1978, there have been several instances of DMD being incorporated into newborn screening programs in Edinburgh, Germany, Canada, France, Wales, Cyprus, Belgium, and the United States (typically as a pilot study on a small subsection of the population). The only nation that was still using creatine kinase levels to screen for DMD in 2012 was Belgium.

Newborn screening is becoming possible for disorders for which early intervention could be beneficial, but none was previously available. This is because treatments are getting better. A peroxisomal disease with a variable clinical presentation, adrenalleukodystrophy (ALD) is one of the disorders that has drawn the attention of those looking to identify patients at an early stage. ALD can take many different forms, some of which do not manifest until adulthood, so adding it to screening programs can be challenging for some nations. The most effective course of treatment is a stem cell transplant, which is a highly risky operation.

3.4.3. Techniques

3.4.3.1. Sample Collection

Most frequently, whole blood samples collected on specially designed filter paper—originally created by Robert Guthrie—are used for newborn screening tests. The filter paper is frequently fastened to a form that asks for certain details about the child and parents. This contains the infant's weight and gestational age, as well as the date and time of birth and sample collection. Along with any additional nutrition the baby may have received (total parenteral nutrition), the form will also include information about whether the baby has received a blood transfusion. The majority of newborn screening cards additionally provide the infant's doctor's contact information if additional testing or care is required. In addition to conducting voluntary urine screening programs where parents collect a sample at 21 days of age and submit it to a provincial laboratory for an additional panel of conditions, the Canadian province of Quebec performs newborn screening on whole blood samples collected as in most other jurisdictions.

When collecting newborn screening samples, the child must be fed at least once within the first 24 to 7 days of the baby's birth. Many times, individual jurisdictions will have more precise guidelines. For example, some states may accept samples taken as early as 12 hours of life, while others may advise waiting until 48 hours or later. Every laboratory will have different standards for what constitutes an acceptable sample and when new ones need to be obtained. Midwives or the hospital can both gather samples. Every day, samples are delivered to the testing laboratory. Newborn screening is required in both the US and Canada, though parents have the option to voluntarily opt out of the screening by writing. While NBS is required in many areas, parents have the option to formally opt out if they would rather not have their child screened. The majority of Europe requires parental consent before screening a newborn. Mandatory screening proponents contend that parents shouldn't be allowed to decline on their children's behalf because the test is in the child's best interests. There has been no reported increase in costs, decrease in the number of children screened or incidence of included diseases in children who did not undergo screening in regions that support informed consent for the procedure.

3.4.3.2. Laboratory Testing

Numerous laboratory techniques are employed, along with bedside testing for congenital heart defects using pulse oximetry and hearing loss using evoked auditory potentials, because newborn screening programs screen for a variety of conditions. Initially, newborn screening relied on basic bacterial inhibition tests to identify a single condition, phenylketonuria, in the early 1960s. One test was needed for newborn screening under this testing methodology in order to identify one condition. With the increased accessibility of mass spectrometry, it became possible to quickly identify several acylcarnitines and amino acids from a single dried blood spot. As a result, a greater range of conditions were identified by newborn screening. Enzyme assays are used to check for deficiencies in biotinidase and galactosemia. Immunoassays are used to diagnose congenital adrenal hyperplasia and hypothyroidism, respectively. They also measure 17α-hydroxyprogesterone.

Both severe combined immunodeficiency and cystic fibrosis are diagnosed using molecular methods.

The Genomic Uniform-screening Against Rare Diseases in All Newborns (GUARDIAN study), BeginNGS and Early Check in the USA, BabyScreen+ in Australia, Generation Study by Genetics England, Screen4Care, Baby Detect in Belgium, and PERIGENOMED in France are just a few of the global next generation sequencing (NGS) initiatives that have been announced as of 2023. One pan-European research study (NEW_LIVES) with two pilot trials planned in Germany and Italy was among the 14 European newborn screening programs surveyed in 2023. The other initiatives included three in Italy, three in the Netherlands, two in Spain, one in Belgium, one in England, one in Germany, one in Greece, and one in France. Out of the 14 initiatives, 11 chose to focus exclusively on NGS for their research: 6 initiatives intended to use whole genome sequencing (WGS) as the first-tier test for NBS; one of these initiatives also intended to test parents using whole exome sequencing (WES) to aid in variant filtering; 3 initiatives use classical NGS gene panels; 2 initiatives will use WES; and 2 initiatives will take a hybrid approach, comparing WGS and WES and WGS, WGS, and classical NGS. gene panels.

3.4.3.3. Reporting Results

Reporting the results on time is the aim. Parents are rarely informed about the submission hospital's paper report, which is sent if the screens are normal. When an anomaly is found, agency staff members—typically nurses—start attempting to get in touch with the doctor, hospital, and/or nursery via phone. They don't give up until they can get the baby evaluated by a suitable specialist doctor (depending on the disease). The specialist will try to confirm the diagnosis by conducting additional corroboratory or disproving tests, or by repeating the tests in a different laboratory or method. Depending on the positive screening results, different tests are run in the confirmatory phase. Analyte-specific assays to validate any elevations found, functional studies to ascertain enzyme activity, and genetic testing to pinpoint disease-causing mutations are examples of confirmatory testing. When a newborn screen comes back positive, there are situations when testing is also recommended for other family members, including the mother of the child or siblings who were not screened for the same condition. This is because some maternal conditions can be detected by the newborn screen results. The specialist will start treatment and inform the family based on the probability of the diagnosis and the risk of delay. The program's effectiveness is routinely assessed, and great efforts are taken to keep the system in place that identifies each baby with these diagnoses.

3.5. MANAGEMENT OF PRETERM AND LOW BIRTH WEIGHT BABIES

Preterm babies are those born before 37 weeks of pregnancy, and low birth weight babies, regardless of gestational age, are those born with a birth weight of less than 2.5 kg. Every year, over 20 million babies are born with low birth weight and an estimated 15 million babies are born preterm. The greatest cause of death for infants and young children under five years old is still prematurity and low birth weight. Infants born prematurely or with low birth weight (LBW) are more susceptible to developmental disorders such as cerebral palsy and retinopathy of prematurity. Prematurity and low birth weight can have long-term effects that increase the chance of developing chronic conditions like obesity and diabetes in adulthood.

3.5.1. Classification of Preterm and Low Birth Weight Babies

The newborn is more likely to experience complications and even die if their birth weight and gestational age are lower, necessitating greater special care. The classification of early and tiny babies—detailed below—should be considered when determining the specific care they will require.

3.5.1.1. Classification Based on Birth Weight

The majority of preterm babies have low or extremely low birth weights, which are categorized below:

Low birth weight: Newborns weighing between 1,500 and 2,499 grams. With some additional attention and assistance, these babies can typically be handled safely at home.

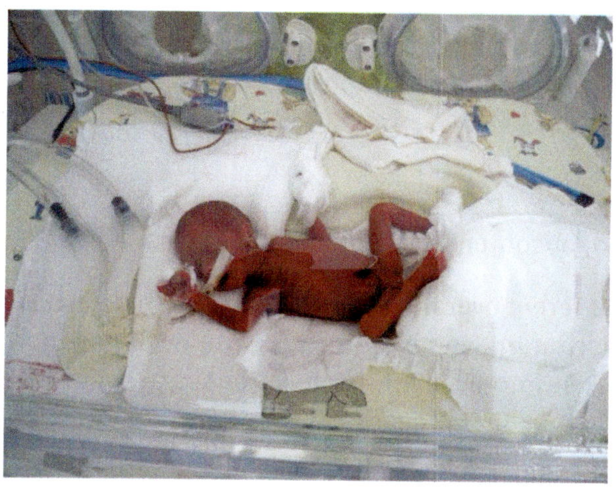

Figure 3.8. *Low birth weight may be a result of preterm birth.*

Source: By Aneta Meszko, Marcin Meszko – Aneta Meszko, CC BY-SA 3.0, https://commons.wikimedia.org/w/index.php?curid=29281512.

Very low birth weight: Babies weighing under 1,500 grams at birth. The inability of such small babies to breathe, swallow, or suckle is a potentially fatal condition, so providing them with appropriate and safe nutrition requires extra care. They also have a harder time keeping their body temperature stable, which puts them at a higher risk of hypothermia. These infants require advanced life support, and they should be sent right away to a hospital that specializes in providing special care for very small infants. However, in certain regions of Ethiopia, rural families may not currently have access to this kind of facility-based care (Figure 3.8).

3.5.1.2. Classification based on Gestational Age

A baby born before 37 full weeks of pregnancy is considered premature. Preterm babies are further categorized as follows based on gestational age:

- **Preterm Baby:** Infants born between 32–36 weeks of gestation, based on the mother's LNMP date, can typically receive safe care at home with additional support and attention.
- **Very Preterm Baby:** Babies whose gestational ages, as determined by the LNMP date, fall between 28 and 31 weeks. For the same reasons as babies with extremely low birth weights, they struggle to feed and regulate their body temperature. If at all feasible, they ought to be referred right away to a hospital for specialized care.

The classifications we just discussed are summarized in Table 3.6, along with the steps you should take.

Table 3.6. Classification of Newborn Babies According to Birth Weight and Gestational Age

Birth Weight and Gestational Age	Classification	Action
Weight less than 1,500 gm	Very low birth weight	Refer URGENTLY to a hospital, making sure to keep the baby warm on the journey
Gestational age less than 32 weeks	Very preterm	Keep the newborn baby warm and refer it soon.
Weight 1,500 to 2,500 gm	Low birth weight	If there is no other problem: counsel on optimal breast feeding, prevention of infection and keeping the baby warm
Gestational age 32–36 weeks	Preterm	As above for low birth weight babies
Weight equal to or above 2,500 gm; gestational age equal to or above 37 weeks	Normal weight and full term	As above for low birth weight and preterm babies

Source: https://www.open.edu/openlearncreate/mod/oucontent/view.php?id=342&printable=1.

Preterm and low birth weight neonates have very different overall needs than term-born neonates when it comes to nutrition, respiratory support, resuscitation, and long-term neurodevelopmental follow-up. When the burden of global mortality is taken into account, preterm births account for 17:7% of deaths under the age of five and 36:1% of all neonatal deaths (Table 3.7).

Table 3.7. Methods for Predicting Preterm Birth Risks and Their Performance Metrics

Sr. No.	Markers	Sample	Period (Weeks)	Detection Limit	Sensitivity (%)	Specificity (%)	PPV (%)	NPV (%)	References
I. Physical method									
1.	Cervical length	NA	22–24	<25 mm	47	89	37	93	[Wildschut, H.I.; Weiner, C.P.; Peters, T.J. 2006]
2.	UCA	NA	18–36	≥111°	65.1	43.6	29.8	77.3	[Luechathananon, S.; Songthamwat, M.; Chaiyarach, S. 2021]

3.	Ferning test	NA	34–37	NA	84.5	78.2	79.5	83.5	[Abdelazim, I.A. 2013]
II. Chemical method									
1.	Nitrazine test	Amniotic fluid	28–36	NA	87.3	80.9	82.1	86.4	[Abdelazim, I.A. 2013]
III. Biomarker-based method									
Specific biomarkers									
1.	fFN	CVF	23–34	≥50 µg/mL	66.7	87.9	36.4	96.2	[Liong, S.; Di Quinzio, M.; Fleming, G.; Permezel, M.; Rice, G.; Georgiou, H. 2015]
2.	PAMG-1	CVF	24–34	≥4 pg/mL	90.0	93.8	78.3	97.4	[Nikolova, T.; Bayev, O.; Nikolova, N.; Di Renzo, G.C. 2014]
					66.7	98.6	75	97.9	[Lotfi, G.; Faraz, S.; Nasir, R.; Somini, S.; Abdeldayem, R.M.; Koratkar, R.; Alsawalhi, N.; Ammar, A. 2019]
3.	IGFBP-1	CVF	20–35	≥30 µg/mL	89.5	94.1	94.4	88.9	[Lembet, A.; Eroglu, D.; Ergin, T.; Kuscu, E.; Zeyneloglu, H.; Batioglu, S.; Haberal, A. 2002]
					83.3	84.4	41.7	97.4	[Eroglu, D.; Yanık, F.; Oktem, M.; Zeyneloglu, H.B.; Kuscu, E. 2007]
					70	74	48	88	[Tanir, H.M.; Sener, T.; Yildiz, Z. 2009]
Nonspecific biomarkers									
1.	Ferritin	Serum		≥37.5 ng/mL	78.7	68.7	71.5	76.3	[Jahedbozorgan, T.; Yaghmaei, M.; Naserieh, M. 2020]
2.	CRP	Serum	≤20	≥5.27 mg/L	75	86.1	37.5	96.87	[Vadillo-Ortega, F.; Estrada-Gutiérrez, G. 2005]

3.	Prolactin	CVF	24–36	>7 ng/mL	78	80	88.64	64.52	[Mehrotra, S.; Solanki, V.; Natu, S.; Chauhan, S.; Sharma, R. 2020]
			20–40	9.5 ng/L	87.03	75	75.80	86.53	[Kariman, N.; Hedayati, M.; Majd, S.A. 2012]
			28–36	30 ng/L	95	78	93	84	[Buyukbayrak, E.; Turan, C.; Unal, O.; Dansuk, R.; Cengizoğlu, B. 2004]
4.	Urocortin-1	Amniotic fluid	13–28	≥57.88 pg/mL	81.8	40.0	40	82	[Karaer, A.; Celik, E.; Celik, O.; Simsek, O.Y.; Ozerol, İ.H.; Yılmaz, E.; Turkcuoglu, I.; Duz, S.A. 2013]
5.	CRH	Serum	24–36	10.45 pg/mL	80	100	100	55.56	[Makrigiannakis, A.; Semmler, M.; Briese, V.; Eckerle, H.; Minas, V.; Mylonas, I.; Friese, K.; Jeschke, U. 2007]
6.	ACTH	Serum	24–36	14.65 pg/mL	80	100	100	55.56	[Makrigiannakis, A.; Semmler, M.; Briese, V.; Eckerle, H.; Minas, V.; Mylonas, I.; Friese, K.; Jeschke, U. 2007]
7.	MMP-8	Amniotic fluid	20 to 36	>30 ng/mL	82.4	78.0	36.0	97.7	[Maymon, E.; Romero, R.; Chaiworapongsa, T.; Berman, S.; Conoscenti, G.; Gomez, R.; Edwin, S. 2001]

UCA: uterocervical angle; PAMG-1: placental alpha macroglobulin-1; fFN: fetal fibronectin; CVF: cervicovaginal fluid, CRH: corticotrophin-releasing hormone, CRP: C-reactive protein; MMP: matrix metalloprotease, ACTH: adrenocorticotrophic hormone.

Source: *Gondane P, Kumbhakarn S, Maity P, Kapat K. Recent Advances and Challenges in the Early Diagnosis and Treatment of Preterm Labor.* Bioengineering. *2024; 11(2):161. https://doi.org/10.3390/bioengineering11020161.*

3.5.2. Preventive and Promotive Care

3.5.2.1. Kangaroo Mother Care (KMC)

KMC, defined as the baby and mother having continuous and prolonged skin-to-skin contact and supporting exclusive breastfeeding or breastmilk feeding, was found to have high certainty evidence for reducing mortality, moderate certainty evidence for reducing infection and hypothermia, low certainty evidence for increasing weight gain, very low certainty evidence for increasing breastfeeding, and no evidence of harm (Figure 3.9).

The use of KMC for medically stable preterm or LBW infants born at home has been recommended to begin in community settings instead of medical facilities, according to updated recommendations. Maintaining KMC for at least eight hours a day was emphasized. Notedly, KMC can be provided by fathers and other family members, but mothers should always give it when at all possible.

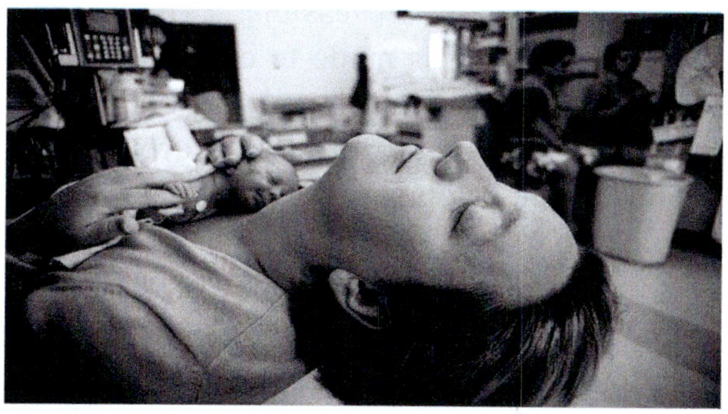

Figure 3.9. *Skin-to-skin contact with the mother can help with thermoregulation.*

Source: By Polihale – Own work, CC BY-SA 3.0, https://commons.wikimedia.org/w/index.php?curid=7071001.

Moreover, unless the infant is critically ill, a new strong, high certainty recommendation was made for the start of KMC as soon as possible after birth (including for hospitalized infants who are not yet clinically stabilized) is in shock, needs artificial ventilation, or is not able to breathe on their own even after resuscitation. The substantial benefits of reduced mortality and hypothermia (high certainty evidence), decreased infections and increased weight gain (low certainty evidence), and the lack of harm were the basis for this recommendation for initial KMC. Including heart rate, breathing, color, temperature, and, if feasible, oxygen saturation, close observation of infants was thought to be crucial, particularly when they were receiving immediate KMC. The GDG encouraged fathers and other caregivers to provide KMC and to implement it globally, including in high-income environments. The instantaneous KMC was acknowledged. That is to say. the need for mother-newborn care units, where parents, siblings, and other family members can spend 24 hours a day with their preterm or LBW babies, and the start of KMC as soon as possible after birth (Figure 3.10).

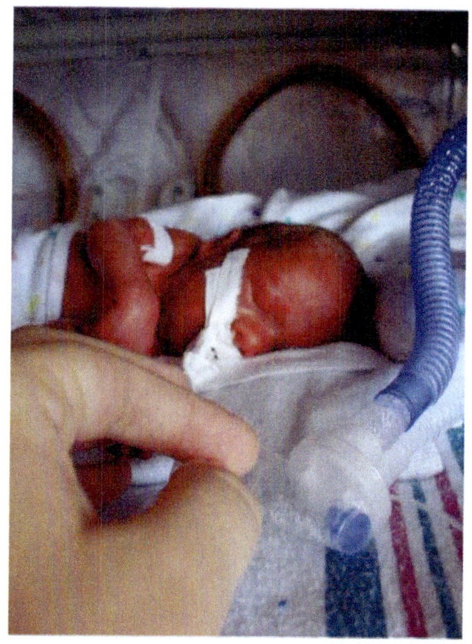

Figure 3.10. *Low birth weight infants may require respiratory support such as intubation and mechanical ventilation due to lung immaturity.*

Source: By ceejayoz – https://www.flickr.com/photos/ceejayoz/3579010939/, CC BY 2.0, https://commons.wikimedia.org/w/index.php?curid=8039784.

3.5.2.2. Probiotics

Probiotics may be taken into consideration for human-milk-fed preterm infants <32 weeks gestation, according to a new, conditional recommendation based on evidence with a moderate level of certainty. In trials involving preterm infants born before 32 weeks of gestation, the balance of evidence demonstrated moderate benefits for reduced mortality, necrotizing enterocolitis, and invasive infection, with no evidence of harm. The variability of the probiotic species assessed in the studies was not entirely clear, and there was little information available regarding long-term negative effects. The GDG did not offer any advice on the kind or composition of probiotics (e.g., powder or drops), dosage, timing, or length of probiotic administration; however, it was recommended that only probiotics specifically designed for preterm or low birth weight infants, which have been approved by national regulatory bodies and come with clear usage guidelines, be used, in conjunction with parental decision-making. Due to insufficient data, neither infants older than 32 weeks nor those who only received formula were advised to follow this recommendation.

3.5.2.3. Emollient Therapy

A new recommendation with low-certainty evidence has been issued for using 'natural' oils (such as sunflower and coconut oil) on premature or low birth weight infants. The recommendation is based on potential benefits such as reduced severe infections and increased weight gain (low-certainty evidence), as well as increased length (moderate-certainty evidence), with no known harms. The guideline development group (GDG) did not recommend using ointments or creams, as there is no proven benefit for critical outcomes. The GDG suggests using sunflower or coconut oils specifically, based on evidence of their effectiveness. Clinicians may use their judgment in determining the duration of use, and oils should be applied gently to avoid damaging the skin.

3.5.2.4. Feeding

Consistent with previous recommendations for all infants, the strong recommendation to exclusively breastfeed preterm or LBW infants until they are six months old has not been altered. Regarding various facets of breast-feeding, seven more revised recommendations were issued.

Feeding Mother's Own Milk: A strong recommendation was made for the use of donor human milk in feeding preterm or LBW infants, particularly those <32 weeks gestation, based on low-certainty evidence showing moderate benefits such as decreased mortality, necrotizing enterocolitis, and infections without any evidence of harm. While supporting mothers to provide their own breastmilk was deemed important, in cases where this is not feasible, a conditional recommendation was made to consider donor human milk. Trials showed moderate benefits in terms of decreased necrotizing enterocolitis and feed intolerance for infants <32 weeks gestation or <1.5 kg, but also found small harms in growth measures such as weight gain, length, and head circumference. It should be noted that donor human milk in these trials was pasteurized, so recommendations on the use of unpasteurized milk could not be made.

Multicomponent fortification of human milk was not always advised for preterm or low-birth-weight (LBW) infants; however, a conditional recommendation was made for very preterm (less than 32 weeks) or very low-birth-weight (less than 10.5 kg) infants fed mother's own or donor human milk, based on low-to moderate-certainty evidence. There was ambiguous evidence regarding the risks of death and necrotizing enterocolitis, while there was evidence for the minor benefits of increased weight, length, and head circumference while in the hospital (low certainty evidence). The GDG concluded that once enteral feeds are well established, commercially available multicomponent fortifiers designed especially for preterm infants should be started (e.g., ≥100 ml/kg daily; "full" enteral feeds are usually defined as 150 ml/kg daily), and the length of time should be determined by clinical judgment.

Based on low-certainty evidence that preterm formula, i.e., mother's milk, and donor human milk are not available, the GDG made a conditional recommendation. For babies <32 weeks gestation or <1.5 kg at birth, commercially available nutrient-enriched formulas designed especially for preterm infants may be taken into consideration. This was supported by evidence of minor benefits, such as increased weight gain and head circumference growth in hospitals, as well as increased psychomotor development, and by the lack of evidence supporting any negative effects from feeding preterm infants nutrient-enriched formula, which consists of protein and energy along with minerals, vitamins, and other nutrients, instead of standard formula. According to the GDG, clinical judgment should be the basis for both initiation and duration.

Based on evidence with a moderate degree of certainty, it was strongly advised that enteral feeding—which includes direct breastfeeding as well as feeding through a cup, naso-, or Oro-gastric tube—be started as soon as possible for preterm or low birth weight (LBW) infants, including those weighing less than 11.5 kg or gestational age of 32 weeks. This was based on evidence of moderate benefits of decreased length of hospital stay and mortality (moderate certainty); there was also evidence of very low certainty of decreased intra-ventricular hemorrhage in trials (n = 14) involving infants <37 weeks gestation or <2.5 kg birth weight, including 6 trials involving infants <32 weeks <1.5 kg; no harms were observed. As soon as possible after birth, infants who are capable of breastfeeding should be placed on the breast; those who are not should be given expressed breast milk and placed on the breast for non-nutritive sucking. The recommendation stressed the need for caution when implementing these suggestions to unstable infants; the start of enteral feeding for these babies should be determined by clinical judgment. When possible, all newborns should be fed human milk; however, if human milk is not available, formula can be given to them instead of parenteral nutrition or delayed enteral feeding, which is not as healthy. A recommendation to limit feed volume was not made because there was no difference in the effect based on the initial feed volume.

Based on low-certainty evidence, a conditional recommendation was made in health facilities that preterm infants <34 weeks gestation may consider scheduled feeding until discharge, instead of responsive feeding. Evidence of very low certainty of small benefits from responsive feeding on shorter hospital stays as well as low certainty of small harms from responsive feeding on reduced weight gain until discharge guided this decision. The GDG recommended that 2–3 hourly scheduled feedings be used, as this is a widely used and practical schedule. The trials that were part of the review employed a variety of feeding schedules. No advice regarding feeding after being released from the hospital could be given. The importance of providing responsive care and nurturing care, regardless of the type of feeding regimen, was emphasized as being essential to the well-being of every preterm or LBW infant.

In premature infants, particularly those born at less than 32 weeks gestation or weighing less than 1.5 kg and requiring alternative feeding methods such as gastric tube or cup feeding, it is conditionally recommended, based on moderate-certainty evidence, to increase feeding advancement by up to 30 ml/kg per day. Studies have shown moderate benefits in terms of time to regain birth weight (high certainty), reduced length of hospital stay, and decreased episodes of apnea (moderate certainty) in trials involving infants born before 37 weeks gestation or weighing less than 2.5 kg. This included 6 trials specifically focusing on infants born before 32 weeks or weighing less than 1.5 kg. The risk of neurodevelopmental disability was found to be of low certainty. All trials compared faster feeding advancement (increases of 30–40 ml/kg per day) with slower advancements (increments of 10–25 ml/kg per day). The Guideline Development Group (GDG) opted to set 30 ml/kg per day as the threshold for fast advancement, aligning with many national guidelines.

3.5.2.5. Micronutrients

Based on moderate certainty evidence, enteral iron supplementation was strongly advised for human milk fed to preterm or low birth weight infants who were not getting iron from another source. The evidence supporting this was limited to moderate benefits of increased length (low certainty evidence), moderately strong evidence of decreased anemia prevalence (moderate certainty evidence), very low certainty evidence of increased ferritin, and no evidence of negative effects. When enteral feeds are fully established, the GDG recommended starting a daily dose of 2–4 mg/kg/day of elemental iron and continuing the administration until the infant receives iron from another source. Furthermore, recommendations for zinc, vitamin A, and vitamin D were conditional, while those for calcium, phosphorus, and several micronutrients were not.

Enteral zinc supplementation may be taken into consideration for human milk-fed preterm or LBW infants who are not receiving zinc from another source, according to a conditional recommendation based on low-certainty evidence. There was evidence for modest to moderate benefits of reduced mortality (low certainty evidence), moderately certain evidence of decreased diarrhea and increased weight, length, and head circumference, and unclear evidence of detrimental effects on mental development (low certainty evidence). When enteral feeds are fully established, the GDG recommended starting a daily dose of 1–3 mg/kg/day of elemental zinc. This dose should be continued until the infant receives zinc from another source.

Enteral vitamin D supplementation may be taken into consideration for human milk-fed preterm or low birth weight (LBW) infants who are not receiving vitamin D from another source, according to a conditional recommendation based on low-certainty evidence. Evidence suggested that there were minor benefits to reduced developmental delay at two years and bronchopulmonary dysplasia at two months (very low certainty evidence), as well as to increased weight and length at six months (moderate certainty evidence). Evidence for mortality was ambiguous (low certainty evidence). When enteral feedings are well established, a 400–800 IU daily dose may be started and continued until the baby gets vitamin D from another source.

For preterm or low birth weight (LBW) infants who are breastfed and have a gestational age of less than 32 weeks or a birth weight of less than 1.5 kg and are not receiving vitamin A from another source, enteral vitamin A supplementation has been recommended conditionally based on low certainty evidence. There was no evidence of harm and only a slight benefit in terms of reduced mortality, bronchopulmonary dysplasia, patent ductus arteriosus, and retinopathy of prematurity (low certainty evidence). When enteral feedings are fully established, the GDG recommended starting a daily dose of 1,000–5,000 IU and continuing it until the infant receives vitamin A from another source.

For preterm or low birth weight babies,

there was insufficient evidence to recommend either multiple micronutrient supplementation or supplementation with calcium and phosphorus.

3.5.3. Management of Complications

Two respiratory interventions were given priority when it came to managing complications in preterm or low-birth weight babies: methylxanthines for apnea and continuous positive airway pressure (CPAP) for respiratory distress. The suggestions for additional interventions remained unaltered.

3.5.3.1. CPAP for Respiratory Distress Syndrome

For preterm infants <37 weeks gestation exhibiting clinical signs of respiratory distress syndrome (RDS), CPAP is strongly advised based on moderate-certainty evidence. Reductions in mechanical ventilation and mortality were two signs of moderate benefits. There was evidence of minor adverse effects with unclear clinical significance concerning elevated pneumothorax. The GDG advised starting CPAP as soon as an RDS diagnosis is made or clinical suspicions are raised. The GDG also issued a conditional recommendation that CPAP therapy be taken into consideration as soon as possible after delivery, based on low-certainty evidence. The GDG concluded that the benefits of immediate CPAP were modest to moderate. Benefits included a decrease in "failed treatment," which was defined as bronchopulmonary dysplasia in preterm infant trials <32 weeks, as well as a decrease in recurrent apnea, hypoxia, hypercarbia, increasing oxygen requirement, or the need for mechanical ventilation. No evidence of harm was present.

The GDG also took into account the requirement that CPAP be implemented by trained personnel using high-quality supplies and equipment, such as monitors and blended, humidified oxygen air. A conditional recommendation for bubble CPAP based on low-certainty evidence was reached after a specific set of CPAP *pressure sources* were examined. These included comparing underwater (water-seal) 'bubble' CPAP with mechanical ventilator CPAP or infant flow driver CPAP, all of which were commercially manufactured (no locally manufactured or locally adapted devices were used). The devices were humidified blended oxygen-air and used short nasal prong interfaces. Based on data from trials involving preterm infants <37 weeks gestation, this decision was made due to the small to moderate benefits of decreased pneumothorax, decreased bronchopulmonary dysplasia, and decreased failed treatment (defined as recurrent apnea, hypoxia, hypercarbia, increasing oxygen requirement, or needing mechanical ventilation). Additionally, there was evidence of minor damage, mostly of unknown cause, including increased nasal injury, which was defined as ulceration, bleeding, septal injury, and scarring, excluding hyperemia or erythema. According to the GDG, the nasal interface (i.e., prongs and cannulas) used with bubble CPAP machines should be chosen carefully, and the infant requires expert nursing care while using the prongs and cannulas.

3.5.3.2. Methylxanthines for Apnea

Caffeine for treatment of apnea in all premature babies. <37 weeks gestation was strongly recommended based on moderate-certainty evidence. Inclusion criteria for the six RCTs relevant to this comparison were gestational age at birth below 37 weeks and evidence of apnea. Evidence of moderate benefits included decreased death, bronchopulmonary dysplasia and neurodevelopmental disability (moderate certainty evidence) and decreased mechanical ventilation (low certainty evidence) in trials of caffeine in preterm infants, with no evidence of harm. The GDG considered that caffeine for the prevention of apnea may be considered in preterm infants <34 weeks gestation, based on low certainty evidence. Inclusion criteria for the seven RCTs relevant to this comparison were gestational age at birth below 34 weeks and no evidence of apnea. Evidence of small to moderate benefits was found for decreased bronchopulmonary dysplasia (moderate certainty evidence) and decreased apneic episodes (low certainty evidence) in trials of preterm infants <34 weeks gestation, and uncertain evidence of harms was found for increased mortality and mechanical ventilation (low certainty evidence). The GDG recommended that if caffeine is not available, other methylxanthines (aminophylline or theophylline) may be considered, given decreased apnea and need for mechanical ventilation in infants given aminophylline and theophylline. While evidence for the use of methylxanthines for the prevention of apnea was available only for preterm infants <34 weeks gestation, the GDG suggested that caffeine (or other methylxanthines) may also be considered for prevention of apnea in preterm infants 34–<37 weeks depending on clinical judgment. Based on the largest trial, the suggested dosing of caffeine was a 20 mg/kg loading dose and 5 mg/kg/day maintenance doses for 6 weeks. The GDG also noted that caffeine is often given until corrected gestational age of > The baby is event-free for at least five days at 34 weeks of gestation.

Additionally, caffeine was strongly recommended for the extubation of preterm infants <34 weeks gestation based on evidence of moderate benefits, including decreased death, bronchopulmonary dysplasia, failed extubation, and neurodevelopmental disability, and no evidence of harm. This recommendation was based on moderate-certainty evidence. The GDG recommended that caffeine be started 24 hours before an anticipated extubation based on the largest trials. If the extubation was not planned, caffeine should be given to the baby within six hours of the procedure. For six days, a loading dose of 20 mg/kg and daily maintenance doses of 5 mg/kg were recommended.

3.5.4. Family Involvement and Support

Many suggestions were developed to help and involve families in the care of infants who are premature or low birth weight. The term "family involvement" refers to the routine care that mothers, fathers, and other family members provide for their newborn while the infant is in the newborn care unit. It could involve family members participating in medical decision-making, hospital infrastructure changes, hospital culture shifts, and mothers, fathers, and other family members giving direct bedside care (e.g., family rooms, rooming in, couplet care, or zero mother-child separation). Additional interventions (also referred to as "cointerventions") used in the studies included financial incentives, skin-to-skin care, KMC, infant massage, psychosocial support, and neurodevelopmental and neurobehavioral care.

A strong recommendation has been made for family involvement in the routine care of preterm or low birth weight babies in health facilities. This recommendation is based on moderate evidence showing benefits such as decreased morbidity, increased weight and length at discharge, improved neurodevelopment, shorter hospital stays, and increased breastfeeding. Additionally, family involvement strategies have been shown to reduce parental anxiety and stress. The recommendation applies to infants born before 37 weeks gestation or weighing less than 2.5 kg, with no evidence of harm.

Home visits were found to have the strongest evidence when five different types of interventions—education and counseling, peer-to-peer support, home visits, digital communication, and discharge preparation—were evaluated for their efficacy in helping families care for preterm or LBW infants. Based on evidence with a moderate level of certainty, home visits by qualified health professionals were highly advised to assist families in caring for their preterm or LBW infant. In trials involving infants under 37 weeks gestation or weighing less than 2.5 kg at birth, there was a slight decrease in the number of hospitalizations (very low certainty evidence) and a moderate decrease in mortality (moderate certainty evidence), with no evidence of adverse effects. Additionally, home visits improved the non-critical outcomes of immunization visits, exclusive breastfeeding rates, attachment between parents and their infant, and reduced parental stress. The GDG recommended additional home visits (i.e., given the paucity of data on these characteristics, extra to the regularly planned postnatal contacts for all babies) should be made and their content, frequency, duration, and intensity should be determined.

Based on very low certainty evidence, a conditional recommendation was made that mothers, fathers, and other family members should receive additional support to care for their preterm or LBW baby. This support should begin in medical facilities at the time of birth and continue during follow-up visits after discharge. Healthcare providers, peer support, and counseling can all be used to offer support, as can education and planning for discharge. In addition to improving breastfeeding and parent-infant interaction, education, counseling, and discharge planning had a significant impact on non-critical outcomes like parental stress, anxiety, and depression.

After reviewing 20 global parental leave policies for parents of preterm or LBW infants, a best practice statement was made. It was recognized that parental leave policies should prioritize the unique needs of mothers and fathers in these situations. The recommendation from the GDG was to implement these policies worldwide, with additional days off work and financial support. However, further research is needed to determine the specifics of how many days of leave and what financial benefits should be provided. The GDG also highlighted the varying needs of parents in these situations, including support for hospital stays, medical appointments, stress, caring for other family members, transportation, and necessary equipment (Baily et al, 2009; Levine et al, 2019; Jasani et al, 2021).

3.6. NEONATAL JAUNDICE

Jaundice in newborns is a condition characterized by a yellowish tint in the whites of the eyes and skin, caused by elevated levels of bilirubin. Additional signs may include increased drowsiness or difficulties with feeding. Possible complications include seizures, cerebral palsy, and kernicterus.

Most of the time, no particular underlying physiological condition is present. In other instances, it is caused by hepatic disease, infection, hypothyroidism, red blood cell depletion, or metabolic disorders (pathologic). It's possible to see a bilirubin level higher than 34 μmol/L (2 mg/dL). When levels in otherwise healthy babies exceed 308 μmol/L (18 mg/dL), jaundice is observed on the first day of life, levels rise quickly, jaundice persists for more than two weeks, or the baby seems ill, then there is cause for concern. If any of the results are concerning, more research is advised to find the underlying cause.

The child's age, the underlying cause, and the bilirubin levels all influence whether treatment is necessary. Exchange transfusions, phototherapy, and more frequent feedings are possible treatment options. Early births typically necessitate more intensive medical care. The average duration of physiological jaundice is less than seven days. In the first week of life, more than half of babies are affected by the condition. Approximately 80% of prematurely born babies are impacted. Jaundice claims the lives of over 100,000 late-preterm and term babies worldwide every year.

3.6.1. Etiology

Neonatal hyperbilirubinemia occurs in two different forms.

3.6.1.1. Unconjugated Hyperbilirubinemia (UHB) or Indirect Hyperbilirubinemia

The more prevalent kind, known as unconjugated hyperbilirubinemia, can be pathological or physiological. A physiological change in the metabolism of newborn bilirubin causes physiological jaundice, which explains 75% of cases of neonatal hyperbilirubinemia. Compared to neonates, whose TSB levels are physiologically higher, healthy adults have a normal TSB level of less than 1 mg/dl. Due to increased red blood cell mass and shortened RBC lifespan, bilirubin load is elevated even in healthy full-term newborns. The enzyme required for bilirubin conjugation, uridine diphosphate glucuronosyltransferase (UGT), is not functioning as well, which further impairs bilirubin clearance. The activity of the UGT enzyme in a newborn is only 1% that of an adult. To further add to the elevated TSB levels, these infants also have increased enterohepatic circulation. In full-term infants, physiological jaundice usually develops after 24 hours, peaks between 48 and 96 hours after birth, and goes away in two to three weeks.

If jaundice appears on the first day of life, TSB is greater than the 95th centile for age based on age-specific bilirubin nomograms, levels increase by more than 5 mg/dL/day or more than 0.2 mg/dL/hour, or jaundice lasts longer than two to three weeks in full-term infants, then it is considered pathological. The etiology of unconjugated hyperbilirubinemia can be separated into the following three groups according to the mechanism of bilirubin elevation:

3.6.1.1.1. Increased Bilirubin Production

Immune-mediated hemolysis – includes incompatibilities with blood groups, such as ABO and Rhesus.

Non-immune mediated hemolysis – includes sequestration conditions such as cephalohematoma, subgaleal hemorrhage, intracranial hemorrhage, polycythemia, and sepsis; RBC membrane defects such as hereditary spherocytosis and elliptocytosis; and RBC enzyme defects such as glucose-6-phosphate dehydrogenase (G6PD) deficiency and pyruvate kinase deficiency.

3.6.1.1.2. Decreased Bilirubin Clearance

Crigler-Najjar type I & II, and Gilbert syndrome.

3.6.1.1.3. Miscellaneous Causes

Additional non-specific causes include congenital hypothyroidism, drugs such as sulfa drugs, ceftriaxone, and penicillins, intestinal blockage, pyloric stenosis, jaundice from breast milk, and jaundice from breastfeeding.

Pathological hyperbilirubinemia in neonates is most commonly caused by exaggerated hemolysis, which can be immune or non-immune mediated. Hemolytic disease of the newborn (HDN) is caused by immune-mediated hemolysis, which is seen in blood group incompatibilities such as ABO/RH incompatibilities. Preformed maternal anti-A and anti-B antibodies of the immunoglobulin (Ig) G subclass cross the placenta in HDN, resulting in hemolysis and unnatural hemolysis in neonates with blood types A, B, or AB because of ABO incompatibility. The direct Coombs test has a low sensitivity and positive predictive value for identifying severe UHB, despite being used to aid in diagnosis. About 15% of pregnancies result in mother and fetus ABO incompatibility, but only 4% of newborns with ABO incompatibility experience HDN as a result of their incompatibility.

When a Rh-negative mother who has previously come into contact with Rh-positive red blood cells—typically from a previous pregnancy or miscarriage—becomes sensitized to the Rh antigen and develops antibodies against it, she is said to have Rh-incompatibility. Sensitization first results in IgM antibodies that are unable to pass through the placenta. But in later pregnancies, the antibody class switch generates IgG antibodies that can pass through the placenta and cause red blood cell hemolysis in the fetus carrying Rh blood. Due to the high immunogenicity of the Rh antigen, severe HDN frequently results, which can cause severe UHB in newborns or hydrops in fetuses. Anti-D immune globulin is advised for all Rh-negative pregnant women by the American College of Obstetricians and Gynecologists (ACOG) at 28 weeks of gestation and again after delivery if the baby is Rh-positive or unknown.

Hemoglobinopathies, sepsis, sequestration, polycythemia, RBC enzyme defects, and RBC membrane defects are examples of non-immune causes of UHB. The most prevalent RBC enzyme defect is glucose-6 phosphatase dehydrogenase (G6PD) deficiency, which is passed down as an X-linked recessive trait. By producing NADPH (nicotinamide adenine dinucleotide phosphate hydrogenase) from NADP (nicotinamide adenine dinucleotide phosphate), G6PD shields RBCs from oxidative damage. G6PD deficient RBCs are hemolyzed in response to oxidant stressors such as disease, specific drugs, dyes, and foods like fava beans. This results in anemia and hyperbilirubinemia. It is known that G6PD deficiency is caused by more than 200 distinct types of mutations. Depending on the variation, different newborns may have different clinical presentations, such as severe hyperbilirubinemia and bilirubin encephalopathy. Another enzyme deficiency that results in hemolysis and can manifest in UHB in neonates is pyruvate kinase deficiency (PKD). It is an autosomal recessive (AR) disorder brought on by a malfunction in the machinery that produces adenosine triphosphate (ATP). RBCs, and young RBCs in particular, have a shorter lifespan in PKD, which causes anemia and UHB.

Hereditary spherocytosis (HS) and hereditary elliptocytosis (HE) are two types of UHB caused by abnormalities in the red blood cell membrane. The most prevalent RBC membrane defect, known as HS or Minkowski Chauffard disease, is brought on by mutations in RBC membrane proteins. Most cases manifest as UHB in the neonatal period and are inherited as autosomal dominant (AD) traits. Another kind of RBC membrane defect that is mostly asymptomatic but sporadically results in UHB in the neonatal stage is hereditary elliptocytosis. Most cases are passed down as AD traits due to mutations in the structural membrane protein of red blood cells. Because the spleen contains the elliptical-shaped RBCs in HE, extravascular hemolysis and elevated TSB result.

Due to an elevated bilirubin load, RBC sequestrations from cephalohematoma, subgaleal hemorrhage, and intracranial hemorrhage are also significant causes or risk factors for UHB in the neonatal period. Another condition linked to a higher risk of UHB in neonates is polycythemia. Intrauterine growth restriction (IUGR), infant of diabetic mothers (IDM), large for gestational age (LGA), smoking by the mother, high altitude, twin to twin transfusion, and placental transfusion (delayed cord clamping/

umbilical cord milking) are clinical conditions linked to polycythemia. Research has indicated that placental transfusion improves both term and preterm infants' neurodevelopmental outcomes and lowers the incidence of postnatal anemia. Although this procedure has grown in acceptance, there is a chance that it will raise the risk of hyperbilirubinemia.

Defects in the uridine diphosphate glucuronosyltransferase (UGT) enzyme, either quantitative or qualitative, are typically the cause of indirect hyperbilirubinemia resulting from reduced bilirubin clearance. Three prototype disorders caused by abnormalities in the UGT enzyme are Gilbert syndrome, Crigler-Najjar syndrome type 1, and Crigler-Najjar syndrome type 2. The most prevalent of these, known as Gilbert syndrome, is caused by a mutation in the UGT1A1 gene, which lowers UGT production and causes unconjugated hyperbilirubinemia. When under stress, Gilbert syndrome usually manifests as mild jaundice without hemolysis or liver dysfunction. It is uncommon to present during the neonatal period, and it is typically linked to G6PD. An AR disorder called Crigler-Najjar syndrome type 1 is brought on by a total lack of UGT activity. In the earliest stages of life, affected patients often exhibit severe hyperbilirubinemia, which can result in bilirubin encephalopathy. Individuals with type 2 Crigler-Najjar syndrome still have some UGT enzyme activity. Because of this, TSB levels are not very high, and bilirubin encephalopathy is not often experienced by patients.

Two other common causes of UHB in newborns are jaundice from breast milk and jaundice from breastfeeding. Breastfeeding jaundice, sometimes referred to as breastfeeding failure jaundice, develops during the first week of life as a result of insufficient breast milk intake, which can cause hypernatremia and dehydration. Intestinal motility is lowered and bilirubin excretion in the meconium or stool is reduced when breastfeeding fails. Breast milk jaundice usually goes away by two weeks of age, having peaked in the second week. It starts late in the first week. Pregnanediol's inhibition of the UGT enzyme and the beta-glucuronidase found in breast milk's deconjugation of conjugated bilirubin in the intestines are the main theories for their causes.

IDM, gastrointestinal obstruction, congenital hypothyroidism, and specific medications are some additional non-medical causes of UHB. The main cause of the higher incidence of jaundice in these infants with IDMs is the polycythemia that they frequently have. Reduced hepatic absorption of bilirubin, decreased UGT activity, and slow gastrointestinal motility are associated with UHB in congenital hypothyroidism. Increased bilirubin recycling is facilitated by gastrointestinal obstruction, which increases enterohepatic circulation. Certain medications may also exacerbate UHB in neonates by interfering with albumin binding and displacing bilirubin from albumin. Additionally, oxidative damage to red blood cells during sepsis can raise the bilirubin load and predispose a newborn to UHB.

Most infants with clinical UHB have a combination of two or more of the previously mentioned factors. Furthermore, an infant is more susceptible to jaundice due to a few known risk factors. Prematurity, Asian ethnicity, male gender, exclusive breastfeeding, and a history of jaundice requiring phototherapy in prior siblings are among these risk factors. Finally, UHB in preterm infants poses a unique set of circumstances. Preterm infants are thought to be more likely to experience jaundice as well as a higher risk of bilirubin encephalopathy and kernicterus. Unfortunately, there is currently a lack of information regarding the scope of the issue and agreed-upon protocols for treating UHB in premature infants. In this population, it's also unclear what the TSB threshold is for starting phototherapy and what the requirements are for exchange transfusion. Antioxidant bilirubin may play a physiological role in newborns. In preterm infants, aggressive treatment aimed at lowering TSB levels may lower antioxidant levels and possibly exacerbate preterm retinopathy. Neural injury and chronic lung disease are also linked to reduced antioxidant status. Because there are no evidence-based guidelines, treating UHB in this population is a difficult task.

3.6.1.2. Conjugated Hyperbilirubinemia (CHB) or Direct Hyperbilirubinemia

Conjugated hyperbilirubinemia, also known as neonatal cholestasis, is caused by impaired hepatobiliary function and is characterized by elevated serum conjugated/direct bilirubin (> 1.0 mg/dL). Because cholestatic jaundice/CHB is nearly always pathologic and requires immediate evaluation and treatment, differentiating it from UHB is essential.

Neonatal cholestasis/CHB has many different causes, which fall into the following categories:

- **Obstruction of Biliary Flow:** Neonatal sclerosing cholangitis, neonatal cholelithiasis, biliary atresia, and choledochal cysts.
- **Infections:** Urinary tract infections (UTIs), septicemia, syphilis, toxoplasmosis, CMV, HIV, rubella, and herpes virus.
- **Genetic Causes:** The conditions that fall under this category are: Alagille syndrome, Dubin-Johnson syndrome, galactosemia, fructosemia, Tyrosinemia type 1, cystic fibrosis, progressive familial intrahepatic cholestasis (PFIC), Aagenaes syndrome, and bile acid synthesis disorders (BSAD).
- **Miscellaneous:** Gestational alloimmune liver disease/neonatal hemochromatosis, cholestasis induced by parenteral nutrition, idiopathic neonatal hepatitis, and hypotension.

The most frequent cause of conjugated hyperbilirubinemia in infants is biliary atresia (BA). The prevalence of BA differs amongst geographical areas. Taiwan, the region with the highest incidence, reports 1 in 6000 live births with it. It affects about one in every 12 live births in the United States. Although the exact cause of BA is unknown, genetics, viruses, toxins, chronic inflammation, and autoimmune damage to the bile ducts all appear to have a part in the disease's pathogenesis. The illness, which affects the intra- and extra-hepatic bile ducts, typically manifests itself as pale stools and jaundice between the ages of two and four weeks. Ultrasonography is used for the initial evaluation, and it may reveal the classic triangular cord sign and an absent gallbladder. To optimize the outcome of a Kasai operation (hepatic portoenterostomy), early diagnosis is essential. Compared to surgery done within 60 days, when more than 70% of patients will establish adequate bile flow, less than 25% of patients are reported to respond if the procedure is postponed for 90 days.

Dilation of the intrahepatic and extrahepatic bile ducts is a symptom of choledochal cysts. Unlike sclerosed ducts in biliary atresia, cysts with normal or dilated intrahepatic bile ducts can be detected by ultrasonography. Nonetheless, choledochal cysts and cystic biliary atresia may look alike. A rare type of cholangiopathy known as neonatal sclerosing cholangitis (NSC) frequently manifests in infancy as hepatosplenomegaly, pale stools, CHB, and elevated serum gamma-glutamyl transferase activity (GGT). Another uncommon condition that can result in severe direct hyperbilirubinemia in newborns is neonatal cholelithiasis.

The most prevalent congenital infection, cytomegalovirus (CMV), can present itself in many ways. The most common signs of hepatic involvement in infected newborns are hepatomegaly and CHB, although most of them are asymptomatic. In the differential diagnosis of neonatal cholestasis, syphilis, toxoplasmosis, herpes, and rubella should be considered, particularly in the presence of other congenital infection stigmata such as thrombocytopenia, coagulopathy, growth restriction, and skin rash. The diagnosis would be aided by a thorough assessment of the mother's medical history as well as particular serologies and cultures. Neonates' UTIs are another major cause of CHB, and part of the diagnostic assessment should include a urine culture. A direct result of bacterial products, alterations in the liver's microcirculation, and bacterially released toxins are considered potential causes of cholestasis in UTI patients.

Alagille syndrome (ALGS) is an AD condition in which there are no interlobular bile ducts due to mutations in the JAG1 or NOTCH2 genes. ALGS is the most common cause of familial intrahepatic cholestasis, occurring in 1 in 30,000 live births. Butterfly vertebrae, congenital heart defects (mostly peripheral pulmonic stenosis), kidney involvement, dysmorphic features (broad forehead, small, pointy chin), and posterior embryotoxic of the eye are characteristic clinical features in addition to cholestasis. GGT levels are abnormally high, frequently 20 times higher than normal. It's interesting to note that CHB in ALGS patients may go away as they age. Rarely do people with cystic fibrosis (CF) exhibit cholestasis symptoms due to aberrant bile occlusion of the bile ducts. In developing countries where immunoreactive trypsinogen is not available for newborn screening, neonatal cholestasis could be the initial indicator of the condition.

The most common genetic cause of cholestatic disease is alpha-1-antitrypsin deficiency, which can mimic biliary atresia in the early stages of infancy. Patients carrying the PiZZ genotype experience hepatocyte apoptosis due to anti-trypsin polymer accumulation in the endoplasmic reticulum, which ultimately causes cholestasis and cirrhosis in later childhood. Cholestasis may also get better with age, just like ALGS. Cholestasis in neonates has been linked to several inborn errors of metabolism, including fructosemia, galactosemia, and tyrosinemia type 1. After consuming galactose from milk, newborns with galactosemia present with cholestatic jaundice, cataracts, hepatomegaly, failure to thrive, renal tubular acidosis, and sepsis caused by *Escherichia coli*. Toxic galactose metabolites build up in several organs as a result of a deficiency in the enzyme galactose-1-phosphate uridyl transferase (GALT). GALT activity in the liver or erythrocytes confirms the diagnosis of galactosemia, which is suggested by the presence of reducing substances in the urine. Hereditary tyrosinemia type 1, an additional AR disorder brought on by a deficiency of the enzyme fumarylacetoacetate hydroxylase, may present with neonatal cholestasis. Renal Fanconi syndrome, hepatomegaly, coagulation abnormalities, and the risk of hepatocellular carcinoma in patients who do not receive treatment are additional features of this disorder.

A collection of three genetic disorders that manifest as cholestasis is known as progressive familial intrahepatic cholestasis (PFIC). They have something in common with gene mutations that affect canalicular hepatobiliary transport.

Type 3 typically appears later in infancy, whereas types 1 and 2 typically appear in the neonatal period. Childhood end-stage liver disease and cirrhosis are common in affected patients. GGT levels are raised in type 3 patients and normal in types 1 and 2. Whereas PFIC2 is brought on by a mutation in the ABCB11 gene, which produces the bile salt excretory protein (BSEP), PFIC1 is brought on by a mutation in the ATP8B1 gene, which produces the FIC1 protein. A mutation in the ABCB4 gene, which produces the multi-drug resistant-3 protein (MDR3), is the cause of PFIC 3. Another kind of idiopathic familial intrahepatic cholestasis syndrome marked by neonatal cholestasis and lymphedema in the lower extremities is called Aagenaes syndrome, also referred to as lymphedema cholestasis syndrome (LCS). It is inherited as an AR trait and is primarily observed in people who are Norwegian in origin. Due to a mutation in the ABCC2 gene, which codes for a non-biliary ion transporter in the liver, there is a rare AR disorder known as Dubin-Johnson syndrome (DJS). The presence of black liver and the excretion of coproporphyrin 1 in the urine are two distinctive characteristics of DJS. A shortage of one of the enzymes necessary for the synthesis of bile acids from cholesterol leads to the condition known as bile acid synthesis disorder (BASD). Although BASDs are a rare cause of cholestasis, many of them can be treated with medication alone.

An important iatrogenic cause of cholestasis, parenteral nutrition-associated cholestasis (PNAC) is most commonly identified in preterm infants receiving parenteral nutrition (PN). About 20% of newborns who have received PN for longer than two weeks have PNAC. Intestinal failure and the length of PN use are two separate risk factors for PNAC. The mechanism is likely multifactorial and not fully understood. The primary cause is believed to be abnormal bile salt metabolisms brought on by prematurity and the negative effects of PN components. Liver injury seems to be exacerbated by additional factors like necrotizing enterocolitis and sepsis. Nearly all cases of neonatal hemochromatosis are caused by gestational alloimmune liver disease (GALD), a fulminant alloimmune disorder that is caused by intra- and extra-hepatic iron deposition that culminates in liver failure.

Maternal IgG immunoglobulin against fetal hepatocytes in GALD crosses the placenta and damages fetal hepatocytes through complement-mediated mechanisms. Individuals may exhibit hypoglycemia, coagulopathy, hypoalbuminemia, cholestatic jaundice, edema, and elevated liver enzymes as indicators of liver failure. There is a nearly 90% chance that GALD will recur in subsequent pregnancies, and it can cause fetal or neonatal death. When, even after a thorough diagnostic workup, the cause of neonatal cholestasis cannot be determined, the condition is referred to as idiopathic neonatal hepatitis. The number of causes of neonatal cholestasis that were previously thought to be idiopathic neonatal hepatitis is increasing, which is contributing to the entity's decreasing size.

3.6.2. Epidemiology

Unconjugated hyperbilirubinemia is a condition that frequently affects newborns. It is estimated that if TSB is greater than 5 mg/dl, 60% of term and 80% of preterm newborns will exhibit clinical jaundice. Nonetheless, it is estimated that only 10% of newborns will need phototherapy to treat their jaundice. After the first day of life, physiological jaundice is thought to be the most common cause of clinical jaundice, accounting for about 50% of cases. In breastfed infants, UCH lasting longer than three weeks occurs in about 15% of cases.

The pathological cause of jaundice is present in only a small percentage of infants with neonatal jaundice. Severe hyperbilirubinemia (TSB>25 mg/dl) affects approximately 1 in every 2500 live births. Of these, G6PD deficiency is the most commonly found cause, followed by ABO incompatibility. Compared to their White and African counterparts, newborns with Southeast and Far East Asian ancestry have higher recorded TSB levels. Neonatal jaundice also seems to be more common in those who live near the Mediterranean Sea, particularly in Greece, and in high altitudes.

The prevalence of chronic bilirubin encephalopathy is estimated to be between 1 in 50,000 and 100,000 live births, while the incidence of acute bilirubin encephalopathy is roughly 1 in 10,000 live births. On the other hand, the estimated incidence of kernicterus is significantly higher in developing countries. Compared to UCH, conjugated hyperbilirubinemia is far less common; it affects about 1 in 2500 term infants. Biliary atresia, which accounts for roughly 25% to 40% of all cases, is the most frequently identified cause of cholestatic jaundice in the neonatal period. Infections and TPN-induced cholestasis are the next most common causes. BA continues to be the most common reason for a pediatric liver transplant, with estimates ranging from 60 to 70% of patients with BA eventually needing a liver transplant in childhood.

3.6.3. Pathophysiology

Heme, a byproduct of hemoglobin breakdown, is catabolized in the reticuloendothelial system (RES) to produce bilirubin. Heme oxygenase first transforms heme into biliverdin, which then releases iron and carbon monoxide. The biliverdin reductase enzyme then transforms biliverdin into bilirubin. This hydrophobic unconjugated bilirubin is carried by the bloodstream to the liver attached to albumin, where the enzyme uridine diphosphate-glucuronosyltransferase (UGT) conjugates it with glucuronic acid in the smooth endoplasmic reticulum. Conjugated bilirubin is soluble in water and is eliminated through bile and the gastrointestinal (GI) tract, where intestinal bacterial flora metabolizes it and excretes most of it in feces. Through the enterohepatic circulation, some conjugated bilirubin is reabsorbed after being partially deconjugated in the GI tract by beta-glucuronidase.

Because of their higher birth hemoglobin levels, shorter RBC life spans, and limited newborn liver conjugating capacity, newborns have higher TSB levels than adults. As a result, compared to adult levels of less than 1 mg/dl, full-term newborns typically have peak serum bilirubin concentrations of 5 to 6 mg/dl. Increased bilirubin production in RES, poor hepatic absorption, insufficient bilirubin conjugation, and/or increased enterohepatic circulation of bilirubin are associated with pathological jaundice in neonates.

Unbound and unconjugated bilirubin binds to the brainstem, hippocampus, cerebellum, globus pallidus, and subthalamic nuclei in cases of severe hyperbilirubinemia after crossing the blood-brain barrier. Bilirubin causes breaks in DNA strands, inhibits the synthesis of proteins and DNA, inhibits some mitochondrial enzymes, and impairs phosphorylation within cells. Additionally, bilirubin disrupts the regular operation of N-methyl-D-aspartate-receptor ion channels and reduces tyrosine uptake. The pathophysiology of bilirubin toxicity, which presents as bilirubin encephalopathy and bilirubin-induced neurologic dysfunction (BIND), is linked to these mechanisms. The degree of brain damage is determined by the length of bilirubin exposure and the amount of bilirubin present in the brain. In the absence of hemolysis, bilirubin toxicity and the TSB level do not, however, correlate well. Preterm babies are particularly susceptible to the harmful consequences of unconjugated free bilirubin. This can be partly attributed to CNS immaturity, relatively lower serum albumin levels, and coexisting conditions such as necrotizing enterocolitis, sepsis, intraventricular hemorrhage, and periventricular leukomalacia.

Abnormalities in the uptake, metabolism, transport, and/or excretion of bile salts and bilirubin lead to conjugated hyperbilirubinemia. These anomalies cause the liver to produce more bile acid, which encourages fibrosis and the growth of bile ducts. Hepatocyte apoptosis and inflammation, which result in cirrhosis and hepatocellular damage, are also caused by bile acid. In cholestasis, insufficient bile secretion causes malabsorption of fat and fat-soluble vitamins, which frequently results in deficiencies of vitamins A, D, E, and K and failure to thrive.

3.6.4. Histopathology

When deeper brain nuclei in autopsy specimens from infants with severe unconjugated hyperbilirubinemia are stained yellow, it is referred to as Kernicterus. These autopsies display several histopathologic characteristics, such as pyknosis-affected nuclei, cytoplasmic vacuolation, and fading of the Nissl substance.

A liver biopsy is often necessary to conclusively diagnose cholestasis and distinguish between Biliary atresia and idiopathic neonatal hepatitis. Histopathological findings in Biliary atresia typically include the enlargement of the hepatic portal tracts with fluid accumulation, fibro-dysplasia, increased bile duct growth, and blockages in the ducts. Multinucleate giant cells and the presence of blood cell production are common features observed in liver samples from individuals with cholestasis. While the abundance of blood cell production in the liver is not specific to any particular condition, it is more commonly seen in cholestasis caused by infections. Distinct histopathological characteristics of other cholestatic diseases include PAS-positive granules indicating alpha-1 antitrypsin deficiency, a lack of bile ducts in Alagille syndrome, and necrosis accompanied by inflammation around the ducts in sclerosing cholangitis.

PFIC1 patients frequently have canalicular cholestasis, one of the familial causes of cholestasis, which is characterized by a distinct lack of ductular proliferation and isolated periportal biliary metaplasia of the hepatocytes. The histopathology of PFIC2 patients is similar, with the exception that extensive lobular and portal fibrosis accompanied by inflammation and changed liver architecture are more prevalent.

3.6.5. History and Physical

A thorough history that covers the neonate's birth, family history, the onset of jaundice, and the mother's serologies is the first step in the evaluation of the jaundiced newborn. When evaluating infants for jaundice, the presence of pruritis in the urine and stool should be evaluated as they may provide insight into the type of jaundice. The American Academy advises identifying risk factors for developing severe hyperbilirubinemia and conducting universal screenings for jaundice in all newborns. Pre-discharge bilirubin in the high-risk zone, jaundice seen in the first 24 hours, blood group incompatibility, gestational age of 35 to 36 weeks, a previous sibling who received phototherapy, cephalhematoma or significant bruising, exclusive breastfeeding, and East Asian race are major risk factors in newborns over 35 weeks gestation. Another established risk factor for the development of severe hyperbilirubinemia is prematureness. Serum bilirubin in the high intermediate range, macrosomic infant of a diabetic mother, polycythemia, male gender, and mother age exceeding 25 years are considered minor risk factors.

It is best to examine newborns during the day to check for jaundice. However, if a newborn has dark skin or has received phototherapy, the clinical assessment may not be accurate. Thus, a transcutaneous bilirubin test (TSB) should always be used to confirm clinically significant jaundice. To determine the cause of pathologic jaundice, a focused physical examination should be carried out. Evaluation is required for signs of dehydration, weight loss, hepatosplenomegaly, petechiae, pallor, cephalhematoma, subgaleal bleed, and extensive bruising. The signs and symptoms of bilirubin encephalopathy, which include poor feeding, lethargy, altered sleep, abnormal tone, or seizures, should also be evaluated in all infants with jaundice. However, it's crucial to remember that up to 15% of newborns with kernicterus experience no symptoms at all during the early stages of the disease. Some etiologies of neonatal cholestasis involve multiple systems, as was covered in earlier sections. Physical examinations should be conducted to identify these symptoms, as they frequently point to a diagnosis and help guide a particular work-up (Baily et al, 2009; Levine et al, 2019; Jasani et al, 2021).

3.6.6. Evaluation

3.6.6.1. Diagnosis of Unconjugated Hyperbilirubinemia

A transcutaneous measurement tool or blood samples for total serum bilirubin can be used to measure bilirubin levels. Transcutaneous bilirubin estimation decreases the number of blood tests required, although it is not as useful in newborns with dark skin or after phototherapy. When the transcutaneous bilirubin (TcB) level is greater than the 95th percentile on the transcutaneous nomogram or 75% of the TSB nomogram for phototherapy, the serum level should be measured. The incapacity to identify the direct fraction of bilirubin necessary for the diagnosis of neonatal cholestasis is another drawback of depending solely on TcB.

The workup that is advised to determine whether a hemolytic disease is the source of unconjugated hyperbilirubinemia includes blood smear, G6PD, complete blood cell count (CBC), maternal/neonatal blood type, and Coombs test. Since serum albumin is thought to be a surrogate marker for free bilirubin, it should always be checked, particularly if the TSB level is getting close to the exchange transfusion levels. The portion of bilirubin that causes bilirubin-induced toxicity is free bilirubin. As a substitute for exchange transfusion, the bilirubin-albumin ratio, or B/A ratio, is an extra tool that may be used to estimate the risk of kernicterus.

For the majority of UCH cases, radiographic imaging is usually not necessary. The most sensitive area of the brain for identifying signal changes on magnetic resonance imaging (MRI) is the posteromedial borders of the globus pallidus. MRI results for bilirubin encephalopathy are highly sensitive. When the disease progresses, hyperintense signals on T1-weighted sequences are seen in infants with bilirubin encephalopathy, which later turns into hyperintense signals on T2-weighted sequences. Reduced levels of choline and N-acetyl-aspartate and elevated levels of glutamate are observed using magnetic resonance spectroscopy (MRS). Notwithstanding, the lack of these results does not rule out the possibility of chronic bilirubin encephalopathy.

3.6.6.2. Diagnosis of Conjugated Hyperbilirubinemia

Serum aminotransferases for signs of hepatocellular injury, alkaline phosphatase and GGT levels for signs of biliary channel obstruction, prothrombin time/INR, and serum albumin for assessment of hepatic synthetic function should all be ordered in patients with conjugated hyperbilirubinemia. Depending on the situation, additional tests such as TORCH titers, urine cultures, viral cultures, serologic titers, results of newborn screening, particular tests for inborn errors of metabolism, alpha-1 antitrypsin phenotype, and particular genetics tests might be required.

Radiology is frequently required as part of the neonatal cholestasis workup. Gallstones, inspissated bile, choledochal cysts, and sludging in the biliary tree can all be detected with hepatic ultrasonography. When biliary atresia is detected with hepatic ultrasound, the triangle cord sign has a high sensitivity and nearly 100% specificity. An additional method that is being utilized more and more to assess neonatal cholestasis is hepatobiliary scintigraphy. Less tracer excretion 24 hours after introduction indicates obstruction and aids in ruling out non-obstructive cholestasis causes as well. It has been demonstrated that earlier phenobarbitone treatment increases the sensitivity of this imaging. Ultimately, a liver biopsy is typically regarded as the most reliable method of identifying neonatal cholestasis. In 90 to 95% of cases, a skilled pathologist's interpretation of the histopathology will help determine the correct diagnosis, and in patients with intrahepatic cholestasis, it may help avoid needless interventions.

3.6.7. Treatment

The age and health state of a newborn determine the appropriate bilirubin levels for phototherapy to begin. Nonetheless, phototherapy is recommended for any newborn whose total serum bilirubin level is higher than 359 μmol/L (equivalent to 21 mg/dL).

3.6.7.1. Treatment of Unconjugated Hyperbilirubinemia

The cornerstones of treatment for individuals with unconjugated hyperbilirubinemia are exchange transfusion and phototherapy.

3.6.7.2. Phototherapy

Phototherapy, a type of treatment that uses colored light to treat neonatal jaundice, converts trans-bilirubin into the water-soluble cis-bilirubin isomer. Instead of using UV light therapy, the phototherapy used here uses a particular blue light frequency. A biliblanket is a device that is placed under the baby's clothing, next to its skin, or it can be applied with overhead lamps, in which case the baby's eyes must be covered.

At Rochford Hospital in Essex, England, phototherapy was first unintentionally discovered when a pathologist, Dr. Perryman, saw that a vial of blood left in the sun had turned green, and a nurse, Sister Jean Ward, noticed that babies exposed to sunlight had lessened jaundice. These findings were combined by Drs. Cremer, Richards, and Dobbs to produce a groundbreaking randomized clinical trial that was published in Pediatrics in 1968. It took an additional 10 years for the practice to gain traction. To shorten the duration of phototherapy, massage therapy may be helpful in addition to phototherapy. It does not, however, seem to lessen the need for phototherapy when treating newborn jaundice.

As per the American national guidelines for 2022, home phototherapy is advised as a substitute for hospital readmission since recent studies conducted in multiple countries have demonstrated that phototherapy can be administered safely and effectively in the family's home. Nonetheless, several reports have raised the possibility that neonatal phototherapy and a higher risk of cancer in the future are related. According to a recent systematic review, phototherapy may be associated with a statistically significant risk of several hematopoietic cancers, including myeloid leukemia.

3.6.7.3. Exchange Transfusions

Similar to phototherapy, the newborn's age and health status determine the appropriate level of exchange transfusion. However, any newborn with a total serum bilirubin level higher than 428 μmol/L (25 mg/dL) should use it.

3.6.7.4. Intravenous Immunoglobulin (IVIG)

When UHB jaundice is caused by immune-mediated hemolysis, IVIG is used to stop RBC hemolysis by coating RBCs' Fc receptors. In immune-mediated hemolysis, the AAP advises IVIG infusion if TSB doesn't drop below 2 to 3 mg/dl of exchange level even after vigorous phototherapy. It's not entirely evident from the data, though, that using IVIG lessens the need for ET. However, in clinical practice, IVIG is frequently utilized to treat unconjugated hyperbilirubinemia.

3.6.7.5. Treatment of Conjugated Hyperbilirubinemia

The specific etiology of conjugated hyperbilirubinemia determines the course of treatment. For the best results, patients with biliary atresia need to have a Kasai operation (hepatic portoenterostomy), ideally within the first two months of their lives. To create a different route for biliary drainage, the Kasai operation entails excising the atretic biliary ducts and fibrous plate and performing a Roux-en-Y anastomosis of the jejunum with the remaining ducts. Certain antimicrobials would be used to treat infectious causes of cholestasis, while cholic acid and chenodeoxycholic acid therapy is frequently effective in treating a variety of BASDs. Improvements in the underlying illness and liver functions are usually the response to metabolic causes of cholestasis. GALD patients seem to respond favorably to double volume exchange transfusion and IVIG. When available, a liver transplant can be curative, but in this age group, it can be technically difficult. Cyclic parenteral nutrition (PN) reduces exposure time and starts enteral feedings as soon as possible to manage cholestasis caused by parenteral nutrition. Reduce the amount of manganese and copper in PN to lessen liver damage.

3.6.8. Differential Diagnosis

Neonatal jaundice has a relatively narrow differential diagnosis because it is easily identified through a physical examination of the infant. Rarely, yellowish skin discoloration caused by high carotene levels can be mistaken for hyperbilirubinemia. However, carotenemia does not involve the mucosa or sclera. Given that foods high in carotenoid content, such as carrots, mangos, green leafy vegetables, sweet potatoes, apricots, and melons, cause carotenemia, it is improbable that a newborn will exhibit this condition. However, the etiology of the two types of neonatal hyperbilirubinemia is quite complex, as was covered in earlier sections. A thorough understanding of these illnesses is necessary for an early diagnosis and suitable care.

3.6.9. Staging

Depending on when it manifests, bilirubin encephalopathy in patients with severe unconjugated hyperbilirubinemia can take various forms. Unconjugated bilirubin's threshold for neurotoxicity is unknown, and infants have been known to develop kernicterus even in the absence of significantly elevated bilirubin levels found during autopsy.

Acute bilirubin encephalopathy: has been described as evolving through three stages:

- Phase 1: During the first one to two days of the illness, phase 1 symptoms include poor feeding, lethargy, hypotonia, or frank seizures.
- Phase 2: Should the infants' condition worsen, they might

enter phase 2, which is marked by elevated muscle tone, particularly in the extensor group, which can result in retrocollis and opisthotonus. Usually, these symptoms appear in the middle of the first week of illness.

- Phase 3: After the first week, this phase is characterized primarily by elevated tone.
- Chronic Bilirubin encephalopathy: Depending on when the symptoms appear, this condition can take two different forms.
- First-year patients with chronic bilirubin encephalopathy exhibit hypotonia, heightened deep tendon reflexes, required tonic neck reflexes, and delayed motor milestones.
- Chronic bilirubin encephalopathy after the first year: This phase is characterized by the following symptoms: hypoplasia of dental enamel, upward gaze abnormality, sensorineural hearing loss, movement disorders (most commonly choreoathetosis), and cerebral palsy of the choreoathetoid type.

3.6.10. Prognosis

The majority of forms of unconjugated hyperbilirubinemia have excellent prognoses with treatment. Bilirubin encephalopathy may develop in patients who receive insufficient or delayed treatment. Developing and low-resource countries have a much higher incidence of bilirubin encephalopathy. According to reports, kernicterus is on the rise in nations where it had all but vanished in the past. The early release of newborns from the hospital of delivery has been the primary cause of this. The only treatment for patients with Crigler-Najjar type 1 is liver transplantation, which comes with a poor prognosis. Bilirubin encephalopathy is common when liver transplantation is not performed.

Depending on the cause, conjugated hyperbilirubinemia has a variable prognosis. Early diagnosis and surgery within the first 60 days of life significantly improve the prognosis and outcome for patients with biliary atresia. In a similar vein, individuals with bile acid synthesis disorder (BASD) have a very good prognosis because their condition responds well to medication. Gestational alloimmune liver disease (GALD) had a dismal prognosis in the past, with up to 80% of cases dying without a liver transplant. However, the prognosis for this illness has significantly improved recently with the introduction of double volume exchange transfusion and IVIG usage. For the majority of other cholestasis types, there is typically not a good prognosis, and many patients will need multidisciplinary interventions.

3.6.11. Complications

Babies who have extreme hyperbilirubinemia run the risk of developing BIND, or bilirubin-induced neurologic dysfunction. Neurotoxicity results from bilirubin's binding to the subthalamic nuclear bodies, globus pallidus, hippocampal regions, and cerebellum. This causes acute bilirubin encephalopathy (ABE), which is characterized by hypotonia, decreased suck, and lethargy. This disease can be cured at this point. On the other hand, if ABE worsens, patients may experience irreversible chronic bilirubin encephalopathy/kernicterus. It shows up as sensorineural hearing loss, posturing, arching, abnormal gaze, seizures, and choreo-athetoid cerebral palsy. Individuals suffering from newborn cholestasis may experience liver failure, cirrhosis, and in rare circumstances, hepatocellular carcinoma. Long-term cholestasis can also result in fat-soluble vitamin deficiencies and failure to thrive.

3.6.12. Consultations

Most patients with unconjugated hyperbilirubinemia can be managed by a pediatric or neonatal provider. Patients may require consultations and follow-ups with a pediatric gastroenterologist, hematologist, and medical geneticist, though, if genetic causes of hyperbilirubinemia are suspected.

The earliest possible referral for patients suspected of having neonatal cholestasis should be made to a pediatric gastroenterologist. The majority of these patients will require a series of tests, and additional referrals will be necessary after the cholestasis's cause is determined. For corrective surgery, infants with biliary atresia must also be referred to a pediatric gastrointestinal surgeon. Similarly, patients with inborn errors of metabolism should see a medical geneticist, a dietician with experience in metabolic disorders, and a metabolic specialist.

Depending on the cause of the newborn jaundice, comprehensive counseling is essential to enhancing the prognosis in the long run. To allay parents' fears and anxieties, it is important to educate them about the good prognosis of the majority of patients with the common causes of unconjugated hyperbilirubinemia. Parents should receive sufficient counseling and education when their child has jaundice from etiologies that have a poor prognosis. Multidisciplinary interventions are frequently necessary. When a child is diagnosed with hereditary hyperbilirubinemia, parents should also be offered genetic counseling and referred to medical geneticists (Baily et al, 2009; Levine et al, 2019; Jasani et al, 2021).

3.7. OTHER NEONATAL DISORDERS

The human genome, which is sometimes referred to as a blueprint, has all of the data and guidelines required to define an individual human. The DNA and related protein molecules that are present in an organism or a cell are collectively referred to as the genome. Each parent contributes one chromosome to each of the 23 pairs of chromosomes that make up the human genome. Chromosomes are thread-like packages of genes and other DNA.

As the functional unit of inheritance, a gene is a particular sequence of DNA. The majority of genes encode the information required to produce proteins, which are molecules that perform all of a cell's essential functions. As a result, minute differences in genes result in minute modifications in proteins. While changes in a single gene or chromosome can account for some human diseases, the majority are complex and may involve several genes and protein pathways. It is thought that a wide range of genes and environmental variables regulate the intricate and coordinated processes required for fetal development. A genetically altered person may be born as a result of one or more of these processes going wrong. Scientific research will reveal details about the biological and regulatory mechanisms underlying human development as well as the crucial pathways through which genetic alterations lead to disease. These studies frequently make use of models derived from other organisms. This data will come from research on humans as well as studies on other model organisms, like yeast or mice, which can shed light on the functioning of important genes in intricate systems.

3.7.1. Diseases Transmitted Through the Placenta or Due to Placental Dysfunction

Numerous different types of organisms, such as viruses, bacteria, spirochetes, and protozoa (e.g., toxoplasmosis). The majority of these infections arise from the mother's infection, with the infectious agents being passed through the placenta—a temporary organ that allows the fetus to take in nutrients and expel waste—via the fetal circulation. The most common symptoms of bacterial infection are amniotic fluid infection and early membrane rupture.

Maternal rubella, also known as German measles, that strikes during the first eight weeks of pregnancy is linked to congenital malformations in over half of the cases; by the 16th week, the percentage drops to about 20% and then continues to decline sharply. A cytomegalovirus infection affects numerous organs, has a high death rate, and, in the case that the fetus survives, can cause severe brain damage. A condition known as toxoplasmosis, which is caused by infection with the intracellular parasite *Toxoplasma gondii*, can be fatal or lead to abnormally small heads, hydrocephalus (an excessive buildup of fluid in the brain cavities), or mental retardation. In an infant, congenital syphilis can affect the skin, liver, spleen, lymph nodes, and kidneys, among other organs. Bone and tooth malformations develop later, and years may pass before signs of a serious central nervous system involvement are noticeable.

Most medications given to mothers have the potential to cross the placenta and have significant effects on the developing fetus, much like infectious agents can. In Europe in the early 1960s, the seemingly innocuous drug thalidomide caused thousands of babies to be born with missing or short limbs. This was a most dramatic and devastating example of this effect. Antibiotics, sedatives, analgesics (pain relievers), antihypertensive medications, and anesthetics can all be harmful to the developing fetus. Antithyroid medication given to the mother has resulted in congenital goiters or thyroid enlargement. It is now evident that whenever a mother is considering medication therapy, the potential negative effects on the fetus must be taken into account.

Serious fetal consequences may also result from the mother abusing alcohol or drugs. Within 72 hours of birth, babies whose mothers are addicted to heroin, morphine, or other opiates frequently experience withdrawal symptoms. The fetal alcohol syndrome is a group of congenital abnormalities that affects many children of alcoholic mothers. These malformations include mental retardation, growth retardation, and microcephaly. The mother provides the fetus with all of its nutrition. In general, the needs of the fetus will take precedence over those of the mother, and the fetus may receive an adequate amount of a particular nutrient even in the presence of maternal deficiency, even though parallel deficiencies in the fetus may reflect maternal deficiency states. For example, mild to moderate iron or calcium deficiencies in the mother are typically not linked to deficiencies in the developing fetus. Conversely, low levels of protein and calories may be linked to smaller fetuses.

Fetal deficiencies can also result from placental dysfunction or abnormal functioning. The severity and timing of placental inadequacy determine the outcomes of placental abnormalities. A fetus experiencing severe placental insufficiency at an early stage of pregnancy may die. It's also possible that fetal growth is being inhibited by placental insufficiency. Placental dysfunction towards the end of pregnancy is linked to early delivery or signs of varying degrees of fetal distress, such as skin staining, fetal wasting, and signs of acute oxygen deprivation.

3.7.2. Injuries Incurred During Birth

The infant may sustain multiple injuries as a result of the physical trauma of delivery. The diffuse soft-tissue swelling of the scalp known as caput succedaneum is not very significant. Serious injury is rare, but difficult delivery can cause more widespread bruising, abrasions, and edema—especially after breech delivery. In one to two percent of babies, bleeding beneath the periosteum (the skull's covering membrane) results in significant swelling; in other cases, it's linked to a minor fracture of the underlying skull; thankfully, spontaneous healing happens quickly. While spinal cord injuries are uncommon, injuries to the peripheral nerves brought on by traction on the head are frequently encountered. These injuries include Erb's paralysis, which results from damage to the fifth and sixth cervical nerves, weakening the arm and shoulder. Phrenic nerve injury can also cause paralysis of the diaphragm, the muscle separating the chest from the abdomen, and facial nerve injury can cause facial palsy. Most of these cases of peripheral nerve injury are fully recovered from.

One very significant type of birth injury is related to oxygen deprivation or anoxia. Low maternal blood pressure, abnormalitics in the uterus, placenta, or umbilical cord that prevent enough blood flow to the fetus or inadequate oxygenation of the mother can all lead to fetal anoxia. Anoxia following delivery can be brought on by shock, blood loss, or insufficient breathing. Clinical signs include blueness of the skin (cyanosis), slowing of the heartbeat, and decreased activity. A newborn may die from severe anoxia, though recovery is more typical. The main concern with anoxia is that, if it lasts longer than a few minutes, it may cause brain damage.

3.7.3. Metabolic Disturbances

Children born into diabetic households are a distinct population with particular metabolic issues. Unknown causes frequently result in intrauterine death. The placenta frequently has anomalies. Large size and large organs at birth are common in newborns, a condition known as macrosomia. Common complications include respiratory distress and hypoglycemia, or low blood sugar. Neonatal hypoglycemia is a relatively common condition, especially in low-birth-weight infants. The central nervous system exhibits abnormalities in 15% of infants with hypoglycemia. Hypoglycemia is usually a temporary condition that improves with treatment.

A temporary increase in the level of bilirubin in the blood is usually the consequence of an imbalance between the rate of red blood cell destruction, the rate at which hemoglobin is converted to bilirubin, and the rate at which bilirubin is excreted in the bile. On the other hand, jaundice can be caused by septicemia, a variety of liver disorders, or blockage of the ducts that carry bile into the digestive system. Moreover, breastfeeding has been linked to abnormally elevated bilirubin levels; this is an extremely rare condition caused by the presence of an unusual substance in the milk.

The underlying cause and the level of excess bilirubin in the blood determine the significance of jaundice. In severe situations, bilirubin may accumulate in brain tissue, which can lead to kernicterus—severe damage to nerve cells. This condition is most common in infants with erythroblastosis fetalis, a blood disorder that is discussed below. It can cause deafness and cerebral palsy. Exchange transfusions, in which the majority of the infant's blood is replaced with blood from donors, are typically effective in preventing brain damage caused by an excess of bilirubin; however, in the most severe cases, multiple transfusions may be necessary.

Within a few days of birth, a condition known as tetany of the newborn manifests as increased neuromuscular irritability, accompanied by twitches, tremors, and convulsions of the muscles. Most of the time, there is a high concentration of inorganic phosphate in the blood and a low concentration of calcium. The disorder seems to be caused by a low blood concentration of magnesium in certain infants. The intravenous administration of calcium usually results in a significant improvement in the infant's condition. Since the condition is temporary, oral calcium supplementation can be stopped after a week or two of treatment.

Unlike the metabolic disorders discussed previously, which are typically temporary conditions affecting newborns, inborn errors of metabolism are chronic illnesses. These arise from a specific metabolic pathway's lack of a functional enzyme. This "enzyme block" causes an excessive build-up of hazardous chemicals that are unable to be processed normally as well as a shortage in the products of the impacted pathway. Genetics determines inborn errors of metabolism, the majority of which are extremely uncommon. Many result in serious illness and brain damage if prompt, efficient treatment is not received. One well-known example is phenylketonuria, which can be identified in the first week of life through a direct blood test (the Guthrie test). After the baby has been identified, a special diet is given to prevent brain damage and promote normal growth. The diet must be followed for at least 10 years, and some medical professionals advise following it forever.

3.7.4. Infections

In addition to common infections like *Escherichia coli, Staphylococcus aureus*, and group B hemolytic streptococci, which are not typically causes of serious infection in older age groups, the newborn infant is susceptible to these common infections. A newborn may contract an infection in the nursery, during delivery, or even inside the uterus. Serious infections such as pneumonia, meningitis (inflammation of the membranes surrounding the brain and spinal cord), and septicemia (bloodstream infection) are frequently encountered. Other than poor feeding, lethargy, pallor, or a slight fever, the infant frequently exhibits minimal symptoms of the illness. The newborn infant has a low level of immunity to infection, so prompt diagnosis and treatment are crucial. When an infection is only suspected, treatment is frequently administered. It has been found that every component of the immune system has congenital defects. The patient's incapacity to fight infection is the most notable aspect of these illnesses. Therefore, untreated cases of agammaglobulinemia (low blood antibody levels) can result in severe infections that kill a patient in infancy or early childhood.

3.7.5. Respiratory Disorders

Newborn infants frequently have a wide range of respiratory function abnormalities. Respiratory distress syndrome (also known as hyaline membrane disease) is one of the worst. RDS affects 0.5 to 1 percent of births overall and is more prevalent in premature infants, as was previously mentioned. Furthermore, it frequently occurs in babies born to diabetic moms and following cesarean delivery (delivery via the mother's abdominal wall). Even though it happens rarely, RDS can also strike full-term babies who don't seem to have any known risk factors. Affected newborns start breathing quickly and shallowly soon after birth, and suitable testing can demonstrate that they are exchanging air (i.e., using up carbon dioxide and absorbing oxygen) inadequately. If professional care is not received, the patient may succumb to their illness in a matter of hours, or it may take several days to fully recover and eventually pass away. The goal of treatment is to reduce the symptoms, which may involve giving oxygen, correcting an associated acidosis, and, if required, using a mechanical ventilation machine to help the baby breathe. Deaths are now less common thanks to modern medical care.

Pneumonia poses a significant risk to infants. When an infant gets an infection from their mother, it usually manifests within hours of delivery; if the infection is acquired after birth, it takes up to 48 hours to manifest. Infants exhibit respiratory distress, and septicemia—a blood infection—is frequently present. The course of treatment involves providing respiratory support and carefully chosen antibiotics at the right dosages. During delivery, an infant may inhale meconium, a semisolid discharge from the infant's bowels, which could obstruct the upper airway. Within two to three days, oxygen therapy, suction-assisted airway clearance, and general respiratory support are typically helpful in accelerating the healing process.

In addition to causing partial or complete lung collapse (pneumothorax), bleeding into the lung, and failure of the lung to expand (atelectasis), leakage of air into the pleural space (between the membrane lining the chest and that enveloping the lungs and other thoracic organs) also results in respiratory failure in the newborn. Often, prompt medical attention is required to guarantee survival.

3.7.6. Cardiovascular Disorders

About seven out of every 1,000 newborns are born with a congenital malformation, which is the primary cause of cardiovascular disturbances in the newborn. They range from those that cannot coexist with life to those that do not lead to disease and do not need medical attention. Occasionally, the cause is identified due to a correlation with a chromosomal abnormality (e.g., Turner's syndrome, and Down syndrome); in a small number of cases, a mother's rubella infection is the cause. Early in fetal development, the lesions appear, and the outcome is typically either an abnormal communication between various parts of the circulation or the heart, or an obstruction of normal blood flow. Heart failure happens when the structural abnormality induces a significant disturbance. Breathlessness, feeding issues, or a blue complexion (cyanosis) are some of the symptoms a baby with heart failure may exhibit. The majority of congenital cardiac defects are accompanied by stethoscope-audible heart murmurs. Ventricular septal defects, or holes between the heart's two lower chambers (the left and right ventricles), are the most prevalent type of congenital lesions. Untreated, many of these close on their own. With the development of echocardiography, the diagnosis of a baby suspected of having congenital heart disease has become more certain and straightforward. The majority of illnesses are treatable with surgery, which is typically postponed until the child is older unless the condition poses an immediate risk to life. One particular cardiovascular condition that is frequently seen in preterm infants is patent ductus arteriosus or the persistence of a crucial fetal circulatory feature. The descending aorta and the pulmonary artery are connected by a fetal blood vessel called the ductus arteriosus. It directs blood toward the placenta, where oxygenation occurs, from the lungs, which are nonfunctional in a fetus. The ductus normally shuts down soon after birth. It acts as a shunt in the opposite direction, directing blood from the aorta to the lungs, when it is patent (open) after birth. As a result, the lungs receive an excessive amount of blood, which leads to pulmonary congestion and breathing problems. It is possible to give medication to induce the ductus to close. If medication therapy doesn't work, the ductus might need to be surgically closed.

3.7.7. Blood Disorders

Blood disorders that affect newborns include those that affect the red blood cells (especially anemias, which are characterized by low levels of functional hemoglobin in the blood) and the clotting factors (e.g., hemophilia). These illnesses, along with others that impact a newborn's blood, are covered in the sections below under the heading "Blood Disease," which deals with conditions related to later infancy and childhood.

A condition known as erythroblastosis fetalis causes the fetus's red blood cells to be destroyed due to an incompatibility between the mother's and the infant's blood types. Incompatibility between a Rh-negative mother and a Rh-positive fetus causes the most severe form. The mother will have circulating antibodies against the Rh factor if she has previously been exposed to Rh-positive red blood cells and became sensitized to them. Her Rh-positive fetus's red blood cells can be destroyed by these antibodies because they can pass through the placenta. Typically, a mother's first Rh-positive fetus is unaffected unless she has received blood transfusions that have sensitized her to the blood. This is since she is not exposed to many fetal red blood cells until after the baby is delivered, at which point a significant amount of fetal red blood cells are transferred into the mother's bloodstream. Future Rh-positive fetuses will be at risk, and the mother may become sensitized as a result of this exposure. Anti-Rh serum should now be given to a Rh-negative mother as soon as possible after she gives birth to a Rh-positive child. Before she becomes sensitized, the serum eliminates any fetal red blood cells in her system, shielding subsequent Rh-positive fetuses from erythroblastosis fetalis.

3.7.8. Gastrointestinal Disorders

One common symptom of newborns is vomiting, which can be caused by intestinal blockage, overfeeding, or it can happen for no apparent reason at all. Vomiting may result from a persistent contraction of the muscle controlling the opening between the stomach and the intestine. Pyloric stenosis is a condition that can arise at any point during the early stages of infancy and typically necessitates surgical intervention.

Typically, the baby passes meconium and has its first bowel movement within 12 hours. A delay could be a sign of bowel obstruction. Congenital intestinal occlusion (atresia) or narrowing (stenosis) are significant causes of obstruction. These can happen anywhere, including the rectum, anus, and duodenum, which is the first part of the small intestine. Some newborns have a tiny pit or dimple instead of a patent anus. Infants diagnosed with Down syndrome are more likely to have duodenal stenosis. Early in infancy, congenital intestinal blockages result in vomiting and constipation; the majority of these can be surgically resolved. The intestinal blockage caused by hard lumps of meconium, known as meconium ileus, almost exclusively affects infants who have cystic fibrosis, an inherited condition that is explained below. The rule is recovery, except certain cases of intestinal perforation.

3.7.9. Kidney and Urinary-Tract Disorders

Despite the wide range of solute content and the resulting large variation in the excretory load imposed, the newborn infant's kidneys are fully capable of maintaining homeostasis, or balance, of fluids and electrolytes under normal circumstances. For example, they adapt readily to the various formulas used in infant feeding. (In this context, electrolytes are defined as substances that acquire an electrical charge, either positive or negative, in solution. However, aberrations in the control of the water and salt balance as well as the acid-base metabolism are frequently observed during stressful times. Due to the newborn's kidneys' limited excretory capacity, medication dosage and fluid therapy must be adjusted.

Congenital anomalies are the most frequent kidney and urinary tract disorders that occur in the neonatal period. Some babies are born with no kidneys at all, or with malformed (dysplastic) kidneys that function poorly. For example, the absence of one kidney is insignificant because one healthy kidney will suffice. Kidney polycystic disease is one example of a severe congenital defect. Numerous large cysts in the kidneys seriously impair renal function in this disorder.

Urinary tract obstructions that occur at birth, such as blockages in the ureter above the bladder or the urethra below it, put the baby at risk for kidney damage and urinary tract infections. When a newborn doesn't pass pee within 12 hours of birth, an obstruction may be the cause. It is uncommon for a newborn to develop nephritis or kidney inflammation. Large amounts of protein are lost in the urine in one well-known type of condition called congenital nephrosis, which leads to the development of severe, widespread edema. Congenital nephrosis and other types of nephritis in infants have a very poor prognosis for recovery.

It can be challenging to diagnose kidney and urinary tract infections in young infants clinically. However, these infections respond well to treatment if identified early and started right away, barring congenital obstructive lesions.

3.7.10. Nervous-System Disorders

Among the most prevalent severe congenital abnormalities are nervous system malformations. Many brain abnormalities can arise, some of which are life-incompatible (e.g., a permanent disability, such as anencephaly-the absence of the cerebral hemispheres), among others. Microcephaly, an abnormally small head caused by limited brain growth, and hydrocephalus, an increase in the volume of cerebrospinal fluid associated with increased pressure, are common brain malformations. The large size of the head is clear evidence of the latter condition. Some infants with hydrocephalus pass away before birth. After birth, the illness could end on its own. The main course of treatment involves either surgically removing any obstruction or diverting spinal fluid to relieve pressure. Therapy aims to stop the damage from getting worse.

A congenital condition known as spina bifida occurs when the spinal column fails to close over a portion of the spinal cord, usually in the lumbar area, leaving that portion of the cord exposed. A portion of the unprotected cord may protrude through the vertebral column defect as nervous tissue, the meninges (the membranous covering of the cord), or both. Hydrocephalus is often present in conjunction with a meningeal protrusion, either with or without neural components. It is common for the spinal cord abnormality to cause impaired nerve function below the level of the lesion, which leads to leg weakness or paralysis and urine incontinence.

Conditions that are acquired, such as those resulting from inadequate oxygen and hemorrhage, were previously discussed in the section on birth traumas. A newborn may develop meningitis, which is an inflammation of the membranes that cover the brain and spinal cord. Unfortunately, because newborns don't always exhibit the same symptoms or findings, diagnosis is frequently delayed. Seizures, or convulsions, are typical in the newborn. These could be brought on by infections, metabolic issues, or harm to the brain sustained during delivery.

3.7.11. Endocrine Disorders

Congenital defects of the endocrine glands, which produce hormones, are rare but can have serious consequences. Congenital hypothyroidism, also known as cretinism, is an especially significant endocrine disease of infancy because it has the potential to cause severe mental retardation if left untreated. It results from a thyroid dysfunction or a metabolic issue with the gland's functioning. With an early diagnosis and appropriate thyroid medication therapy, all disease signs and symptoms quickly go away, leading to a dramatic improvement. In nations with advanced healthcare systems, a newborn's blood sample is used to perform a chemical test for cretinism. Thus, effective treatment can start soon after birth.

A set of disorders known as congenital adrenal hyperplasia occurs when there is an abnormality in the synthesis of normal adrenocortical steroid hormones, which are secreted by the cortex, or outer substance, of the adrenal glands. Adrenocorticotropic hormone, or ACTH, is a pituitary hormone that stimulates the cortex of the adrenal glands excessively, which causes abnormal gland enlargement and an excess of androgenic (masculinizing) adrenal hormones. Consequently, the genitalia of females may develop abnormally in utero, and there may be signs of an excessive androgenic effect in either sex during infancy, including accelerated growth, early pubic hair appearance, and phallus enlargement.

3.7.12. Musculoskeletal Disorders

Foot and hip abnormalities are common congenital musculoskeletal defects. Talipes equinovarus, also known as classic clubfoot, is a congenital twisting of the foot in which the front of the foot is bent inward toward the heel and the heel bends upward. Splints and plaster casts are typically used in correction to force the foot into the proper position; in extreme cases, surgery may be required. The front of the foot is turned outward and bent upward in talipes calcaneovalgus. This type of clubfoot is typically caused by the uterus's mechanical pressure holding the foot in an odd position. The majority of the time, passive stretching exercises can resolve this issue; however, in more difficult cases, casts or splints may be necessary.

Congenitally dislocated hips are most common in girls born at term by breech delivery and are linked to lax joints. When detected early enough in the clinical examination process, the condition is usually treatable with modest measures. If it goes unnoticed until a two-year-old begins to walk with a limp, significant surgery might be required.

3.7.13. Skin Disorders

Because of its immature glands and thin epidermis, an infant's skin is especially prone to infection and blistering. Diaper rashes, also called napkin rashes, are extremely common and can worsen if more infections spread to the skin areas that come into contact with a wet diaper.

Numerous common birthmarks exist. Most are caused by either an excess of pigment in the skin, known as nevi, or developmental abnormalities of the blood vessels, known as hemangiomas. The "strawberry" hemangioma, which is red, raised, and unsightly, is a common concern for parents. It may grow larger in the early weeks, but by the time a child reaches seven years old, it gradually disappears. A common pigmented birthmark in infants of black or Oriental stock, a Mongolian blue spot appears like a light bruise and is typically found on the back or buttocks. After the age of seven, it fades and becomes less noticeable.

3.7.14. Chromosomal Disorders

A normal person has 46 chromosomes, but occasionally a fetus can have extra chromosomes due to developmental defects. While Down's syndrome (mongolism) predisposes the fetuses to miscarriages or stillbirths, most other abnormalities result in survival. There is one case of Down syndrome for every 600 births. The child in question has a round skull, a flat face, oblique eyes, a small, drooping mouth, a short, broad neck, and hands. They also carry an extra copy of chromosome number 21. For those who have Down syndrome, moderate to severe mental retardation is the primary issue. Most are unable to live independent lives as adults. They also experience a higher frequency of severe congenital defects and an excess of respiratory infections in their early years of life. Nonetheless, the majority of them grow up to be fairly healthy adults in developed nations, despite having a lower life expectancy than the average person.

Chromosome disorders pertaining to sex are also prevalent. Since they have a greater effect on the gonads' development than on the external genitalia, many of these conditions are not diagnosed until after puberty, when the child or parents start to worry about the absence of sexual characteristic development. Girls typically have two X chromosomes for sex. There is only one X chromosome in people with Turner's syndrome. Because the girls are small and have other obvious distinguishing characteristics, the syndrome may be identified early in life. Nevertheless, only a thorough examination of the blood cells' chromosomes will allow for the confirmation of the diagnosis. These girls stay small and don't develop secondary sexual traits unless they receive more hormones. A girl with the condition is still infertile because of her small gonads, vagina, and uterus.

One X and one Y sex chromosome make up a typical boy. There is an extra X chromosome in people with Klingelherr's syndrome. Even though the disorder is just as common as Down syndrome, it is typically not identified until the testicles stop growing during puberty. Although the boys' health is good, infertility is common.

It is commonly known that men are more likely than women to suffer from general mental illnesses and that in certain families, men are afflicted more frequently than women. There are some distinct types of mental impairment associated with the male X chromosome. Using the right laboratory procedures, a "fragile site" on the X chromosome can be found in some of the affected males. It is said that these men have the fragile X syndrome (Baily et al, 2009; Levine et al, 2019; Jasani et al, 2021).

A Closer Look

Neonatal Meningitis

Males predominate in cases of neonatal bacterial meningitis, which affects 2/10,000 full-term and 2/1,000 low-birth-weight (LBW) neonates. It happens in roughly 15% of newborns with sepsis and sporadically takes place in isolation.

- Etiology of Neonatal Bacterial Meningitis

These are the prevailing pathogens

- Group B streptococcus (GBS—predominantly type III)
- *Escherichia coli*, especially strains that have the K1 polysaccharide present.
- Listeria monocytogenes

Additional pathogens that have been reported include coagulase-negative staphylococci, nonenterococcal group D streptococci, alpha-hemolytic streptococci, *Staphylococcus aureus*, gram-negative enteric organisms (such as *Citrobacter diversus*, *Enterobacter* species, and *Klebsiella* species), *Haemophilus influenzae*, *Neisseria meningitidis*, and *Streptococcus pneumoniae*.

The most common cause of neonatal bacterial meningitis is bacteremia, which arises from neonatal sepsis; the risk of meningitis increases with the colony count in the blood culture. Scalp lesions may also cause neonatal bacterial meningitis, especially if developmental defects result in communication between the skin's surface and the subarachnoid space, thereby increasing the risk of diploic vein thrombophlebitis. There is rarely a direct extension from a contiguous otic focus (such as otitis media) to the central nervous system (CNS).

- Symptoms and Signs of Neonatal Bacterial Meningitis

Often, the only symptoms that are present are those that are typical of neonatal sepsis, such as apnea, respiratory distress, jaundice, and temperature instability. More precisely, CNS symptoms (such as irritability, vomiting, focal seizures, lethargy, and vomiting) point to neonatal bacterial meningitis. More specific for the diagnosis is so-called paradoxical irritability, in which a parent's comforting and cuddling irritates the newborn instead of relieving their pain due to the movement of inflamed meninges. About 25% of people have a bulging or full fontanelle, and only 15% have nuchal rigidity. These results are less common the younger the patient. There may also be anomalies related to the cranial nerves, specifically those related to the third, sixth, and seventh nerves.

Group B streptococcus meningitis (GBS meningitis) often presents initially as a systemic illness with prominent respiratory signs and can occur during the first week of life, often accompanying early-onset neonatal sepsis. However, GBS meningitis frequently develops after this time, usually within the first three months of life, as an isolated illness marked by the absence of prior perinatal or obstetric complications and the presence of more specific meningitis symptoms (such as fever, lethargy, or seizures). When gram-negative enteric bacilli cause neonatal bacterial meningitis, ventriculitis usually follows. Bacteria can cause both severe vasculitis and meningitis. Cysts and abscesses are most likely to be caused by Diversus and *Cronobacter sakazakii* (formerly *Enterobacter sakazakii*). Brain abscesses can also be caused by the bacteria Serratia and *E. coli* K1. Increased intracranial pressure (ICP), which is frequently accompanied by vomiting, a protruding fontanelle, and occasionally an enlarging head size, is the first clinical sign of a brain abscess. Deterioration in a neonate with meningitis who is otherwise stable points to a progressive increase in intracranial pressure (ICP) brought on by hydrocephalus, an abscess that has burst into the ventricular system, or both.

- Diagnosis of Neonatal Bacterial Meningitis
    - Cell counts in the cerebrospinal fluid (CSF), protein and glucose levels, Gram stain, and culture.
    - Testing with the polymerase chain reaction (PCR).
    - Occasionally, brain MRIs, CT scans, or ultrasonography.

Any neonate suspected of having sepsis or meningitis should have a lumbar puncture (LP) to obtain a CSF examination and make a definitive diagnosis of neonatal bacterial meningitis. Nonetheless, performing LP on a newborn can be challenging, and there is a chance that it will result in hypoxia. LP is dangerous when there is a poor clinical state (such as respiratory distress, shock, or thrombocytopenia). The neonate should be treated as though meningitis is present if LP is delayed. Days after the illness onset, the presence of inflammatory cells and abnormal glucose and protein levels in CSF can still suggest the diagnosis, even if the clinical condition improves. To prevent the introduction of epithelial rests and the subsequent development of epitheliomas, LP should be performed using a trocar-equipped needle.

Culture the CSF regardless of whether it is acellular or bloody. Depending on the population under study, anywhere from 15 to 35% of neonates with negative blood cultures also have positive CSF cultures. If bacterial meningitis is suspected and CSF cultures are negative, multiplex PCR panels can be used to test CSF for multiple common pathogens (e.g., if the culture may have been affected by prior antibiotic use). If there is doubt about the clinical response, LP should be repeated in 24 to 48 hours. If gram-negative organisms are involved, LP should be repeated in 72 hours to guarantee sterilization.

Rerunning the CSF analysis aids in prognostic prediction and therapy duration guidance. A repeat LP at 24 to 48 hours in neonates with GBS meningitis may have predictive value, according to certain experts. If the neonate is doing well at the end of therapy, LP should not be repeated.

Normal CSF values are debatable and partly dependent on age. Generally speaking, the CSF of both term and preterm infants without meningitis contains ≤ 20 white blood cells/mcL (0.02 × 10^9/L), with polymorphonuclear leukocytes potentially making up a fifth of these cells. Term infants have levels of CSF protein that are more variable when meningitis is not present. < 100 mg/dL (1 g/L), whereas preterm infants have levels up to 150 mg/dL (1.5 g/L). CSF glucose levels in the absence of meningitis are > 75% of the serum value determined concurrently. These concentrations could be as low as 20–30 mg/dL (1.1 to 1.7 mmol/L)). It has been demonstrated that normal CSF values do not rule out a diagnosis of meningitis by identifying bacterial meningitis through culture in neonates with normal CSF indices.

A newborn who is not responding well to antibiotic therapy may have ventriculitis. When a ventricular puncture results in a white blood cell count higher than that of the LP, when ventricular fluid culture or Gram stain is positive, or when ventricular pressure increases, the diagnosis is made. Dilated ventricles also confirm ventriculitis. Ultrasonography, MRI, or CT with contrast may help diagnose when a brain abscess or ventriculitis is suspected.

- Prognosis for Neonatal Bacterial Meningitis

The mortality rate from neonatal bacterial meningitis approaches 100% if treatment is not received. The prognosis is based on birth weight, organism, and clinical severity after treatment. 5 to 20% of neonates with treated bacterial meningitis die from the illness. The mortality rate for organisms that cause necrotizing meningitis or vasculitis can be as high as 75%. In 20 to 50% of infants who survive, neurologic sequelae (such as hydrocephalus, hearing loss, and intellectual disability) develop; the prognosis is worse when gram-negative enteric bacilli are the cause.

The quantity of organisms in the CSF at diagnosis also has an impact on prognosis. There is a direct correlation between the duration of positive CSF cultures and the occurrence of complications. Neonatals with GBS typically have their CSF cultures sterilized during the first 24 hours of antibiotic therapy. With a median duration of two days, those with gram-negative bacillary meningitis stay positive for longer.

The mortality rate from GBS meningitis is notably lower than that from early-onset GBS sepsis.

- Treatment of Neonatal Bacterial Meningitis:
    - **Empiric Antibiotic Therapy:** Initial empirical therapy is still up for debate and is dependent on the patient's age. Many experts advise ampicillin plus an aminoglycoside for newborns. If meningitis caused by a gram-negative organism is suspected, a third-generation cephalosporin (such as cefotaxime) is also added until culture and sensitivity results are available. However, regular use of cefotaxime for empirical therapy may hasten the development of resistance, and long-term use of third-generation cephalosporins increases the risk of invasive candidiasis. Ampicillin works against bacteria like Listeria, GBS, and enterococci. Gentamicin treats numerous gram-negative infections and works in concert with these organisms. The majority of gram-negative pathogens are sufficiently covered by third-generation cephalosporins.

Hospitalized neonates with resistant organisms may have previously received antibiotics (e.g., for early-onset sepsis); fungal disease may also be considered in a neonate who appears septic after an extended period of hospitalization. Depending on the risk of meningitis, sick newborns with hospital-acquired infections should first be treated with vancomycin plus an aminoglycoside, either with or without a third-generation cephalosporin or a carbapenem that acts against *Pseudomonas aeruginosa*, such as cefepime or meropenem.

Once CSF culture results and sensitivities are known, antibiotic dosages are modified. Before the release of culture results, the results of the Gram stain should not be utilized to restrict coverage.

- **Organism-Specific Antibiotic Therapy:** The suggested course of action for GBS meningitis in infants. < 1 week of age is penicillin G 100,000 units/kg IV every 6 hours or ampicillin 100 mg/kg IV every 8 hours for infants ≤ 7 days or 75 mg/kg every 6 hours for infants > Seven days. Gentamicin is also administered for synergy at an age-appropriate dosage. If there is a clinical improvement, the infecting organism is susceptible to the penicillin being used, and CSF sterilization is verified, the medication can be discontinued.

For *L. or enterococci. monocytogenes*, ampicillin and gentamicin are usually administered for the duration of the illness.

Treatment for gram-negative bacillary meningitis is challenging. A high percentage of sequelae affect survivors of the conventional regimen of ampicillin plus an aminoglycoside, which results in a mortality rate of 15 to 20%. In newborns with confirmed gram-negative meningitis, a third-generation cephalosporin (such as cefotaxime) should be administered instead. Both an aminoglycoside and a third-generation cephalosporin or extended-spectrum beta-lactam (such as meropenem) may be used until sensitivities are established if antibiotic resistance is a concern.

Parenteral therapy should be administered for a minimum of 14 days in cases of gram-positive meningitis and a minimum of 21 days in cases of complicated gram-positive or gram-negative meningitis. Antibiotic instillation intraventricularly is not advised.

- Adjunctive Measures: Adjunctive measures used to treat neonatal sepsis should also be used to treat neonatal meningitis because the two conditions may be seen as part of the same continuum. Neonatal meningitis is not treated with corticosteroids. Early childhood neurologic complications, such as sensorineural hearing loss, should be closely monitored in patients.

Summary

- Accurately defining and reporting perinatal deaths (ie, fetal and infant deaths) is a critical first step in understanding the magnitude and causes of these important events.
- Resuscitation at the time of birth is different from all other forms of resuscitation because of the physiological transition from fetal to neonatal life. The vast majority of neonates will make this transition without any significant medical interventions.
- The vast majority of newborns respond to resuscitation when ventilation is provided effectively. Therefore, neonatal resuscitation guidelines support the establishment of effective ventilation, including placing an advanced airway before starting chest compressions.
- Infants who are born severely compromised and remain bradycardic with a HR >60 beats min^{-1} despite effective ventilation and chest compressions may respond to adrenaline (epinephrine).
- Each newborn baby is carefully checked at birth for signs of problems or complications. The healthcare provider will do a complete physical exam that includes every body system.
- The Apgar score helps find breathing problems and other health issues. It is part of the special attention given to a baby in the first few minutes after birth. The baby is checked at 1 minute and 5 minutes after birth for heart and respiratory rates, muscle tone, reflexes, and color.
- A baby's birth weight is an important marker of health. Full-term babies are born between 37 and 41 weeks of pregnancy. The average weight for full-term babies is about 7 pounds (3.2 kg). In general, very small babies and very large babies are at greater risk for problems.
- A complete physical exam is an important part of newborn care. The healthcare provider carefully checks each body system for health and normal function. The provider also looks for any signs of illness or birth defects.
- Newborn screening (NBS) is a public health program of screening infants shortly after birth for treatable conditions, but not clinically evident in the newborn period. The goal is to identify infants at risk for these conditions early enough to confirm the diagnosis and provide intervention that will alter the clinical course of the disease and prevent or ameliorate the clinical manifestations.
- The lower the birth weight and gestational age of the newborn, the higher the risk of complications and death and the more special care he or she needs.
- Among interventions for the management of complications in preterm or LBW infants, two respiratory interventions were prioritized: continuous positive airway pressure (CPAP) for respiratory distress and methylxanthines for apnea.
- Neonatal jaundice is a yellowish discoloration of the white part of the eyes and skin in a newborn baby due to high bilirubin levels. Other symptoms may include excess sleepiness or poor feeding. Complications may include seizures, cerebral palsy, or kernicterus.

- Infectious diseases of the fetus are caused by many different types of organisms, including viruses, bacteria, spirochetes, and protozoa (e.g., toxoplasmosis).

References

1. Abdelazim, I.A. Fetal fibronectin (Quick Check fFN test®) for detection of premature rupture of fetal membranes. *Arch. Gynecol. Obstet.* **2013**, *287*, 205–210.
2. Aziz K, Chadwick M, Baker M, Andrews W. Ante- and intra-partum factors that predict increased need for neonatal resuscitation. *Resuscitation*. 2008;79:444–452. doi: 10.1016/j.resuscitation.2008.08.004
3. Baily, M.A. and Murray, T.H. (2009).*Ethics and Newborn Genetic Screening*. Johns Hopkins University Press. ISBN 978-0-8018-9151-9
4. Berazategui JP, Aguilar A, Escobedo M, et al.; ANR study group. Risk factors for advanced resuscitation in term and near-term infants: a case-control study. *Arch Dis Child Fetal Neonatal Ed*. 2017;102(1):F44–F50.
5. Buyukbayrak, E.; Turan, C.; Unal, O.; Dansuk, R.; Cengizoğlu, B. Diagnostic power of the vaginal washing-fluid prolactin assay as an alternative method for the diagnosis of premature rupture of membranes. *J. Matern.-Fetal Neonatal Med.* **2004**, *15*, 120–125.
6. Cheng A, et al. Part 6: resuscitation education science: 2020 American Heart Association Guidelines for Cardiopulmonary Resuscitation and Emergency Cardiovascular Care *Circulation*. 2020; In press.
7. Eroglu, D.; Yanık, F.; Oktem, M.; Zeyneloglu, H.B.; Kuscu, E. Prediction of preterm delivery among women with threatened preterm labor. *Gynecol. Obstet. Investig.* **2007**, *64*, 109–116.
8. Escobedo MB, Aziz K, Kapadia VS, Lee HC, Niermeyer S, Schmölzer GM, Szyld E, Weiner GM, Wyckoff MH, Yamada NK, Zaichkin JG. 2019 American Heart Association Focused Update on Neonatal Resuscitation: An Update to the American Heart Association Guidelines for Cardiopulmonary Resuscitation and Emergency Cardiovascular Care. *Circulation*. 2019;140:e922–e930. doi: 10.1161/CIR.0000000000000729
9. Finn, D.; Roehr, C.C.; Ryan, C.A.; Dempsey, E.M. Optimising Intravenous Volume Resuscitation of the Newborn in the Delivery Room: Practical Considerations and Gaps in Knowledge. *Neonatology* **2017**, *112*, 163–171.
10. Holmes AV. Establishing successful breastfeeding in the newborn period. Pediatr Clin North Am. 2013 Feb;60(1):147-68.
11. Jahedbozorgan, T.; Yaghmaei, M.; Naserieh, M. Comparison of serum ferritin levels in pregnant women with preterm and term deliveries. *Immunopathol. Persa* **2020**, *6*, e25.
12. Jasani B, Torgalkar R, Ye XY, et al. Association of umbilical cord management strategies with outcomes of preterm infants: a systematic review and network meta-analysis. *JAMA Pediatr.* 2021;175(4):e210102.
13. Karaer, A.; Celik, E.; Celik, O.; Simsek, O.Y.; Ozerol, İ.H.; Yılmaz, E.; Turkcuoglu, I.; Duz, S.A. Amniotic fluid urocortin-1 concentrations for the prediction of preterm delivery. *J. Obstet. Gynaecol. Res.* **2013**, *39*, 1236–1241.

14. Kariman, N.; Hedayati, M.; Majd, S.A. The role of vaginal prolactin in diagnosis of premature rupture of membranes. *Iran. Red Crescent Med. J.* **2012**, *14*, 352.

15. Kattwinkel J, Perlman JM, Aziz K, Colby C, Fairchild K, Gallagher J, Hazinski MF, Halamek LP, Kumar P, Little G, et al. Part 15: neonatal resuscitation: 2010 American Heart Association Guidelines for Cardiopulmonary Resuscitation and Emergency Cardiovascular Care. *Circulation.* 2010;122(suppl 3):S909–S919. doi: 10.1161/CIRCULATIONAHA.110.971119

16. Keir, A.; Froessler, B.; Stanworth, S. QUESTION 2: Are intravenous fluid boluses beneficial in late preterm or term infants with suspected haemodynamic compromise? *Arch. Dis. Child.* **2016**, *101*, 201–202.

17. Keir, A.K.; Karam, O.; Hodyl, N.; Stark, M.J.; Liley, H.G.; Shah, P.S.; Stanworth, S.J.; NeoBolus Study Group. International, multicentre, observational study of fluid bolus therapy in neonates. *J. Paediatr. Child. Health* **2019**, *55*, 632–639.

18. Kochanek KD, Murphy SL, Xu JQ, Arias E; Division of Vital Statistics. *National Vital Statistics Reports: Deaths: Final Data for 2017* Hyattsville, MD: National Center for Health Statistics; 2019(68). https://www.cdc.gov/ nchs/data/nvsr/nvsr68/nvsr68_09-508.pdf. Accessed February 28, 2020.

19. Lavonas EJ, et al. Part 7: systems of care: 2020 American Heart Association Guidelines for Cardiopulmonary Resuscitation and Emergency Cardiovascular Care *Circulation*. 2020; In press.

20. Lawrence RM, Lawrence RA. Breastfeeding: more than just good nutrition. Pediatr Rev. 2011 Jul;32(7):267-80.

21. Lembet, A.; Eroglu, D.; Ergin, T.; Kuscu, E.; Zeyneloglu, H.; Batioglu, S.; Haberal, A. New rapid bed-side test to predict preterm delivery: Phosphorylated insulin-like growth factor binding protein-1 in cervical secretions. *Acta Obstet. Gynecol. Scand.* **2002**, *81*, 706–712.

22. Levine GN, O'Gara PT, Beckman JA, Al-Khatib SM, Birtcher KK, Cigarroa JE, de Las Fuentes L, Deswal A, Fleisher LA, Gentile F, Goldberger ZD, Hlatky MA, Joglar JA, Piano MR, Wijeysundera DN. Recent Innovations, Modifications, and Evolution of ACC/AHA Clinical Practice Guidelines: An Update for Our Constituencies: A Report of the American College of Cardiology/ American Heart Association Task Force on Clinical Practice Guidelines. *Circulation*. 2019;139:e879–e886. doi: 10.1161/CIR.0000000000000651

23. Liong, S.; Di Quinzio, M.; Fleming, G.; Permezel, M.; Rice, G.; Georgiou, H. New biomarkers for the prediction of spontaneous preterm labour in symptomatic pregnant women: A comparison with fetal fibronectin. *BJOG Int. J. Obstet. Gynaecol.* **2015**, *122*, 370–379.

24. Little MP, Järvelin MR, Neasham DE, Lissauer T, Steer PJ. Factors associated with fall in neonatal intubation rates in the United Kingdom–prospective study. *BJOG*. 2007;114:156–164. doi: 10.1111/j.1471-0528.2006.01188.x

25. Lotfi, G.; Faraz, S.; Nasir, R.; Somini, S.; Abdeldayem, R.M.; Koratkar, R.; Alsawalhi, N.; Ammar, A. Comparison of the effectiveness of a PAMG-1 test and standard clinical assessment in the prediction of preterm birth and reduction of unnecessary hospital admissions. *J. Matern.-Fetal Neonatal Med.* **2019**, *32*, 793–797.

26. Luechathananon, S.; Songthamwat, M.; Chaiyarach, S. Uterocervical angle and cervical length as a tool to predict preterm birth in threatened preterm labor. *Int. J. Women's Health* **2021**, *13*, 153–159.

27. Magid DJ, et al. Part 2: evidence evaluation and guidelines development: 2020 American Heart Association Guidelines for Cardiopulmonary Resuscitation and Emergency Cardiovascular Care *Circulation*. 2020; In press.

28. Makrigiannakis, A.; Semmler, M.; Briese, V.; Eckerle, H.; Minas, V.; Mylonas, I.; Friese, K.; Jeschke, U. Maternal serum corticotropin-releasing hormone and ACTH levels as predictive markers of premature labor. *Int. J. Gynecol. Obstet.* **2007**, *97*, 115–119.

29. Maymon, E.; Romero, R.; Chaiworapongsa, T.; Berman, S.; Conoscenti, G.; Gomez, R.; Edwin, S. Amniotic fluid matrix metalloproteinase-8 in preterm labor with intact membranes. *Am. J. Obstet. Gynecol.* **2001**, *185*, 1149–1155.

30. Mehrotra, S.; Solanki, V.; Natu, S.; Chauhan, S.; Sharma, R. Study of Prolactin in Cervicovaginal Secretion in Women with Preterm Labor and Normal Pregnancy. *J. South Asian Fed. Obstet. Gynaecol.* **2020**, *12*, 34–37.

31. Moon RY, Hauck FR, Colson ER. Safe Infant Sleep Interventions: What is the Evidence for Successful Behavior Change? Curr Pediatr Rev. 2016;12(1):67-75.

32. Nikolova, T.; Bayev, O.; Nikolova, N.; Di Renzo, G.C. Evaluation of a novel placental alpha microglobulin-1 (PAMG-1) test to predict spontaneous preterm delivery. *J. Perinat. Med.* **2014**, *42*, 473–477.

33. Niles DE, Cines C, Insley E, Foglia EE, Elci OU, Skåre C, Olasveengen T, Ades A, Posencheg M, Nadkarni VM, Kramer-Johansen J. Incidence and characteristics of positive pressure ventilation delivered to newborns in a US tertiary academic hospital. *Resuscitation*. 2017;115:102–109. doi: 10.1016/j.resuscitation.2017.03.035

34. Shalish, W.; Olivier, F.; Aly, H.; Sant'Anna, G. Uses and Misuses of Albumin during Resuscitation and in the Neonatal Intensive Care Unit. In *Seminars in Fetal and Neonatal Medicine*; Elsevier: Amsterdam, The Netherlands, 2017.

35. Søreide E, Morrison L, Hillman K, Monsieurs K, Sunde K, Zideman D, Eisenberg M, Sterz F, Nadkarni VM, Soar J, Nolan JP; Utstein Formula for Survival Collaborators. The formula for survival in resuscitation. *Resuscitation*. 2013;84:1487–1493. doi: 10.1016/j.resuscitation.2013.07.020

36. Stewart D, Benitz W., COMMITTEE ON FETUS AND NEWBORN. Umbilical Cord Care in the Newborn Infant. Pediatrics. 2016 Sep;138(3)

37. Tanir, H.M.; Sener, T.; Yildiz, Z. Cervical phosphorylated insulin-like growth factor binding protein-1 for the prediction of preterm delivery in symptomatic cases with intact membranes. *J. Obstet. Gynaecol. Res.* **2009**, *35*, 66–72.

38. Tricco AC, Lillie E, Zarin W, O'Brien KK, Colquhoun H, Levac D, Moher D, Peters MDJ, Horsley T, Weeks L, Hempel S, Akl EA, Chang C, McGowan J, Stewart L, Hartling L, Aldcroft A, Wilson MG, Garritty C, Lewin S, Godfrey CM, Macdonald MT, Langlois EV, Soares-Weiser K, Moriarty J, Clifford T, Tunçalp Ö, Straus SE. PRISMA Extension for Scoping Reviews (PRISMAScR): Checklist and Explanation. *Ann Intern Med*. 2018;169:467–473. doi: 10.7326/M18-0850

39. Vadillo-Ortega, F.; Estrada-Gutiérrez, G. Role of matrix metalloproteinases in preterm labour. *BJOG Int. J. Obstet. Gynaecol.* **2005**, *112*, 19–22.

40. Visscher MO, Adam R, Brink S, Odio M. Newborn infant skin: physiology, development, and care. Clin Dermatol. 2015 May-Jun;33(3):271-80.

41. Warren JB, Phillipi CA. Care of the well newborn. Pediatr Rev. 2012 Jan;33(1):4-18.

42. Wildschut, H.I.; Weiner, C.P.; Peters, T.J. *When to Screen in Obstetrics and Gynecology*; Elsevier Health Sciences: Amsterdam, The Netherlands, 2006.

43. Wyckoff MH, Aziz K, Escobedo MB, Kapadia VS, Kattwinkel J, Perlman JM, Simon WM, Weiner GM, Zaichkin JG. Part 13: neonatal resuscitation: 2015 American Heart Association Guidelines Update for Cardiopulmonary Resuscitation and Emergency Cardiovascular Care. *Circulation*. 2015;132(suppl 2):S543–S560. doi: 10.1161/CIR.0000000000000267

44. Wyckoff MH, Wyllie J, Aziz K, de Almeida MF, Fabres J, Fawke J, Guinsburg R, Hosono S, Isayama T, Kapadia VS, et al; on behalf of the Neonatal Life Support Collaborators. Neonatal life support: 2020 International Consensus on Cardiopulmonary Resuscitation and Emergency Cardiovascular Care Science With Treatment Recommendations. *Circulation*. 2020;142(suppl 1):S185–S221. doi: 10.1161/CIR.0000000000000895

Chapter

GROWTH AND DEVELOPMENT

4

Contents

INTRODUCTION

There are four stages in a child's growth and development:

- Infancy
- Preschool years
- Middle childhood years
- Adolescence

An infant usually loses 5–10% of their birth weight in the first few days after delivery. Approximately two weeks of age is when an infant should begin to gain weight and grow rapidly. An infant's weight should double from birth by the time they are 4 to 6 months old. Growth is slower in the latter part of the first year of life. In between one and two years of age, a toddler will only put on roughly 5 pounds (2.2 kilos). Between the ages of two and five, weight gain will stay around five pounds (2.5 and kilograms) annually. A child grows steadily between the ages of two and ten. When puberty first appears, usually between the ages of 9 and 15, there is a final growth spurt.

These variations in growth rates match the child's nutritional requirements. In comparison to a preschooler or school-age child, an infant requires more calories per unit of body weight. A child's nutritional needs rise once more as they approach adolescence. A child in good health will grow according to their own curve. Every child may, however, consume different amounts of nutrients. Offer a diet that is appropriate for the child's age and includes a wide range of foods. It is best to start eating healthily in infancy. This can aid in the prevention of illnesses like obesity and high blood pressure.

Orientation and Directional Terms

Term	Definition	Illustration
Cognitive development	Cognitive development means the development of the ability to think and reason. Children ages 6 to 12, usually think in concrete ways (concrete operations).	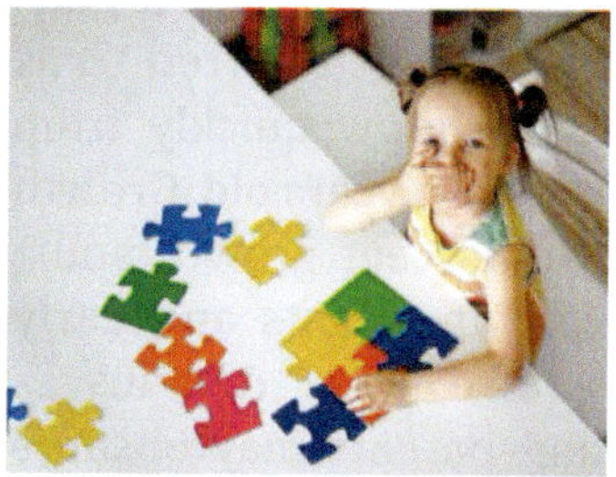
Infant	A baby, from birth to age 1 year.	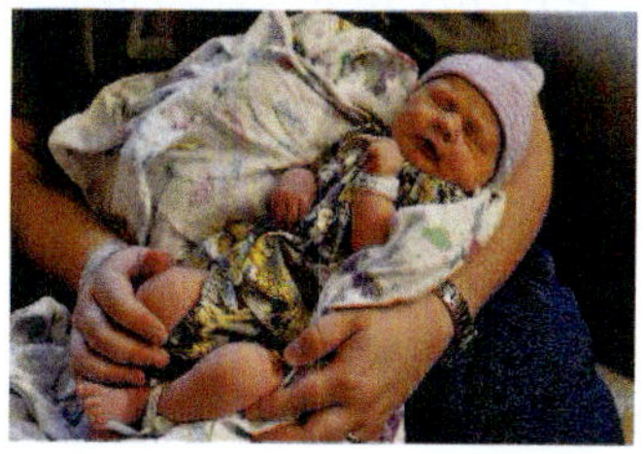
Adolescence	A period of life in which the biological and psychosocial transition from childhood to adulthood occurs.	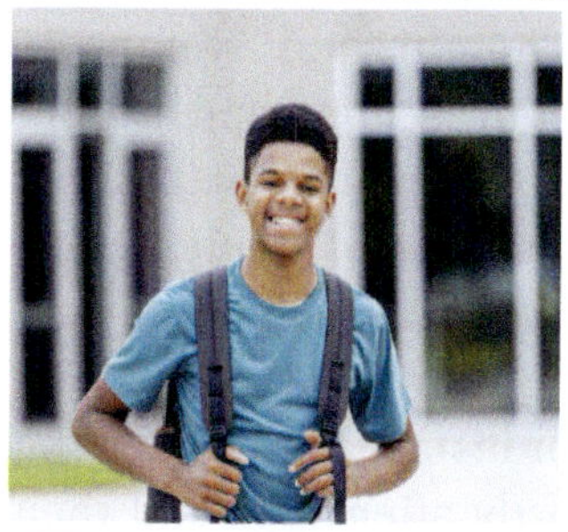
Body mass index	A measure to determine the amount of body fat and amount of lean body mass.	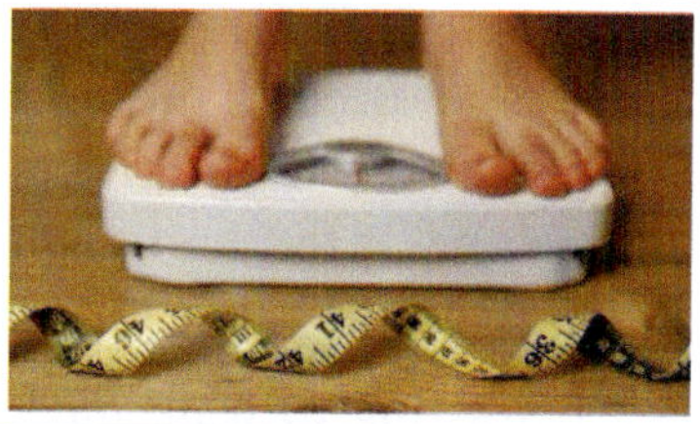
Teething	Teething is when your baby's teeth start to come through their gumline. Another word for it is odontiasis.	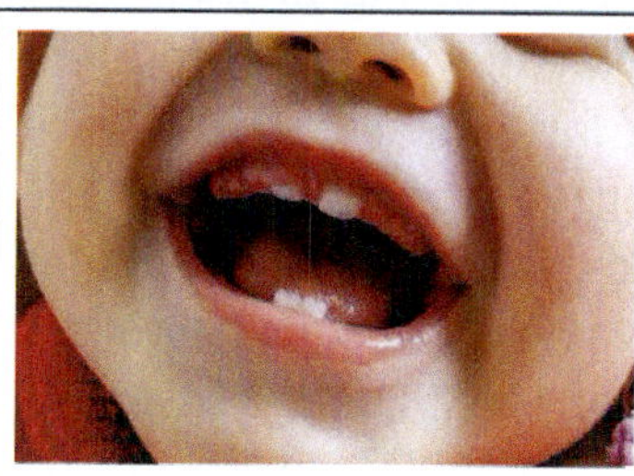

4.1. PHYSICAL GROWTH OF INFANTS AND CHILDREN

An increase in the size of the body's organs and length, weight, or height is referred to as physical growth. Children grow quickly from birth until they are one or two years old. Growth then slows until the adolescent growth spurt follows this fast growth in infants and early toddlers. Children require fewer calories as their growth slows, and parents may observe a decrease in appetite. Parents may experience anxiety when their two-year-old child exhibits highly unpredictable eating patterns. Even though they appear to eat almost nothing, some kids still seem to be growing and thriving. In actuality, they typically eat less one day and more the next to make up for it.

Growth in both height and weight is consistent during the preschool and school years. Until the next significant growth spurt happens in the early stages of adolescence, children typically grow by the same amount every year. Organs develop at varying speeds. The reproductive system, for instance, experiences a brief growth spurt shortly after birth and then very little change until shortly before sexual maturation (puberty). On the other hand, the early years of life are when the brain grows almost exclusively. By the end of the first year, the kidneys are functioning at the adult level.

Youngsters who are starting to walk have a cute body type, with the back curving and the belly protruding forward. They could also have a very bow-legged appearance. By the age of three, the body starts to appear leaner and more muscular as muscle tone increases and the percentage of body fat decreases. At this age, the majority of kids can physically control their bladder and bowels. Physicians track the children's weight gain concerning their height and report on the children's growth in comparison to other children of the same age. Using standard growth charts from the World Health Organization, doctors document all growth parameters in a chart from birth to two years of age (WHO). Doctors use growth charts from the Centers for Disease Control and Prevention (CDC) to record growth parameters after the age of two (Figure 4.1).

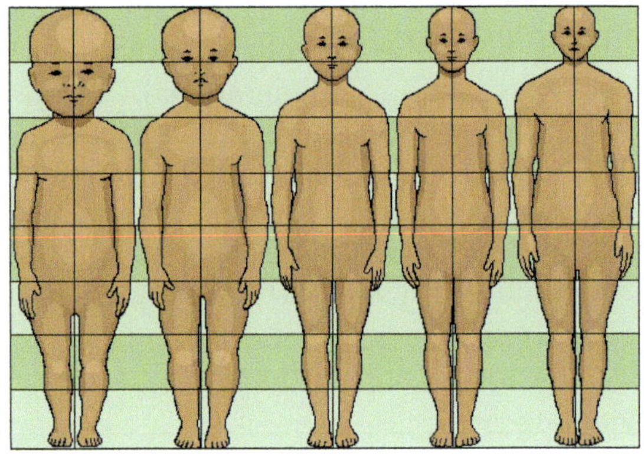

Figure 4.1. *Shown from left to right: Human body proportions at birth, at 2 years, at 6 years, at 12 years, and at 19 years.*

Source: https://wtcs.pressbooks.pub/infanttoddlerdev/chapter/Chapter 4-physical-development-in-infancy-toddlerhood/.

4.1.1. Length and Height

The lengths of infants are measured. Children who can stand are used to measure height. Babies are measured on their backs with an appropriate tool, such as a supine stadiometer, which is a measuring table; children who can stand are measured with a vertical or standing stadiometer. Generally speaking, at five months and 12 months of age, the length of full-term infants increases by roughly 30% and more than 50%, respectively. A baby's height at five years old is roughly double its birth length, having grown an average of 10 inches (25 centimeters) in the first year. By the time they are 2 years old, most boys have half of their adult height. Around the age of 19 months, most girls reach half of their adult height.

4.1.2. Weight

During the first few days of life, full-term newborns usually lose 5 to 8% of their birth weight. By the end of the first 2 weeks, they have gained this weight back. After that, babies usually gain one ounce every day for the first two months and one pound every month after that. The birth weight usually doubles by the time the child is five months old, and by the time they are a year old, it has tripled. The number of children and adolescents in the United States who suffer from obesity (excess body weight) has continued to rise since the 1980s. Some kids develop obesity at a young age. The classification of overweight and obesity is based on the body mass index (BMI). Extended BMI-for-age growth charts for boys and girls with extremely high BMIs are available from the CDC.

4.1.3. Head Circumference

The measurement around a child's head's largest area is called head circumference. The tape measure is placed by doctors around the back of the head, above the ears and eyebrows. This measurement is crucial because it tells doctors whether the child's brain is developing normally and because the size of the head corresponds to the size of the brain. Up until the age of three, children's head circumference is regularly measured.

The brain is 25% larger at birth than it will be as an adult, and the head circumference is roughly 14 inches (35 centimeters). The brain is 75% the size of an adult's at one year old. The brain is 80% of its adult size by the age of three. The brain is 90% of its adult size by the age of seven.

4.1.4. Teeth

Teeth erupt at different times, mostly due to genetic factors. However, conditions like Down syndrome, hypopituitarism, hypothyroidism, and rickets can also cause a delay in tooth eruption. About five to nine months of age is typically when lower front teeth erupt. Usually between the ages of 8 and 12 months, the upper front teeth erupt. By the time they are 12 months old, babies typically have 6 teeth, 18 months, and 16 teeth, and by the time they are 2½ years old, they have all 20 baby (deciduous) teeth. Between the ages of 5 and 13, permanent (adult) teeth replace baby teeth. In girls, permanent teeth typically erupt earlier. Teething refers to the symptoms (like drooling and fussiness) brought on by tooth eruption (Shonkoff and Phillips, 2000; Roggman et al, 2008; Davies, 2011; Ridley, 2011; Sharma et al, 2021).

4.2. DEVELOPMENT

Size growth is referred to as physical growth. Development is an increase in capacity and function. Environmental, dietary, and genetic factors influence both processes. Developmental descriptions frequently break down into distinct domains, such as language, cognition, gross and fine motor skills, and social and emotional development. Although there is a lot of overlap, these designations are still helpful.

Research has determined ranges of normalcy as well as average ages at which particular milestones are reached. A typical child's development in each of the several domains varies, as evidenced by the toddler who talks in complete sentences but walks slowly. The pace and pattern of development are determined by the interaction of genetic factors and environmental factors, which include nutrition, stimulation, disease, and psychological factors. Development is continuously assessed as parents, educators, and medical professionals assess children. There are numerous tools available for more focused development monitoring. Multiple domains of evaluation are facilitated by the Denver Developmental Screening Test II. The scoring sheet effectively illustrates the crucial idea of a range of normalcy and shows the average ages for reaching specific milestones. One can also use other tools.

4.2.1. Principles of Development

There are a few fundamental development concepts to remember:

- Change is visible throughout the lifespan and development is continuous (though this text ends with adolescence). Furthermore, early experiences influence later development.
- Development is multidirectional. We demonstrate improvements in certain domains of development but losses in others.
- Development is multidimensional. We are subject to change in three general domains/dimensions: social and emotional, cognitive, and physical.
- The physical domain encompasses variations in weight and height, changes in gross and fine motor skills, changes in sensory abilities, the nervous system, and the susceptibility to illness and disease.
- The changes in wisdom, intelligence, perception, memory, problem-solving, and language are all included in the cognitive domain.
- The psychosocial or social and emotional domain is concerned with how changes in emotion, self-perception, and interpersonal relationships with friends, family, and peers occur.

The three domains are interdependent. A change in one domain could have a cascading effect, causing changes in the other domains as well.

- Plasticity, or the capacity to adapt and the malleability of many of our traits, is what defines development. Although early experiences are crucial, children have extraordinary resilience, or the capacity to overcome hardship.
- Development is multicontextual. Nature (genetics) and nurture (environment) both have an impact on us; our behavior, beliefs, and values are products of the environment in which we live as well as the time and place of our birth. Understanding that actions, motives, feelings, and decisions are all a part of a larger picture is crucial in this situation.

Let us now examine a framework for analyzing development.

4.2.2. Periods of Development

Consider the developmental stages you would expect a child development course to cover. Perhaps you have three stages on your list: childhood, adolescence, and adolescence. Developmentalists, or those who study development, divide this phase of life into the following five stages:

- Prenatal Development (conception through birth)
- Infancy and Toddlerhood (birth through two years)
- Early Childhood (3 to 5 years)
- Middle Childhood (6 to 11 years)
- Adolescence (12 years to adulthood)

The distinct features of the various childhood and adolescent stages are reflected in this list. Therefore, even though an 8-month-old and an 8-year-old are both regarded as children, their motor skills, social skills, and cognitive abilities are very different. Both their dietary requirements and their main psychological issues are different.

4.2.2.1. Prenatal Development

After conception, development starts. The mother's health is the main priority as all of the body's major structures are developing. The main concerns are understanding nutrition, labor and delivery, and teratogens, or environmental factors that can cause birth defects (Figure 4.2).

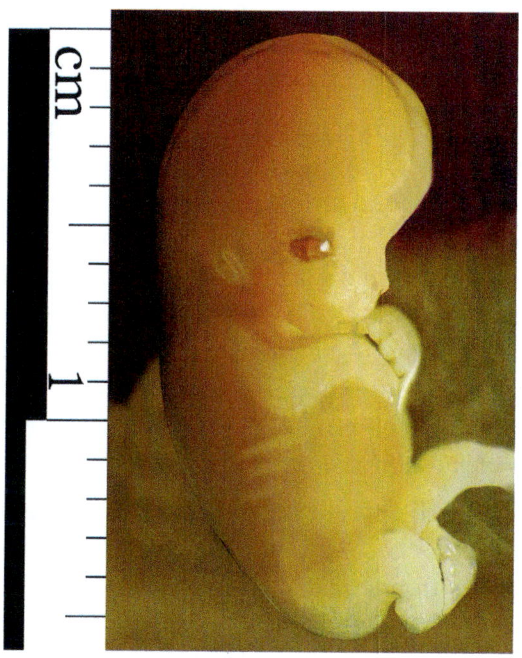

Figure 4.2. *A tiny embryo depicting some development of arms and legs, as well as facial features that are starting to show.*

Source: By The original uploader was GoldenBear at German Wikipedia. - Life Issues Institute, 1721W Galbraith Road, Cincinnati, OH 45239, 513.729.3600, www.lifeissues.org, CC BY-SA 3.0, https://commons.wikimedia.org/w/index.php?curid=22862400.

4.2.2.2. Infancy and Toddlerhood

The physical, emotional, behavioral, and mental development of children between the ages of 0 and 36 months is known as infant and toddler development.

Every developmental stage in infants (0 to 12 months) and toddlers (12 to 36 months) is marked by distinct milestones. There is considerable variation in the range of times within which the majority of healthy infants and toddlers achieve each milestone. For instance, when a baby or toddler starts to crawl, walk, or talk can depend on a variety of factors, including culture, environment, socioeconomic status, and genetics. Children in environments deficient in social stimulation, undernutrition, or access to quality healthcare may not develop as quickly as children in more enriched environments. When milestones are missing or noticeably delayed, there is reason for concern regarding the development of infants and toddlers because these circumstances may indicate an underlying medical or mental illness. It is critical for a child's health to identify issues at an early developmental stage. While parents are frequently the first to voice concerns, educators and childcare providers may notice issues that parents have missed or have been too scared to address. They might also be able to recognize children who have been mistreated or ignored and show abnormal development.

4.2.2.2.1. Infancy

After a typical birth, the majority of babies are awake and interacting with their environment within hours. All bodily systems are functional despite their immaturity. Babies are capable of yawning, blinking, coughing, suckling, swallowing, and passing waste. Although vision takes several years to reach adult levels, hearing is well developed. Research on infants shows that they are already able to distinguish between straight lines and shapes that resemble faces. It is also evident that newborns have a startle reflex, which causes them to react to loud noises and unexpected movements. Even the smallest babies can hold onto someone's finger thanks to the grasping reflex. Infants also exhibit a strong sense of taste and smell; they will turn away from offensive odors and indicate a preference for sweet flavors over bitter ones.

Heads are physically large compared to the rest of the body. The range of the average birth weight is approximately 2.5 to 4 kg (5 to 10 pounds), and the range of the average birth length is 45–53.3 cm (18 to 21 inches). Following a 5 to 7% weight loss at birth, infants typically gain 142 to 170 grams (5 to 6 ounces) per week on average. In the days that follow, babies settle into their own routines, sleeping, crying, becoming aware, and then going back to sleep. Sleeping on their backs lowers the risk of sudden infant death syndrome (SIDS). Young infants sleep in the fetal position. When they first start to need 6 to 10 feedings a day, many babies sleep for three to four hours in between meals.

For babies, the two main ways they communicate are by crying and fussing. According to research, "baby talk," which is thought to be crucial for language development, is well-received by infants. In response to touch, infants will turn toward their mothers' voices in particular and seek out the breast or bottle. They prefer to be held close to the heart, and swaddling—firmly enshrouding them in blankets—is frequently comforting. Shushing noises can also help calm a distressed baby because they resemble sounds made in the womb.

Newborn reflexes start to fade between two and three months. If this doesn't happen, there might be a neurological issue. At this age, babies stop crying and start to smile at people. As they get to know their own fingers and toes, they amuse themselves. Babies love games like pat-a-cake and bye-bye, and their favorite toys are rattles and mobiles. It's common to feel attached to one's parents or primary caregiver. Babies begin to experience separation anxiety at eight or nine months of age, and they become upset when their parents or other primary caregivers are gone.

By four months of age, an infant's vision has improved, and he or she can focus on bright objects and is drawn to primary colors, especially red. Infants who saw both symmetrical and asymmetrical faces in a study indicated a preference for the symmetry of faces that adults had deemed to be "attractive." Yet, infants preferred asymmetry between the ages of five and eight months. Eight-month-old babies who tended to favor consonant musical tones responded differently to rhythm changes. Since children pick up skills through imitation, monitoring a child's healthy development greatly depends on how well an infant or toddler can imitate others. A smile in return is one of the earliest indications of infant imitation. Infants later pick up on imitating other people's sounds and facial expressions.

Normal infants grow to a relatively equal head and chest circumference. In the prone position, infants learn to flip from one side to the other. They advance to crawling and then sitting by themselves. Standing by yourself comes after pulling up on someone's hands or furniture. Many babies have taken their first steps by the end of the first year. After the cooing of early infancy, older babies start to make simple sounds with their voices and say words like mama, dada, and bye-bye. The baby can now use a spoon and a baby cup, as well as pick up tiny food fragments. Babies attempt to turn pages in books and brush their own hair. They might attempt to dance and sing because they like songs and rhymes. At this age, babies are very gregarious and want to be part of the family. They will join in the applause once they understand it. Additionally, some babies show their independence by kicking, resisting, or yelling. While this independence is strongly discouraged in certain cultures, it is accepted in others.

4.2.2.2.2. Toddler Years

Infants grow into toddlers by the end of their first year of life. Toddlers' physical growth slows between the ages of one and three as they develop their motor and communication skills. Normal development still heavily relies on imitation, which frequently manifests as role-playing at home or at school or as dressing up as princesses or superheroes. Normal toddlers exhibit boundless enthusiasm, energy, and curiosity as well as the beginnings of sophisticated thinking and learning skills. Emotional expression can take many forms, from openly giving hugs and kisses to sobbing and losing your temper. Older toddlers comprehend the notions of pride, shame, and guilt and express them when appropriate. Young children frequently think they are the center of the universe. Though they might not want to share or take shifts, they do understand the idea of ownership.

The head circumference continues to grow at a rate of 1–3 cm (half an inch) every six months, indicating healthy brain development. Most toddlers will have doubled in height and quadrupled in weight by the time they are three years old. Even though the back appears swayed and the abdomen protrudes until age three, its body starts to resemble an adult's. When rushing, even well-walked toddlers can trip and fall. Toddlers benefit greatly from push-and-pull toys and big balls as they develop their motor skills and coordination. The toddlers can sit on a small chair by themselves or climb into a large chair.

A toddler draws with their entire arm at the age of one. These abilities have advanced to finger and thumb manipulation by the age of three. Most toddlers are potty trained by the end of the third year, but accidents can still happen if they are sleeping or deeply engaged in an activity. Many toddlers have mastered the use of doorknobs by the age of two. If there are no child safety precautions in place, a toddler may leave a room or house without an adult's knowledge. Toddlers are naturally curious and have this ability, which makes them prone to wandering. They thus need adult supervision at all times, especially when they are in public or in unfamiliar areas.

The toddler likes to play hide-and-seek and hide things because they now get the idea of object permanence. Toddlers enjoy playing with other kids, but they might not cooperate or abide by the rules. Having the capacity to simultaneously hold toys or objects in both hands is a crucial sign of healthy brain development. The toddler should be able to recognize objects and body parts, put one object inside another, and manipulate mechanical objects so they work as intended. The toddler can comply with basic instructions. The toddler's language skills develop quickly, moving from simple words to complete sentences. The toddler can have conversations with others by the time they are three years old, though some of the words may not make sense. Toddlers start to grasp the idea of cause and effect, but they can't always tell when something could be dangerous. A toddler's appetite starts to wane and they often insist on eating just one or two of their favorite foods. They can undress and help put on clothes by handling bulky buttons, zippers, and Velcro fasteners. The toddler can wash their hands and give themselves an imperfect brushing of their teeth. Toddlers may attempt to delay going to bed, but they may sleep 10 to 12 hours every night.

Most toddlers have moved past the "terrible twos" and are now friendlier and more cooperative by the time they are three years old. Of the total height, males have reached 53% and females have reached 57%. A three-year-old typically weighs between 30 and 38 pounds (13 to 17.6 kg). The body is more erect and the head is now proportionate to the rest of the body. The majority of three-year-olds have grown out of their baby teeth and have 20/40 vision. Hoping and jumping are preferred methods of propulsion. The child exhibits hand dominance and can operate the pedals of small riding toys. Many toddlers can count from 1 to 10 or 20, recognize common shapes, and identify primary colors. A three-year-old's vocabulary typically consists of 300–1,000 words, and they may have nursery rhymes, stories, and favorite songs committed to memory. Rarely, children as young as three years old have mastered reading (Shonkoff and Phillips, 2000; Roggman et al, 2008; Davies, 2011; Ridley, 2011; Sharma et al, 2021).

4.2.2.3. Early Childhood

Early childhood development is the time before and during early childhood that is marked by rapid changes in physical, psychological, and social development.

4.2.2.3.1. Pediatric Growth

Pediatric growth is measured in terms of length or height, weight, BMI (beginning at age 2), and head circumference (used from 0 to 2 years of age). Numerous factors, such as genetic, environmental, hormonal, nutritional, and psychosocial ones, influence it. Size at birth is influenced by many factors, including maternal nutrition, alcohol, tobacco, and drug use, and it can also be laterally influenced by genetic syndromes and the height of family members. Normal growth is also influenced by a variety of endocrine factors and hormones, including thyroid hormones, glucocorticoids, growth hormone, insulin-like growth factors, and reproductive hormones.

- **Normal Physical Parameters and Ranges:** By comparing kids of a similar age and gender, percentile growth charts—like the ones produced by the Centers for Disease Control and Prevention (CDC) and displayed on this page—are used to monitor growth. The 95th, 90th, 75th, 50th, 25th, 10th, and 5th percentiles are the main percentile lines. The normal range of growth is defined by the CDC growth reference charts as falling between the 5th and 95th percentiles.

Shifting percentiles after two years of age may be the first indication of an underlying issue, even though it is normal for babies to do so during the first two years of life as a result of transitioning from an intrauterine to an external environment. During the first two years of life, babies grow at their fastest rate, or height velocity. Furthermore, a child's growth curve can be interpreted and the expected height potential can be computed using the mid parental height (MPH). Males and females use the following computations, respectively:

Male = (father's height + mother's height + 13 cm)/2

Female = (father's height-13 cm + mother's height)/2.

- **Abnormal/Delayed Development:** When kids don't reach developmental milestones at the same rate as their peers in the community, it's called developmental delay. Rather than being a diagnosis, it is more of a term used to describe a wide range of psychological and physical characteristics.

- **Growth Delay:** When a child's growth crosses at least two percentiles beyond the first two years of life on a growth chart, when they are small for gestational age at birth and show no signs of gaining weight, or when they have abnormal height velocity for their age, they should be evaluated for abnormal linear growth. Furthermore, a child should be evaluated for short stature if their height is two standard deviations (SD) or less from the average height for their age or from the MPH. Short stature may have a pathological or normal cause. Constitutional growth delay and hereditary or familial short stature are two common causes of growth delay. When a child's MPH predicts their final height appropriately and their parents' heights fall within the lower 10th percentile, this is known as familial short stature. A child with a constitutional growth delay is one whose delayed puberty results in a growth delay that will eventually catch up once puberty starts. Once a child reaches the age of three, bone age measurements can be used to differentiate between a normal and pathological cause. Early childhood pathological causes typically involve malnourishment and failure to thrive, which can occur during fetal development or postpartum.
- **Development Delay:** Intellectual disability (ID) and global developmental delay (GDD) are two categories of developmental delay. While intellectual disability is defined as deficiencies in reasoning, adaptive functioning, or other intellectual aspects and usually manifests later in life, global developmental delay is defined as a delay in two or more domains of development.

There are many different causes of both ID and GDD, including genetic mutations (Prader-Willi disease, fragile X syndrome, etc.). to teratogen exposure during pregnancy (Fetal Alcohol Syndrome). The causes of ID and GDD in a person can frequently be the same.

4.2.2.3.2. Physical Development

The term "physical development" refers to the growth of the brain, the ability to move, and all other pertinent developmental stages that support movement. Early childhood development encompasses the progressive acquisition of fine and gross motor skills, balance, coordination, and control over movement. Early childhood physical development milestones include:

- Development and regulation of limbs, joints, muscles, etc.
- Fine and gross motor skills
- Mastery of a variety of physical abilities, including manipulating tools, physical literacy, agility, and dynamic skills.
- Sensory development
- Inhibition of primitive reflexes.

Physical development and a child's capacity to grow and thrive are related. Children's physical development can be improved by giving them enough opportunities for movement and physical play during their early years. The children's lack of physical activity is closely associated with several health and behavioral problems, such as postural disorders and challenges with potty training.

- **Early Childhood Education and Development of the Body:** Early childhood education and care, or ECEC, is essential to the physical development of young children. Given the high percentage of kids enrolled in early childhood education, parents and preschools share equal responsibility for raising robust, healthy kids. Young children's cognitive, social, and physical development is strongly positively impacted by the quantity and caliber of physical education in early childhood education. Early childhood is a time of fast learning, growth, and development, and each child develops at a different rate and at a different speed. Ensuring the normal physical development of preschool-aged children requires incorporating physical training that is tailored to their age- and anatomy-related developmental characteristics. Given its substantial impact on a wide range of developmental outcomes, including behavioral, cognitive, and emotional ones, physical space is becoming increasingly important in early childhood education and care.

4.2.2.3.3. Cognitive Development

The most active stage of a person's brain development occurs during early childhood. The child's future academic and cognitive success depends on ensuring optimal cognitive development in the early years. The expansion and improvement of mental capacities, thought processes, and problem-solving techniques are referred to as cognitive development. Early on, sensory abilities and visual perception help young children quickly pick up, process, and comprehend information from their experiences and surroundings. Research on children's cognitive development emphasizes the significance of brain development and the need for a stimulating environment to foster the development of cognitive abilities. Infants' capacity to process information from their senses—visual, tactile, auditory, and olfactory—as well as their ability to plan and control their movements, is largely due to the rapid brain development that occurs during the first few years of life.

Kohlberg's theory of moral development phases is one of the most well-known concepts outlining the gradual development of morality and moral reasoning in children. This theory holds that moral development happens in six stages, with the pursuit and maintenance of justice serving as the primary emphasis. The social environment, family dynamics, early childhood education and care, and physical activity are all significant determinants of how young children develop cognitively.

4.2.2.3.4. Language and Communication Development

Cries are a newborn baby's primary means of communication, and the types of cries they make depend on their needs, which can include hunger, pain, or even boredom. Early consonant sounds like /k/ and /g/ are developed in babies by the second and third months of their lives. Babbling begins in the second half of the first year, when babies start making repetitive sounds like mamamama or babababa. More vocalization by infants is associated with improved communication abilities. Each child has different early communication skills. Early language and communication development is influenced by a wide range of factors, such as individual differences, lived experiences, cultural context, and general developmental progressions.

Early language and communication development is greatly aided by appropriate techniques and supportive environments. Promoting early language and communication development can be done in many ways. The Turn and Talk approach is a popular strategy for fostering young children's language development. Using this approach, kids are urged to discuss a subject with their classmates to improve their language skills.

4.2.2.3.4. Social and Emotional Development

The definition of social competence is behavior that promotes effective social interaction. While social competence is developed in children from an early age, social competence is displayed and the process of becoming socially competent develops later. Regular adult supervision by caregivers other than parents creates a secure environment for children to form peer relationships while adults are keeping an eye on them. Toddlers and young children may share similar interests and needs when it comes to social interaction, such as running after balls, jumping off steps, and playing games like run-chase. Children who have the chance to engage with people other than their parents are more likely to have social interactions. Empirical data suggests that children who spend more time with their peer groups develop social skills related to friendships and interactions. Maladaptive behaviors are the result of unfavorable social interaction experiences. Aggression or bullying are examples of maladaptive social behaviors; avoidance, withdrawal, or passive acquiescence are examples of other maladaptive social behaviors.

4.2.2.3.5. Emotional Development

These abilities begin to develop at a young age and are a lifelong process in emotional development. Early in life, children experience the development of basic emotions like happiness, fear, sadness, anger, curiosity, and surprise. The emotional development of young children is greatly influenced by their relationships with their primary caregivers. Soon after birth, they attempt to mimic the facial expressions of their primary caregivers, which serves as their initial means of communication. Through positive interactions with their parents and other primary caregivers, children gradually learn how to control their emotions.

4.2.2.4. Middle Childhood

Middle childhood is defined as the ages of 6 to 11, and a lot of what happens to kids during this time is related to their involvement in the early school years. Today's world consists of picking up and honing new academic skills as well as evaluating oneself and others based on comparisons of one's own abilities and accomplishments. Through team sports, test results, and other recognition programs, schools compare their students and make these comparisons public. At this stage of development, growth rates slow down and children can improve their motor skills. Through interactions with friends and classmates, children also start to learn about relationships in the social sphere outside of their families.

4.2.2.5. Adolescence

Usually occurring between puberty and adulthood, adolescence is a transitional stage of both physical and psychological development (typically corresponding to the age of majority). Although adolescence is typically linked to adolescence, it can manifest physically, psychologically, or culturally at any time before or after these years. Preadolescence is when puberty usually starts, especially in females. Both physical and cognitive development can continue well into adolescence, especially in males. The precise definition of adolescence has not been agreed upon by scholars, and age only serves as a rough indicator. Certain definitions begin at age 10 and conclude at age 30. An adolescent is defined by the World Health Organization as a person who is between the ages of 10 and 19.

4.2.2.5.1. Biological Development

- **Puberty in General:** Puberty is a multi-year period marked by fast physical and psychological development that ends with sexual maturity. For girls, puberty typically starts at age 11, and for boys, it starts at age 12. Although environmental factors like diet and exercise also play a role, heredity is the primary determinant of each person's unique puberty timeline. Precocious and delayed puberty can also be caused by these factors (Figure 4.3).

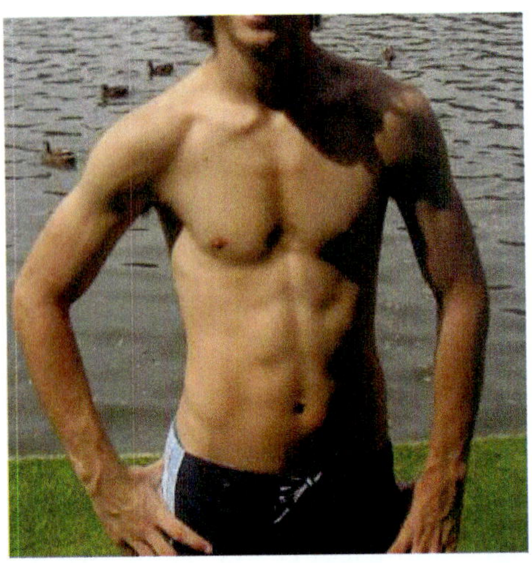

Figure 4.3. *Upper body of a teenage boy. The structure has changed to resemble an adult form.*

Source: By Yemenite Camel, CC BY 3.0, https://commons.wikimedia.org/w/index.php?curid=4198496.

Distinct physiological changes in an individual's height, weight, body composition, and circulatory and respiratory systems are some of the most important aspects of pubertal development. Hormonal activity is a major factor influencing these modifications. Hormones have two roles in the body: they are both active and organizational. As puberty approaches, hormone changes during adolescence set off physical and behavioral changes in the body.

The process of puberty is lengthy and starts with an increase in hormone production, which leads to several physical changes. It is the period of life marked by a significant shift in the hormonal balance toward adulthood as well as the emergence and development of secondary sex traits (such as a deeper voice and larger Adam's apple in boys and the development of breasts and more curved and prominent hips in girls). The pituitary gland causes a spike in hormones to be released into the bloodstream, which sets off a series of events. As a result, both the male and female gonads are activated, causing them to grow and develop quickly. The triggered gonads then start producing large amounts of hormones. The ovaries mainly release estrogen, while the testes release testosterone. These hormones are produced at a progressively higher rate until sexual maturation is reached. Gynecomastia in boys can occur as a result of obesity, tissue reactivity, or sex hormone imbalance.

Male facial hair typically grows in a specific order during puberty: between the ages of 14 and 17, the corners of the upper lip are usually where facial hair first appears. It then covers the entire upper lip to form a mustache. The development of hair in the region beneath the lower lip and on the upper cheeks comes next. Eventually, the hair covers the entire lower face, the sides, and the lower edge of the chin to create a full beard. This particular order may differ for some people, as it does for the majority of biological processes in humans. In late adolescence, around the ages of 17 and

18, facial hair is frequently present, though it may not appear until much later. Some men wait 10 years after puberty before growing full facial hair. For an additional two to four years after puberty, facial hair gets coarser, darker, and thicker.

For males, the primary indicator of puberty is sperm arche, or the first ejaculation, which typically happens at the age of 13. It's menarche, or the start of menstruation, for females, which usually happens between the ages of 12 and 13. Hereditary factors play a role in determining a girl's menarche age, but diet and lifestyle also have an impact. A girl needs to reach menarche with a specific percentage of body fat, regardless of her genetic makeup. As a result, girls who consume large amounts of fat in their diet and do not exercise tend to start menstruating earlier than girls whose diet is lower in fat and who engage in activities that burn fat (e.g., gymnastics and ballet). Girls who are undernourished or who grow up in cultures where physical labor is expected of them also start menstruating later in life.

Puberty can occur at a time that has significant psychological and social repercussions. Boys who mature early tend to be taller and stronger than their peers. They have the benefit of drawing attention from possible mates and getting chosen first in sports. Adolescent boys frequently exhibit positive body images, increased self-assurance, security, and independence. Boys who mature later in life may have a negative body image and lack confidence as a result of comparing themselves to more mature friends and peers. But early puberty is not always a good thing for boys; the hormone surge that comes with early sexual maturation in boys can also lead to increased aggression. Pubescent boys may experience more social pressure to fit in with adult norms because they seem older than their peers; society may also perceive them as more emotionally mature even though their social and cognitive development may not keep up with their outward appearance. Research has indicated that boys who are early maturing have a higher likelihood of engaging in risky behaviors and being sexually active.

One common feature of maturing females is increased self-consciousness, which can occasionally result from early maturation in girls. Pubescent girls may experience increased levels of insecurity and dependence due to their bodies developing ahead of time. As a result, girls who mature sexually before their peers are more likely to suffer from eating disorders (like anorexia nervosa). The goal of almost half of diets for American high school girls is weight loss. Girls may also experience sexual advances from older boys before they reach a mature emotional and mental stage. Early-maturing girls are more likely to be exposed to alcohol and drug abuse in addition to having earlier sexual experiences and more unintended pregnancies than late-maturing girls. Individuals with similar experiences typically do worse academically than their less experienced peers.

Boys typically finish puberty around the ages of 16–17, while girls typically reach their full physical development around the ages of 15–17. It is unusual for someone to grow taller than the post-pubertal age. About four years after the onset of the first physical symptoms of puberty, girls reach reproductive maturity. Boys, on the other hand, mature more slowly but keep growing for roughly six years following the onset of noticeable pubertal changes (Figure 4.4).

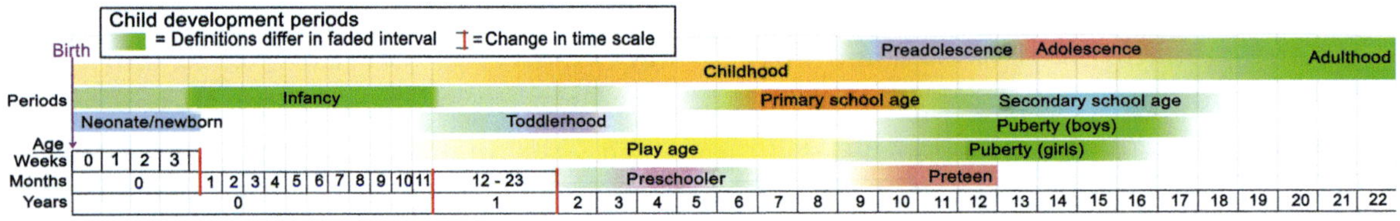

Figure 4.4. *Approximate outline of development periods in childhood and early adulthood development. Adolescence is marked in red at top right.*

Source: By Mikael Häggström – Own work, Public Domain, https://commons.wikimedia.org/w/index.php?curid=7209351.

- **Growth Spurt:** There are three distinct stages in the physical development of girls during their teenage years. Breast buds and pubic hair develop at the beginning, which usually corresponds with the start of rapid growth. The second stage of sexual maturity coincides with the peak period of physical growth, which happens about a year later. Girls enter the third stage, which usually includes menarche, 1 to 1.6 years after secondary sex characteristics first appear. They will have experienced an adult fat distribution and a noticeable hip broadening by this point, having completed their growth spurt. Furthermore, breast development is finished, and axillary hair—the hair in the armpits and pubic area—becomes darker and more widely distributed. It can be challenging to pinpoint the precise start of male sexual development as opposed to that of girls.

Puberty normally lasts five years for boys and three and a half years for girls (menarche). They have already gone through their growth spurt at this point, and their body has clearly changed, with wider hips and a more adult-like distribution of fat. By this point, breast development will also be finished. The curve of general body growth at adolescence in boys can be correlated with four developmental stages. The fat spurt is often the first indication of sexual maturation in boys. The growing boy puts on weight and almost gets chubby, with a distribution of fat that is a little more feminine. This most likely happens because the testes' Leydig cells, which are more prevalent, stimulate the production of estrogen before the Sertoli cells start to produce appreciable amounts of testosterone. Boys may look physically awkward and obese during this stage. Stage II is noticeable about a year after the scrotum starts to enlarge. Subcutaneous fat is redistributed and pubic hair growth begins during this period. Stage III begins 8 to 12 months after the height gain reaches its peak velocity. During this phase, the breasts fully develop and the hips clearly widen, with a fat distribution more akin to that of an adult. For the majority of people, these three phases add up to a full growth spurt. Axial hair starts to grow at this point, and only the upper lip of the face has facial hair. Along with a persistent decline in subcutaneous fat and a visibly harder and more angular body form, there is also a surge in muscle growth. Although the distribution of pubic hair looks more mature, it has not yet reached the medial region of the thighs. The scrotum and penis are almost adult size. It can be challenging to determine when boys reach stage IV, which happens anywhere from 15 to 24 months after stage III. This marks the end of the height growth spurt. A further increase in muscular strength is present, along with adult pubic and axillary hair distribution and color, as well as facial hair on the chin and upper lip.

A fast rise in a person's height and weight during puberty caused by the simultaneous release of androgens, thyroid hormones, and growth hormones is known as the adolescent growth spurt. On average, males go through their growth spurt two years later than females. Teenagers grow at a rate that is almost exactly the same as a toddler during their peak height velocity, or the period of most rapid growth—roughly 10.3 cm (4 inches) for boys and 9 cm (3.5 inches) for girls annually. Adolescents not only see changes in height but also a notable increase in weight. Adolescent weight gain accounts for almost half of an individual's adult body weight. Males in their teens and early adult years may keep gaining muscle naturally even after puberty.

Although the accelerated growth in various body parts occurs at different times for each adolescent, it follows a fairly consistent pattern. The extremities—the head, hands, and feet—grow first, then the arms and legs, and finally the torso and shoulders. One of the reasons an adolescent's body may appear out of proportion is because of this uneven growth.

Bones harden and become more brittle during puberty. The process known as epiphysis causes the ends of the long bones to close at the end of puberty. These skeletal alterations may differ depending on one's ethnicity. For instance, in the United States, the bone density of black adolescents increases significantly more than that of white adolescents, which may explain why there are fewer bone fractures and a lower risk of osteoporosis among black women.

The body's distribution of muscle and fat changes during puberty is another important set of physical changes. It is a different process for men and women. Before puberty, there are almost no differences in the distribution of fat and muscle between the sexes; during puberty, boys grow muscle much faster than girls, though muscle development is rapid for both sexes. On the other hand, although body fat increases in both sexes, it does so considerably more in girls. Girls often experience an increase in body fat in the years immediately preceding puberty. In post-pubertal boys, the ratio of muscle to fat is approximately three to one, whereas in girls it is approximately five to four. This could clarify why there are gender variations in athletic performance.

Adolescents' growing hearts and lungs have an impact on their circulatory and respiratory systems during pubertal development. Strength and exercise tolerance increase as a result of these modifications. The development of larger hearts and lungs, higher systolic blood pressure, a lower resting heart rate, a greater ability to carry oxygen to the blood, a greater capacity to neutralize the chemical products of muscular exercise, higher blood hemoglobin, and a greater number of red blood cells are all characteristics that distinguish men from women.

Adolescent biology is largely influenced by environmental factors, although there are some genetic differences between the sexes. For instance, girls may experience inadequate nutrition from diets that frequently lack essential nutrients like iron, and they may also tend to reduce their physical activity during preadolescence. The physical development of females is subsequently impacted by these environmental factors.

- **Reproduction-Related Changes:** The traits associated with the sex organs directly relate to primary sex characteristics. Growth of the testes and scrotum occurs first in the male puberty stages, and then the penis grows. The prostate, bulbourethral gland, and seminal vesicles all grow and develop at the same time as the penis. Since many boys experience their first ejaculation as a result of masturbation, the first seminal fluid ejaculation typically happens approximately a year after the onset of accelerated penis growth. However, this is frequently determined culturally rather than biologically. Boys typically become fertile before they reach adulthood.

Changes in the primary sex characteristics of females include the development of the vagina, uterus, and other reproductive system components. Menarche, or the start of the menstrual cycle, is a relatively late development that happens after a protracted hormonal cycle. Regular ovulation occurs about two years after menarche, so a girl is usually not fully fertile for several years after menarche. Therefore, unlike men, women typically have a mature physical appearance before being able to conceive.

All changes unrelated to sexual reproduction are considered changes in secondary sex characteristics. Males experience these changes in the form of pubic, facial, and body hair, as well as voice deepening, roughening of the skin around the thighs and upper arms, and increased sweat gland development. Secondary sex changes in females include nipple elevation, pubic and underarm hair development, hip widening, elevated breasts, and expanded areolae. The British pediatrician who developed the classification system, Tanner, is the name given to the five stages that characterize the changes in secondary sex traits that occur during puberty.

- **Changes in the Brain:** The human brain continues to develop even after puberty and into one's 30s, particularly in the frontal lobe. Neuroscientists disagree on when exactly brain development fully ends, but it is believed to extend beyond the age of 30. While the brain is still developing, individuals may exhibit behaviors associated with immaturity. However, there is no proven link between the development of the prefrontal cortex during adolescence and irrational behaviors. The brain reaches 90% of its adult size by age six, with minimal growth during adolescence.

The amount of gray matter in the brain exhibits an inverted U pattern during adolescence, while the amount of white matter increases linearly. The brain's amount of gray matter is reduced and superfluous neuronal connections are removed through a process known as synaptic pruning. But this doesn't mean the brain stops working; on the contrary, myelination—the covering of axons—increases and the number of inactive pathways decreases, making the brain more functional.

Primary function areas of the brain, like motor and sensory areas, are the first to be pruned. Later in development, the brain regions engaged in more intricate functions start to lose material. These comprise, among other areas, the lateral and prefrontal cortices. The prefrontal cortex, which is involved in higher-order cognitive processes like decision-making and cognitive control, experiences some of the most notable changes in the brain during development. Adolescence is a time of increased myelination and synaptic pruning in the prefrontal cortex, which enhances information processing efficiency and fortifies neural connections between the prefrontal cortex and other brain regions. This results in enhanced impulse control and a better assessment of risks and rewards. To be more precise, the ventromedial prefrontal cortex is crucial for decision-making, whereas the dorsolateral prefrontal cortex is important for impulse control and forward planning. A change in the orbitofrontal cortex is critical for assessing risks and rewards.

Glutamate, dopamine, and serotonin are the three neurotransmitters that are crucial for the development of the adolescent brain. An excitatory neurotransmitter is glutamate. Most of the neural connections that are cut during the synaptic pruning that takes place during adolescence have receptors for excitatory neurotransmitters like glutamate. Because of this, the brain's synaptic balance is more inhibitory than excitatory by the time an adult reaches early adulthood.

Dopamine is linked to enjoyment and making decisions while paying attention to the surroundings. Adolescence is characterized by an increase in dopamine input to the prefrontal cortex and an increase in dopamine levels in the limbic system. The equilibrium between excitatory and inhibitory neurotransmitters, along with elevated dopamine levels during adolescence, could potentially impact adolescents' propensity for taking risks and their susceptibility to boredom.

One neuromodulator that affects mood and behavior is serotonin. The limbic system's development is crucial for processing social information and emotional experiences as well as for deciding what constitutes a reward or punishment. Adolescents are more sensitive to rewards and stress due to variations in the limbic system's levels of the neurotransmitters dopamine and serotonin. Adolescents may become more vulnerable due to the ensuing rise in emotional variability. Serotonin's effects extend beyond the limbic system. During adolescence, the gene expression of several serotonin receptors changes significantly, especially in the human frontal and prefrontal cortex.

4.2.2.5.2. Cognitive Development

The period of adolescence is one of fast cognitive development. Adolescence, according to Piaget, is the period of life when a person's thoughts begin to become more abstract and their egocentric thoughts become less prevalent, enabling them to reason and think more broadly. The development of executive functions, or the cognitive abilities that allow for the regulation and synchronization of thoughts and behavior, has been shown by behavioral and fMRI studies. These abilities are typically linked to the prefrontal cortex. The ideas, concepts, and thoughts that are formed during this stage of life have a significant impact on one's future and help to shape their character and personality.

Rapid cognitive growth is the result of biological changes in the brain's structure and connectivity, as well as an increase in experience, knowledge, and shifting social demands. While each person experiences certain changes at a different age, the changes listed below start at puberty or soon after, and some skills continue to develop as the adolescent gets older. According to the dual systems model, impulsivity and other adolescent behaviors are caused by a maturational imbalance between the brain's socioemotional system and cognitive control systems. The baseline of teenage cognitive development is the subject of some studies, such as the ABCD Study.

- **Theoretical Perspectives:** Understanding the cognitive changes that occur during adolescence can be done in at least two ways. The constructivist theory of cognitive development is one of them. It adopts a quantitative, state-theory methodology based on Piaget's work and postulates that the cognitive development of adolescents occurs relatively quickly and dramatically. The second viewpoint, known as information processing, comes from research on artificial intelligence and aims to explain cognitive development in terms of the expansion of particular thought processes.

- **Improvements in Cognitive Ability:** People are about as capable of making critical decisions and using critical thinking as adults are by the time they are 14 years old. In five domains, these advancements take place in adolescence:
  - **Attention:** Selective attention, the ability to concentrate on one stimulus while blocking out others, shows improvements. The capacity to focus on two or more stimuli at once, known as divided attention, also gets better.
  - **Memory:** Higher levels of performance have been noted in both short-term and long-term memory.
  - **Processing Speed:** Teenagers think faster than younger people do. Between the ages of five and middle adolescence, processing speed increases significantly; between the ages of 14 and 15, it starts to level off and does not seem to change until late adolescence or adulthood.
  - **Organization:** Adolescents can think more effectively by using mnemonic devices and other techniques because they are more conscious of how they think.
  - **Metacognition:** A better understanding of one's own thought processes leads to increased self-control and social awareness.

Research conducted after 2005 suggests that the brain continues to change efficiently well into adulthood. A "point of maturity" in the twenties is somewhat arbitrary, as many significant brain regions are known to be fully developed by the age of 14 or 15, making the definition of "maturity" elusive and subject to debate.

Prefrontal cortex pruning has been observed to persist into the sixth decade of life, leveling off by the time an individual is 14 or 15 years old. White matter is said to increase until approximately the age of 45, at which point it is gradually lost due to aging. The idea that the brain finishes developing in the twenties is called into question if myelination persists into one's forties and fifties.

- **Hypothetical and Abstract Thinking:** Adolescents have a more abstract way of thinking compared to children, allowing them to think about possibilities that go beyond what currently exists. This increased capability in deductive reasoning enhances their ability to engage in hypothetical thinking and plan for the future. Adolescents can anticipate the consequences of their actions and consider alternative explanations for events, making them more adept at debating and challenging assumptions. Additionally, they develop a more advanced understanding of probability.

The emergence of more abstract, methodical thinking is another noteworthy feature of adolescent cognitive development. For instance, teenagers are better able to understand the higher-order abstract logic found in proverbs, puns, metaphors, and analogies than younger children are. Their enhanced ability enables them to recognize the various ways that language can be used to communicate ideas, including sarcasm, metaphor, and satire. (Oftentimes, kids under the age of nine are completely incapable of understanding irony. This also makes it possible to apply sophisticated logic and reasoning to social and ideological issues like politics, philosophy, religion, morality, friendship, faith, justice, and honesty, among other social and ideological concerns.

- **Metacognition:** Metacognition, or the process of thinking about thinking, is the third increase in cognitive capacity. It frequently entails keeping an eye on one's own cognitive activity while thinking. Teenagers who are more aware of their own thought processes can exercise self-control and learn more efficiently. It has a bearing on social cognition as well, leading to heightened self-awareness, intellectualization, and introspection (though this latter term refers to thinking critically about one's own ideas rather than the Freudian interpretation as a defense mechanism). Teenagers are far more adept than younger ones at comprehending that mental activity is not entirely within a person's control. The capacity for introspection can result in two types of adolescent egocentrism, namely the personal fable and the imaginary audience, which cause two different types of thinking difficulties. These probably peak at 15, along with a generalized self-consciousness.

A more complex theory of mind is involved in perspective-taking, which is connected to metacognition and abstract thought. Adolescents develop the ability to take a social perspective when they can comprehend how the ideas or deeds of one person can affect those of another, even when they are not directly involved.

- **Relativistic Thinking:** Adolescents are less inclined than children to accept facts as unchanging truths and more inclined to challenge the claims made by others. They discover that the rules they were taught as absolute are actually relativistic through experiences they have had outside of their immediate family. They start to make the distinction that younger children do not: they start to distinguish between rules that are based on culturally relative standards (such as dating only until a certain age) and those that are established out of common sense (such as not touching a hot stove). This may result in a time when authority is questioned across the board.
- **Risk-Taking:** Many studies have been conducted on the cognitive and emotional mechanisms underlying teenage risk-taking, as the majority of injuries suffered by teenagers are linked to risky behavior (drug and alcohol abuse, careless or distracted driving, unprotected sex, etc.). In answering this question, it is critical to determine whether risky behaviors are more common among adolescents (prevalence), whether risk-related decisions are made by adolescents in a way that is similar to or different from that of adults (cognitive processing perspective), or whether adolescents use the same processes but arrive at different conclusions because they value different things.

According to the behavioral decision-making theory, both adults and adolescents should consider the possible benefits and drawbacks of a decision. Nonetheless, studies have indicated that teenagers appear to value rewards—especially social ones—more than adults do.

The idea that adults and adolescents view risk similarly but arrive at different conclusions because of their differing values appears to be supported by the research. There are those who contend that an increased inclination towards risk-taking during adolescence could have evolutionary advantages. Teenagers wouldn't have the confidence or drive to leave their family of origin, for instance, if they weren't willing to take risks. Furthermore, from a population standpoint, it is advantageous to have a subset of people who aren't afraid to try new things and take risks, as this will balance out the more traditional aspects of the knowledge that older adults tend to hold.

Adolescents now place a higher value on dating and sexual attraction, and taking chances is necessary to win over possible partners. This suggests that risk-taking may also have reproductive benefits. Additionally, studies suggest that baseline sensation seeking may influence risk-taking behavior at all stages of life. Sexual activity carries some risk because of the possible outcomes, especially for young people. The aspects of unprotected sex, poor birth control, multiple partners are risk factors.

Higher rates of parental abuse and lower rates of parental support and monitoring are two aspects of teenage lives that are linked to risky sexual behavior.

- **Inhibition:** Adolescents exhibit reduced behavioral inhibition, including deficiencies in extinction learning, which is linked to their heightened propensity for risk-taking. This has significant ramifications for risky behavior, like illicit drug use or unsafe sex, since teenagers are less likely to refrain from actions that could have unfavorable long-term effects. This phenomenon also has implications for behavioral treatments grounded in the theory of extinction, like drug addiction treatment or cue exposure therapy for anxiety. It has been proposed that adolescent propensity to relapse to drug-seeking even after behavioral addiction treatment may be explained by impaired inhibition, specifically extinction (Shonkoff and Phillips, 2000; Roggman et al, 2008; Davies, 2011; Ridley, 2011; Sharma et al, 2021).

4.2.2.5.3. Social Development

- **Identity Development:** The teenage life cycle includes a stage called identity development. Most people start looking for their identity during their teenage years. Adolescents are more willing to "try on" various behaviors and looks during this time to figure out who they are. Adolescents frequently cycle through several identities in an effort to discover who they are and what makes them feel most like themselves. It can be challenging to develop and maintain an identity during adolescence for a variety of reasons, including social status, environment, and family dynamics. Research indicates that this process of changing the content and structure of one's ideas about oneself is normative and that it may be better defined as identity development than formation. Self-clarity and self-esteem constitute the two primary facets of identity development. High levels of self-awareness and self-control during mid-adolescence will result in better decisions during the transition to adulthood since decisions made during adolescence can influence later life. Self-concept, sense of identity, and self-esteem are the three broad approaches that researchers have employed to comprehend identity development. Adolescence produces a more responsible generation of young adults. Teenagers focus more on their appearance and devote more time and energy to it as their bodies change. Teens make an attempt to look presentable, in contrast to children. An adolescent's identity development is significantly influenced by their upbringing and environment. Research conducted by the American Psychological Association has demonstrated that adolescents from less affluent backgrounds struggle more to form their identities.
- **Self-Concept**: The ability to define one's opinions and beliefs with confidence, consistency, and stability is referred to as one's self-concept. Cognitive development

in the early stages of adolescence leads to increased self-awareness, awareness of others and their opinions and thoughts, the capacity to think abstractly about future possibilities, and the capacity to weigh several options at once. Because of this, self-descriptions in teens differ greatly from those of young children, who typically define themselves based on their physical characteristics. Instead, adolescents define themselves in relation to their beliefs, values, and opinions.

- Adolescents can imagine a variety of future selves, as well as the outcomes of their decisions and long-term possibilities. Investigating these options could lead to sudden shifts in how the adolescent presents themselves as they select or reject traits and behaviors, attempting to steer the real self away from the feared self and toward the ideal self—who they wish to be. These distinctions seem to encourage achievement through behavior consistent with the ideal and different from the feared possible selves, even though they are uncomfortable for many.
- As adolescents become aware of the contextual factors influencing both their own behavior and other people's perceptions, they start to differentiate their self-concept further and start to qualify their traits when asked to describe themselves. By the middle of adolescence, differentiation seems to be fully developed. The personality traits that teenagers use to define themselves peak in the seventh and ninth grades. Because they are contextual in nature, they may contradict one another. During these years, adolescents often experience distress due to the recognition of inconsistent content in their self-concept. However, this distress may have a positive effect on their structural development.
- **Sense of Identity:** Teenage egocentrism manifests as a conscious wish to fit in with their peer groups and be accepted by others. In contrast to the contradictory facets of self-concept, identity stands for a consistent sense of self that is stable in all situations and encompasses both past experiences and future objectives. While Erik Erikson maintained that not everyone fully achieves identity, everyone has a self-concept. Erikson's theory of developmental stages encompasses the identity crisis, wherein young people need to consider various options and incorporate various aspects of themselves before firmly establishing their beliefs. He emphasized that the identity challenge is never completely resolved once and for all at one point in time, but he also defined the resolution of this process as a stage of identity achievement. Teenagers start by using their membership in the crowd to define who they are. Teens can explore new identities, grow apart from their parents, and form bonds with peers through their clothes. Teenagers' quest to discover who they are has been greatly aided

by fashion, which is constantly changing along with the nuances of their personalities. Teenagers deliberately experiment with different looks to see what works best for them to define who they are. The adolescent can come to terms with who they are through trial and error in comparing both their perceived image and the image others react to and see.

- **Environment and Identity**: The development of an adolescent's identity is greatly influenced by their surroundings. Research indicates that the more privileged an individual's upbringing, the more successfully they develop their identity, even though the majority of studies on adolescents are done on middle-class, white children. An adolescent's identity formation is a critical stage in their development. Recent research indicates that, compared to the middle of the 20th century, the transition to adulthood is now happening over a longer period of years, based on demographic patterns. As a result, the stage of life known as youth—which includes late adolescence and early adulthood—has gained prominence. Consequently, this has led to the importance of several factors during this development. Adolescents' social identities are shaped by a multitude of factors, including social media, coping mechanisms, and commitment. Each of these elements is impacted by the surroundings in which an adolescent is raised. A child raised in a more affluent household is generally exposed to greater opportunities and better circumstances. Teenagers from underprivileged areas or neighborhoods with high crime rates are more likely to grow up in unfavorable environments. Adolescence is a delicate time in a person's development, and decisions made during that period can be significantly impacted by experiences they had during that period. Even though they are not exposed to negative environments, kids who grow up in affluent suburban communities are more likely to engage in activities that strengthen their identities and promote successful identity development.

Identity and sexual orientation. An erotic inclination toward people of one or more genders is defined as sexual orientation; this tendency is most commonly characterized as sexual or erotic attraction. Psychologists have been attempting to comprehend how adolescent sexual orientation develops in recent years. There are many different developmental pathways that a person can take, according to some theorists, and an individual's particular path may depend on their sex, sexual orientation, and when they reach puberty.

A four-stage model for the development of homosexual sexual identity was put forth by Troiden in 1989. The first stage, referred to as sensitization, typically begins in childhood and is characterized by the child's realization of the attraction of same-sex relationships. Identity confusion, the second stage, usually appears a few years later. At this point, the young person starts having sex with a same-sex partner because they are so overcome with inner conflict over their sexual orientation. Adolescents enter the third stage of identity assumption, which typically occurs a few years after they leave home, at which point they start coming out to their family and close friends and define themselves as gay, lesbian, or bisexual. The young adult embraces their sexual identity as a way of life during the last stage, referred to as commitment. As a result, this model predicts that the coming out process starts in childhood and lasts until the early to mid-20s. In recent years, alternative theories have been investigated in response to contests to this model.

Adolescence is when most gay/lesbian and transgender teenagers start to identify and understand their sexual identities. Once an identity has been established, many teenagers may decide to come out during this time in their lives; many others may experience a phase of doubt or denial, which may include trying out heterosexual and homosexual experiences. The average age at which a person becomes aware of their sexual orientation is around 10, according to a study of 194 lesbian, gay, and bisexual youth under the age of 21. However, the process of coming out to peers and adults typically occurs around 16 or 17, respectively. It can be challenging for some young people to accept and develop a positive LGBT identity for a variety of reasons. When young people who are unsure of their gender identity or sexual orientation are surrounded by peers who adhere to heteronormative norms, peer pressure plays a significant role and can lead to significant distress as they feel like they don't fit in. Although coming out can also help people adjust psychologically, there are risks involved. It's true that there's often a risk of violence, hurtful jokes, and exclusion when coming out in a heteronormative peer environment. As a result, bullying and rejection from peers or family members account for up to four times the suicide rate among LGBT adolescents compared to their heterosexual peers.

- **Self-Esteem**: Self-esteem is the last significant component of identity formation. One's ideas and sentiments regarding their identity and self-concept are referred to as their self-esteem. The majority of self-esteem theories contend that people of all ages and genders have a strong desire to uphold, defend, and improve their sense of self. Contrary to popular assumption, there is no empirical proof that self-esteem significantly declines during adolescence. While baseline self-esteem is remarkably stable throughout adolescence, barometric self-esteem fluctuates quickly and can lead to significant distress and anxiety. Many argue that more specialized measures could reveal more about the adolescent experience, and there have been doubts raised about the validity of global self-esteem scales. Girls who have supportive friendships are more likely to have high self-esteem; for them, having a friend is primarily about having someone to turn to for moral and social support. When girls don't get accepted by their friends or can't find someone to do things and have interests in common with, they experience low self-esteem. Boys, on the other hand, are more focused on defining their relationship to authority and claiming and demonstrating their independence. Because of this, they are more likely to have high self-esteem from their ability to successfully influence their friends; however, the main cause of low self-esteem in teenage boys is a lack of romantic competence, such as the inability to win or keep the affection of the opposite or same-sex (depending on sexual orientation). Men and women alike experience low self-esteem following the end of a romantic relationship, which makes them more vulnerable to other symptoms associated with this condition. Suicide is thought to be three to four times more common in men and twice as likely to occur in women. Depression and hopelessness are just two of the many symptoms.

- **Relationships:** In general, an adolescent's social development is greatly influenced by the relationships they have with their family, friends, and peers. Adolescents frequently develop strong emotional bonds with friends as their social circles expand quickly and they learn to differentiate between friends and acquaintances. This is not harmful, but it is a form of peer pressure if these friends put someone in situations that could be harmful. Since adolescents are easily influenced by the people they form close relationships with, adolescence is a crucial time in social development. It's also a delicate time because this is the first-time people can really make decisions for themselves. An adolescent's social development depends greatly on their relationships because of the tremendous influence that peers can have on them. These connections become important because they start to teach the teenager about personalities—what they are, how they develop, and why a person has that particular personality type. Psychological comparisons can be used as a process to explain the formation of implicit personality theory as well as an indicator of how the theory is developing. To put it another way, we would be laying the groundwork for developing a general theory of personality by contrasting the traits of one individual with those of another (and, dot. such a theory would provide a helpful foundation for comprehending particular individuals). This emphasizes the significance of communication and relationships in one's development and is comparable to the use of social comparison in the formation of one's identity and self-concept, which includes one's personality. Reference groups are used in social comparison about identity development and psychology. Adolescent peers make up these reference groups. This implies that the teens' reference groups are made up of the people they choose or accept as friends and the people they talk to frequently. As a result, these people can have a significant influence on the adolescent's future. Relationships have the biggest impact on a person's social development, according to research.

- **Family**: One's role in a family rapidly changes during adolescence. Early adolescence, when they are increasingly seen as equals by parents, is when children can show significant influence over family decisions despite their tendency to assert themselves strongly as young children. The challenge for the adolescent is to become more independent while maintaining a loving relationship with their parents. Puberty is frequently accompanied by a marked rise in parent-child conflict and a weakening of the family unit. Arguments frequently center on little matters of control, which teenagers may have previously believed their parents had total control over, like curfew, appropriate attire, and the teenager's right to privacy. Disagreement between parents and adolescents also rises when friends have a stronger influence on one another and introduce new influences to the adolescent that might go against the values of the parents. Parental and teenage arguments have also become more frequent as a result of social media. Although social media was once safe for parents to use, it has now turned into a dangerous place for kids. While teenagers aspire for independence, parents often worry about what their child is doing on social media platforms because of the growing number of predators on these platforms. The fact that a lot of parents are not familiar with social networking sites in the first place adds to their mistrust. Knowing how to maximize the benefits of online communication while minimizing its risks is a significant challenge for the parent-adolescent relationship. Even though parent-child disputes do increase during adolescence, these are still comparatively small matters. Most teenagers still hold the same attitudes and values as their parents when it comes to the major issues in their lives.

Siblings are a source of support and conflict for kids during their formative years. Depending on the gender of the siblings, adolescence may have different effects on this relationship. Intimacy between same-sex sibling pairs rises in the early stages of adolescence and then stays steady. Sibling pairs with mixed sexes behave differently; in the early stages of adolescence, they drift apart, but from middle adolescence onward, there is an increase in intimacy. Children's first relationships are with their siblings, and these relationships will always shape their social and self-perception. Maintaining healthy sibling relationships can benefit teenagers in many ways. In addition to being able to function as peers, siblings can boost each other's confidence and sociability. Though the effects of this can vary depending on the older sibling's activities, older siblings can guide younger siblings.

A major factor that could impact adolescence is a shift in the family dynamic, particularly in the case of divorce. Divorce is common, accounting for up to 50% of marriages, and it exacerbates the already significant changes that occur during adolescence. Soon after a divorce, custody battles frequently reveal parental ambivalence and out-of-control behavior. There is typically less contact between the adolescent and their noncustodial parent after a divorce. Divorce can benefit families in severe situations of abuse and instability in the home because it reduces conflict. Nonetheless, the majority of studies point to a detrimental impact on adolescence and subsequent development. According to a recent study, children of divorce who go through additional family transitions in late adolescence perform worse in math and social studies over time when compared to peers who grow up in stable post-divorce families. The adolescent epistemological trauma theory, which was presented in a recent study, proposed that stressful life experiences, like parental divorce, during the formative years of late adolescence foretell lifelong effects on adult conflict behavior, which can be lessened by efficient behavioral assessment and training. When a person is in their twenties or early thirties, the negative effects of parental divorce from childhood or adolescence persist. Romantic relationships and conflict style are among these detrimental effects; as adults, they are more likely to employ avoidance and competition as conflict management strategies. (Shonkoff and Phillips, 2000; Roggman et al, 2008; Davies, 2011; Ridley, 2011; Sharma et al, 2021).

The home environment and parents continue to play a significant role in shaping the behaviors and choices of adolescents, even in the face of shifting family roles during adolescence. Teens who are close to their parents are less likely to partake in risky behaviors like drinking, smoking, fighting, and/or unprotected sexual activity. Parents also have an impact on adolescent education. According to a study, teenagers who identify as authoritative parents at the age of 14 are more likely to finish secondary school by the age of 22 because they feel supported and encouraged by their parents, who in turn encourage them to finish their education so they don't let them down.

- **Peers**: Development on both a social and general level depends on peer groups. During adolescence, peer relationships become more intense and influential than in previous stages, and communication with peers increases significantly, impacting the teen's decisions and choices. Regardless of the traits of those friends, children's development can be positively impacted by high-quality friendships. As kids start to form relationships and friendships with different people, it helps them as teenagers and lays the groundwork for peer groups and adolescence. Peer groups are particularly crucial during adolescence, a developmental stage marked by a sharp rise in peer time and a decline in adult supervision. Adolescents also tend to identify with larger groups of peers based on shared characteristics and associate with friends of the opposite sex far more than they did as children. Adolescents frequently turn to their friends as coping mechanisms in a variety of circumstances. Adolescents use their friends as a coping mechanism when faced with social stresses, according to a three-factor structure of dealing with friends that includes avoidance, mastery, and nonchalance.

Adolescents can develop and assess their social skills, as well as explore their feelings and identity, through communication within peer groups. Members of peer groups have the chance to hone social skills like empathy, sharing, and leadership. Teenagers select their peer groups based on traits they share with those groups. Adolescents learn to accept who they are becoming by making use of these relationships. Adolescents' own self-concept incorporates group norms and values. Through acquiring new communication skills and considering their own opinions and values, along with those of their peers, an adolescent can share and express emotions and other concerns without being afraid of being rejected or judged. Peer groups can positively impact an individual in a number of ways, including motivation and performance in the classroom. Peers can help each other develop socially, but they can also get in the way of it. Peer pressure can have detrimental effects, such as pushing people to experiment with drugs, alcohol, vandalism, and theft. Peer pressure susceptibility rises in the early stages of adolescence, peaks at age 14, and then starts to decline. Teenagers in Spain have provided additional evidence that peers impede social development. Emotional reactions to problems, as opposed to solution-based ones, and emotional instability have been connected to physical aggression against peers. A wide range of persistent psychological issues, particularly depression, are associated with both relational and physical aggression, as well as social rejection. Teens who have been bullied consequently frequently experience issues that result in additional victimization. Adolescents who have experienced bullying are more likely to bully others and to experience bullying themselves in the future. In contrast, this relationship is less stable when cyberbullying occurs, which is a relatively recent problem among teenagers.

Teenagers typically form smaller-scale relationships with cliques and larger-scale relationships with crowds. In their early adolescence, teenagers frequently form close-knit, exclusive cliques consisting of peers of the same sex. Despite the widespread belief that cliques are always bad, they actually have the potential to benefit teenagers by assisting in their socialization and identity development. For instance, a clique of extremely athletic male peers may foster a greater sense of loyalty and rivalry within the group. Cliques have also evolved into a kind of collective parent, i.e., advising teenagers on appropriate and inappropriate behavior. Cliques frequently combine into mixed-sex groups as teenagers start dating one another in their late adolescence. Then, as socialization becomes more couple-oriented, these small friend groups disintegrate even more. More broadly, teenagers tend to identify with crowds—that is, with gatherings of people who are involved in the same activity or interest. Stereotyping young people as jocks or nerds is often based on crowd identities. Crowds at large, multiethnic high schools are frequently drawn according to their ethnicity. Adolescents experiment with new identities and widen their social circles by using online technology, such as adding more friends on Facebook and other social media platforms. Some teenagers use these newer platforms to improve their relationships with their peers, but there are drawbacks as well, like the previously mentioned cyberbullying and detrimental effects on the family.

- **Romance and Sexual Activity**: During adolescence, romantic relationships tend to become more common. 53% of teenagers have experienced a romantic relationship lasting at least one month within the preceding 18 months by the time they are 15 years old. In a 2008 study conducted by YouGov for Channel4, 20% of 14–17-year-olds surveyed revealed that they had their first sexual experience at 13 or under in the United Kingdom. A 2002 American study found that those aged 15–44 reported that the average age of first sexual intercourse was 17.0 for males and 17.3 for females. Over the adolescent years, relationships typically last longer as well. The development of cognitive skills required to sustain a romantic bond (e.g., caregiving, appropriate attachment) and sexual maturation can account for this steady increase in the likelihood of a long-term relationship, even though these skills are not fully developed until late adolescence. Teens who are in committed relationships can build self-worth and acquire the skills needed for successful relationships in the future. All things considered, healthy romantic relationships between teenagers can have long-term advantages. Good romantic relationships are positively correlated with social competence, self-worth, and confidence as well as higher levels of commitment in early adulthood. Adolescents who possess high self-esteem are likely to view themselves as more successful partners, while those who have had unfavorable experiences may have low self-esteem when it comes to romantic relationships. Teenagers frequently date people who are similar to them in terms of popularity, race, ethnicity, and physical attractiveness. Nonetheless, some characteristics make some people, especially teenage girls, want diversity. Boys usually date partners who are the same age or younger, while girls typically date partners who are the same age or older. Most adolescents date people who are roughly their own age.

Sexual maturation occurs during adolescence and shows up in social interactions as well. While casual sexual encounters, also known as "hookups," are common among adolescents, the majority of sexual experiences during this developmental stage occur in romantic relationships. Teens can use social media and technology to look for romantic relationships because they believe it's a safe space for them to experiment with dating and self-discovery. These interactions on social media could lead to the start of another relationship. Hugs, kisses, and handshakes are symbols of fulfillment and devotion. Genital stimulation, a sign of heavy sexual activity, is frequently linked to violence, depression, and unsatisfactory relationships in young adolescents. Sexual activity that occurs in a romantic relationship during late adolescence is not affected by this effect. There may be a subset of people who are predisposed to both early sexual activity and emotional distress because of research that indicates there are genetic causes of early sexual activity that are also risk factors for delinquency. After adjusting for genetic risks, however, older adolescents' romantic relationship-based sex was actually associated with lower levels of deviant behavior than their relationship-free sex (hook-ups). (Shonkoff and Phillips, 2000; Roggman et al, 2008; Davies, 2011; Ridley, 2011; Sharma et al, 2021).

In relationships between teenagers, dating violence can happen. When asked about their experiences in relationships, 12–25% of teenagers said they had witnessed physical violence, and 25–30% said they had encountered psychological aggression. While most physical aggression does not lead to a medical visit, there have been reports of hitting, throwing objects, and slaps. In relationships, physical aggression usually decreases from high school through college and early adulthood. Unlike adult relationships, there is no discernible difference in the rates of male and female aggressors in heterosexual couples.

Adolescent females from minority groups are more likely to experience intimate partner violence (IPV). According to recent research, many young urban girls are highly vulnerable to becoming victims of multiple forms of intimate partner violence. When diagnosing depression in teens from urban minority communities, practitioners should look for signs of intimate partner violence (IPV), both physical and non-physical, as early detection can help identify youth who need support and intervention. Adolescent victims, like adult victims, may seek medical attention for issues unrelated to IPV incidents but are reluctant to report abuse. Therefore, regardless of the primary complaint, screening ought to be a standard component of medical care for teenagers. It is important that adults take IPV in adolescents seriously, even though policy lags behind. Many adults minimize cases of IPV in adolescents or assume they don't happen because relationships at young ages are seen as puppy love.

Adolescents face additional risks in today's society as their sexuality starts to change. While some of these, like emotional distress (fear of exploitation or abuse) and STIs/STDs, including HIV/AIDS, are not inherently associated with adolescence, others, like teenage pregnancy (through contraceptive failure or non-use), are viewed as social issues in the majority of western societies. Teens who are sexually active have a one in four chance of getting a STI. Teenagers in the US frequently opt out of sexual activity altogether because they erroneously think it lowers their risk of contracting STIs. Clinicians nationwide are reporting an increase in herpes and human papillomavirus (HPV) diagnoses. HPV is known to cause genital warts and is estimated to afflict 15% of teenagers. More girls between the ages of 15 and 19 than any other age group contract gonorrhea. Individuals under the age of 21 account for 25% of newly diagnosed cases of HIV. 81% of parents want schools to start having conversations with their kids about condom and contraception use, according to a survey conducted in March by the Kaiser Family Foundation. Additionally, they think that STI testing ought to be available to students. Teachers also wish to discuss these subjects with their students. However, even though 9 out of 10 sex education teachers nationwide agree that contraceptives should be taught in the classroom, more than 25% say they have received clear directives from administrators and school boards not to (Table 4.1).

Table 4.1. Child Growth-a Case Study

Differences between WHO percentiles and smoothed centile curves at 24 months of age for length-for-age, weight-for-age, weight-for-length, body mass index-for-age, and head circumference-for-age, for boys and girls

	Sex	3rd	25th	50th	75th	97th
Weight-for-age (kg)	Boys	0.1	0.5	0.7	0.8	1.2
	Girls	0.3	0.3	0.5	0.8	1.4
Length-for-age (cm)	Boys	1.8	1.8	1.7	1.7	1.7
	Girls	1.8	1.8	1.8	1.8	1.8
Weight-for-length (kg/cm)	Boys	−0.4	−0.1	0.1	0.2	0.3
	Girls	−0.4	0	0.2	0.4	0.8
BMI-for-age (kg/m^2)	Boys	0	0	0.2	0.4	0.6
	Girls	−0.2	0	0.1	0.3	0.6
HC-for-age (cm)	Boys	−0.5	−0.3	0.1	0.3	0.2
	Girls	−0.5	−0.3	−0.1	0	0.2

HC—head circumference; BMI—body mass index.

Percentages of infants above the 90th percentile and below the 10th percentile of the WHO standards for weight-for-age, length-for-age, BMI-for-age, and head circumference-for-age, at neonatal period, 6 months, 12 months, and 24 months of age.

		At Neonatal Period		At 6 Months		At 12 Months		At 24 Months	
	Sex	Above 90th (%)	Below 10th (%)	Above 90th (%)	Below 10th (%)	Above 90th (%)	Below 10th (%)	Above 90th (%)	Below 10th (%)
Weight-for-age (kg)	Boys	14.12	10.73	9.59	8.90	4.79	22.60	3.60	14.39
	Girls	13.89	7.78	8.22	16.44	27.59	17.24	1.41	13.38
Length-for-age (cm)	Boys	17.51	4.52	2.07	14.48	4.11	21.23	3.65	18.98
	Girls	16.67	5.56	2.05	13.01	2.78	20.14	3.52	22.54
BMI-for-age (kg/m^2)	Boys	9.04	2.82	13.79	5.52	6.16	14.38	5.84	8.03
	Girls	10.0	7.22	14.38	9.59	5.56	11.81	4.93	7.75
HC-for-age (cm)	Boys	40.68	0	18.49	2.74	5.48	7.53	5.04	4.32
	Girls	38.33	0	16.44	2.05	12.41	3.45	5.63	4.23

HC—head circumference; BMI—body mass index.

Source: Garzón M, Papoila AL, Alves M, Pereira-da-Silva L. Comparison of growth curve estimates of infants in São Tomé Island, Africa, with the WHO growth standards: A birth cohort study. International Journal of Environmental Research and Public Health. 2019; 16(10):1693. https://doi.org/10.3390/ijerph16101693.

4.3. ISSUES IN DEVELOPMENT

4.3.1. Nature and Nurture

What characteristics—such as height, weight, personality, diabetes, etc.—make people who they are? the outcome of genetics, the environment, or both? The "nature/nurture" controversy has been debated by academics for decades. Those who support nature would contend that heredity is the primary factor responsible for the development of any given feature. Nurture proponents contend that our environments have the greatest influence on who we are. All facets of human development are still up for debate, but most academics concur that the two forces are constantly interacting. It is challenging to determine whether a particular behavior is purely the product of nature or nurture.

4.3.2. Continuity Versus Discontinuity

The answer to the question of whether human development is best understood as a process of more abrupt change or as a slow, gradual one often depends on the developmental theorist answering the question and the subject matter being studied. Stage theories include the ideas of Piaget, Freud, Erikson, and Kohlberg. Stage theories, also known as discontinuous development, postulate that developmental change frequently takes place in discrete, qualitatively distinct stages that follow a predetermined, universal sequence.

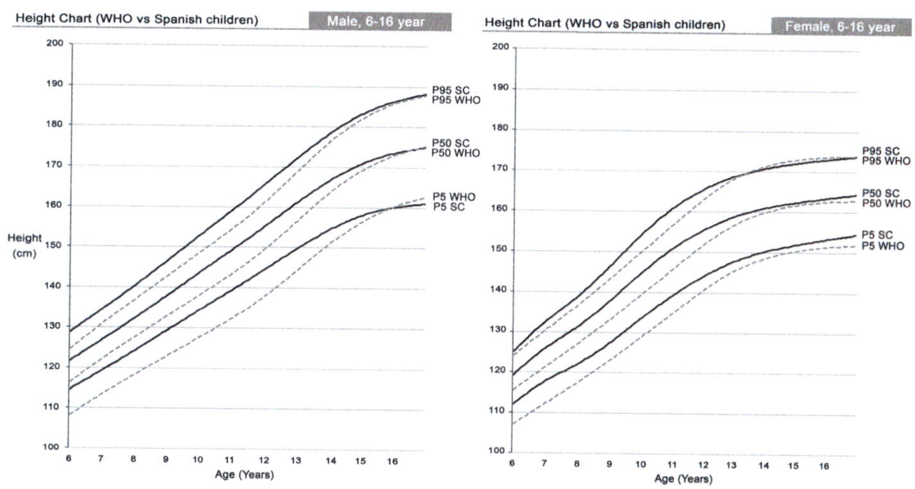

Figure 4.5. *Comparison of the 2007 WHO height percentile and children from eastern Spain. Two-sample Anderson Darling test for goodness of fit of the curves: male 5th percentile (AD: 3.84; p = 0.010); Male 50th percentile (AD: 3.03; p = 0.026); male 95th percentile (AD: 3.24; p = 0.020); female 5th percentile (AD: 5.39; p = 0.002); female 50th percentile (AD: 3.60; p = 0.013); female 95th percentile (AD: 3.08; p = 0.025).*

Source: Pérez-Bermejo M, Alcalá-Dávalos L, Pérez-Murillo J, Legidos-García ME and Murillo-Llorente MT (2021) Are the growth standards of the world health organization valid for Spanish children? The SONEV study. Front. Pediatr. 9:700748. doi: 10.3389/fped.2021.700748 (Shonkoff and Phillips, 2000; Roggman et al, 2008; Davies, 2011; Ridley, 2011; Sharma et al, 2021).

Children and adults differ at every developmental stage in terms of traits and attributes. Stage theorists therefore believe that development is more erratic. Others believe that development is a slower, more gradual process known as continuous development. These people include behaviorists, Vygotsky, and information processing theorists. For example, they would perceive the adult as having more sophisticated skills that the child had in some other way, rather than brand-new abilities. The development of more sophisticated skills is influenced by environmental experiences and brain development (Figure 4.5).

4.3.3. Active Versus Passive

Some theorists see humans as having a much more active role in their own development; how much control do you have over your own developmental path, or are you at the mercy of your genetic inheritance and your environment? For example, Piaget thought that children actively investigate their environment and create new conceptual frameworks to make sense of what they encounter. Many behaviorists, on the other hand, believe that humans have a more passive role in development.

4.3.4. Research Methods

Understanding the fundamentals of the methods used to gather data is crucial to learning any science. Following a set of guidelines intended to foster doubt or skepticism while characterizing, explaining, or testing any phenomenon is the hallmark of scientific research. Because academicians and researchers seem to be constantly changing their stories, some people are reluctant to trust them. But that's precisely what science entails—a constant quest to learn more about the topics at hand and to understand the mechanisms and causes behind events. Science is a means of embarking on an endless adventure. Development has seen adjustments to dietary guidelines, explanations of aging-related psychological states, and parenting guidance. Therefore, consider studying human development to be a lifetime endeavor.

Write down two things you know about childhood in the space of a few minutes. Now, how do you know this? You likely know this because of your personal experiences (experience reality), beliefs held by others, or cultural norms (agreement reality). Personal inquiry has a number of issues. Read the following sentence aloud:

Paris in the

the spring

Are you sure that is what it said? Read it again:

Paris in the

the spring

You just encountered one of the issues with personal inquiry—the propensity to see what we believe—if you read it a different way the second time (adding the second the). Because our perceptions are frequently shaped by our assumptions, when we believe something, we frequently see it even when it is not there. This issue could simply be the consequence of cognitive "blinders," or it could be a more deliberate attempt to bolster our own opinions. The propensity to ignore contradicting evidence in favor of evidence that supports our position, is known as confirmation bias. Science is falsifiable, and scientific investigation entails attempts to reject or refute a theory or set of assumptions. This is how science differs from non-science. A theory is not scientific if it cannot be refuted. Furthermore, a lot of what we do in personal inquiry is make inferences from our own experiences or validate our own beliefs by talking with like-minded others about what we believe to be true.

Science provides a more methodical approach to comparisons that prevent bias.

4.3.4.1. Scientific Methods

The following steps are involved in one scientific investigation method:

- Determining a research question
- Reviewing earlier research on the subject (also referred to as a literature review).
- Choosing an information-gathering strategy.
- Conducting the study
- Interpreting results
- Making conclusions, outlining the study's shortcomings and making recommendations for additional research.
- Making your results accessible to others (to exchange knowledge and have your work reviewed by others).

Once others have used your findings to further investigate the area of interest, a literature or knowledge base will have been established. According to this paradigm of scientific inquiry, conducting research is a linear process that is directed by a particular research question. Additionally, in order to comprehend and present the results of the study, statistics or quantification are usually used. Studies carried out in this way are reported in a number of scholarly journals.

Steps like these may be included in another research model known as qualitative research.

- Begin with a broad area of interest
- Gain entrance into a group to be researched
- Take field notes on the environment, the people, the activities, the structure, and any other relevant topics.
- During interviews, pose open-ended, general "grand tour" questions to your subjects.
- Modify research questions as the study continues
- Note patterns or consistencies
- Investigate new areas that the people you are observing think are important.
- Report findings

Theoretical concepts are "grounded" in participant experiences in this kind of research. Informing the researcher about their world, the people in the setting are the teachers, and the researcher is the student. To prevent their biases and presumptions from compromising reporting accuracy, researchers should be conscious of them, accept them, and place a bracket around them. Occasionally, a topic is first explored through qualitative research, and then additional quantitative studies are used to verify or clarify the findings.

Let's take a closer look at a few research methods or techniques that are used to evaluate, describe, and explain. Every one of these designs has advantages and disadvantages, and they are occasionally combined with other designs in a single study.

4.3.4.2. Observational Studies

Observational studies entail observing and documenting participant behavior. This could happen in a natural environment, like watching kids play in a park, or it could happen in a lab playroom behind a one-way glass. The researcher may use a checklist to record the frequency and length of events (such as the number of conflicts between 2-year-olds) or they may watch and document as much as they can about an event (e.g., by watching kids in a classroom and noting the specifics of the layout of the space as well as the actions and words of the kids and teachers). Generally speaking, the advantage of observational studies is that they don't rely solely on self-reporting; instead, the researcher can observe how people behave. People frequently don't always act like they say they do. The inability of observational studies to provide a causal explanation for a relationship is one of their main weaknesses. However, when researching children, observational studies are helpful and frequently employed. The Hawthorne effect is the tendency for children to alter their behavior when they are aware that they are being observed, which can lead to poor survey performance.

4.3.4.3. Experiments

In an attempt to explain how particular factors or events produce outcomes, experiments are made to test hypotheses, or specific statements about the relationship between variables, in a controlled environment. Anything whose value varies is called a variable. In research, concepts are operationalized, or converted into variables, so the investigator must define precisely what will be measured.

Cause and effect can only be established if three requirements are satisfied. It is helpful to use experimental designs to satisfy these requirements.

Dependent and independent variables need to be connected. Put another way, when one is changed, the other also changes. The researcher's addition or modification of an element is known as the independent variable. The result or factor that is impacted by the addition of the independent variable is known as the dependent variable. For instance, exercise would be the independent variable and stress would be the dependent variable if we were examining how exercise affects stress levels.

It is necessary to identify the cause. The researcher must confirm that the observed effect is not being caused by any unknown or external variables. The experimental setup facilitates this. In an experiment, we would ensure that the diets of the subjects remained the same during the exercise regimen. If not, exercise may not be the primary cause of the shift in stress levels; rather, it may be the diet.

Starting with a sample (or subset of the population), subjects are randomly assigned to either the experimental group or the control group in a basic experimental design. The group that will be exposed to an independent variable or condition that the researcher is introducing as a possible explanation for an event is known as the experimental group. The control group will not be exposed to the independent variable, but it will have the same experiences as the experimental group to serve as a comparison. The two groups are measured once more to determine whether there has been any change following the experimental group's exposure to the independent variable. In that case, we would be in a better position to propose that the change in the dependent variable was caused by the independent variable.

The ability of the experimental design to aid in the establishment of cause-and-effect relationships is its main benefit. This design's drawback is how hard it is to apply a lot of what occurs in a lab to real-world situations.

4.3.4.4. Case Studies

Case studies entail a thorough investigation of a single case or circumstance. To find out as much as possible about a person or situation, information can be gathered through testing, interviews, observation, and other methods. When looking into unusual situations, like brain trauma or children raised in isolation, case studies can be useful. Additionally, as part of their routine practice, clinicians who conduct case studies frequently use them to obtain information about a client or patient who is seeking treatment. Case studies offer rich detail about circumstances or conditions and can be used to investigate areas about which little is known. However, because cases in case studies are not chosen at random and no control group is included for comparison, the results cannot be extrapolated to broader populations.

4.3.4.5. Surveys

Because they are so commonly used, most people are familiar with surveys. Because surveys can be completed online, over the phone, in person, or by mail, they improve accessibility for participants. In a survey, a group of subjects are asked a predetermined set of questions. Subjects are required to select from a response set that may include options like "strongly disagree, disagree, undecided, agree, strongly agree" or "0, 1–5, 6–10, etc." in a highly structured survey. We call this the Likert Scale. Sociologists, marketing researchers, political scientists, therapists, and other professionals frequently use surveys to quickly collect data on a wide range of independent and dependent variables. Surveys can provide surface-level information on many different topics, but they might not provide a deep understanding of human behavior.

Of course, there are several ways to design a survey. Forced choice and semi-structured questions, where the researcher permits the respondent to provide details or a description of specific events, are examples of these. One of the hardest things to do when creating a good survey is to ask the right questions with objectivity so that respondents can answer clearly instead of always selecting "undecided." It is useless to know that 30% of respondents are unsure, so careful thought and work should go into creating survey questions. The fact that each response on a forced choice item is coded makes it easy to enter and use statistical software to analyze the results. When respondents provide long answers that need to be analyzed differently, the analysis process takes significantly longer. Surveys help report on practices, and analyzing expressed beliefs, attitudes, and opinions. Nevertheless, their accuracy may be limited because they rely more on self-reports or what people claim to do than on observation. (Ridley, 2011).

A Closer Look

Sudden Unexpected Infant Deaths (SUID)

Approximately 3,500 infant deaths that are unexpected occur in the United States each year (SUID). These infant deaths—which happen to be under a year old—have no apparent cause at the moment.

The three SUID types that are frequently reported are:

1. When a healthy baby passes away suddenly and unexpectedly and there are conflicting results from the medical and forensic investigations (including autopsies), the diagnosis of SIDS is made. Approximately 1,400 infants died of SIDS in 2020, making it the leading cause of death for infants under the age of one year. Between the ages of 4 and 6 weeks, the risk of SIDS is highest. Potential causes of SIDS are routinely investigated because the condition is diagnosed when no other cause of death can be identified. According to a popular theory, babies who pass away from SIDS may have problems in the part of the brainstem that controls breathing. The theory goes that when a baby has breathing difficulties while they sleep, they don't wake up and die from SIDS. The following are risk factors for SIDS that doctors have identified, even though the exact cause is unknown:
   - low birth weight
   - siblings who have had SIDS
   - sleep apnea
   - of African-American or Eskimo decent
   - low socioeconomic status (SES)
   - smoking in the home
2. **Unknown Cause:** The unexpected death of a baby younger than a year old, for which there is no explanation because the cause of death was not thoroughly investigated.
3. **Accidental Suffocation and Strangulation in Bed:** The following situations can result in an infant being accidentally suffocated in bed: the infant being rolled over or against by someone else while they sleep, the infant becoming wedged between a mattress and a wall, or the infant being strangled when their head or neck gets trapped between crib railings.

Dr. Susan Beal noted in the 1970s that babies who slept face-down had a higher infant mortality rate. Following the safe sleep guidelines (1992) publication of the American Academy of Pediatrics, which recommended that infants sleep on their backs (a non-prone position), the combined SUID rate significantly decreased. The SIDS death rate is currently less than one-fourth of what it was (130 per 100,000 live births in 1990 versus 40 in 2015) thanks to a significant Back to Sleep Campaign that took place in 1994. Many risks, resulting from the interplay of biological and social factors, affect the majority of SIDS victims. However, research has made stomach sleeping, a significant risk, widely known.

Summary

- Physical growth refers to an increase in body size (length or height and weight) and in the size of organs. From birth to about age 1 or 2 years, children grow rapidly. After this rapid infant and early toddler growth, growth slows until the adolescent growth spurt.
- Length is measured in infants. Height is measured in children who can stand. Infants are placed on their backs on a suitable device, such as a measuring table (called a supine stadiometer), and children who can stand are measured using a vertical or standing stadiometer.
- Full-term newborns typically lose 5 to 8% of their birth weight during the first few days of life. They regain this weight by the end of the first 2 weeks. After this period of time, newborns typically gain about 1 ounce per day during the first 2 months, and 1 pound per month after that. This weight gain typically results in a doubling of birth weight by age 5 months and a tripling by 1 year.
- Head circumference is the measurement of the largest area of a child's head. Doctors place the tape measure above the eyebrows and ears and around the back of the head. This measurement is important because the size of the head reflects the size of the brain, and this measurement lets doctors know whether the child's brain is growing at a normal rate.
- The timing of tooth eruption varies, mainly for hereditary reasons. However, tooth eruption may also be delayed by disorders such as rickets, hypopituitarism, hypothyroidism, or Down syndrome.
- Development is growth in function and capability. Both processes depend on genetic, nutritional, and environmental factors. Descriptions of development are often divided into specific domains, such as gross motor, fine motor, language, cognition, and social/ emotional growth. These designations are useful, but substantial overlap exists.
- Conception occurs and development begins. All of the major structures of the body are forming and the health of the mother is of primary concern. Understanding nutrition, teratogens (or environmental factors that can lead to birth defects), and labor and delivery are primary concerns.
- Early childhood development is the period of rapid physical, psychological and social growth and change that begins before birth and extends into early childhood.
- The ages of 6 through 11 comprise middle childhood and much of what children experience at this age is connected to their involvement in the early grades of school. Now the world becomes one of learning and testing new academic skills and by assessing one's abilities and accomplishments by making comparisons between self and others.
- Adolescence is a transitional stage of physical and psychological development that generally occurs during the period from puberty to adulthood (typically corresponding to the age of majority). Adolescence is usually associated with the teenage years, but its physical, psychological or cultural expressions may begin earlier or end later. Puberty typically begins during preadolescence, particularly in females.

References

1. Berl, M. M., Duke, E. S., Mayo, J., Rosenberger, L. R., Moore, E. N., & VanMeter, J., et al. (2010). Functional anatomy of listening and reading comprehension during development. *Brain and Language, 114*(2), 115–125. https://doi.org/10.1016/j.bandl.2010.06.002.

2. Bishop, D. V., Anderson, M., Reid, C., & Fox, A. M. (2011). Auditory development between 7 and 11 years: An event-related potential (ERP) study. *PLOS ONE, 6*(5), e18993. https://doi.org/10.1371/journal.pone.0018993.

3. Davies, D. (2011). *Child Development: A Practitioner's Guide* (3rd ed.). Guildford Press.

4. Ford, A. L. B., Elmquist, M., Merbler, A. M., Kriese, A., Will, K. K., & McConnell, S. R. (2020). Toward an ecobehavioral model of early language development. *Early Childhood Research Quarterly, 50*, 246–258. https://doi.org/10.1016/j.ecresq.2018.11.004.

5. Friederici, A. D., Brauer, J., & Lohmann, G. (2011). Maturation of the language network: From inter- to intrahemispheric connectivities. *PLOS ONE, 6*(6), e20726. https://doi.org/10.1371/journal.pone.0020726.

6. Giedd, J. N., & Rapoport, J. L. (2010). Structural MRI of pediatric brain development: What have we learned and where are we going? *Neuron, 67*(5), 728–734. https://doi.org/10.1016/j.neuron.2010.08.040.

7. Hu, Z., Chan, R. C., & McAlonan, G. M. (2010). Maturation of social attribution skills in typically developing children: An investigation using the social attribution task. *Behavioral and Brain Functions, 6*, 10. https://doi.org/10.1186/1744-9081-6-10.

8. Jolles, D. D., & Crone, E. A. (2012). Training the developing brain: A neurocognitive perspective. *Frontiers in Human Neuroscience, 6*, 76. https://doi.org/10.3389/fnhum.2012.00076.

9. Mattei, D., & Pietrobelli, A. (2019). Micronutrients and brain development. *Current Nutrition Reports, 8*(2), 99–107. https://doi.org/10.1007/s13668-019-0268-z.

10. McCall, R. B., Groark, C. J., Hawk, B. N., Julian, M. M., Merz, E. C., Rosas, J. M., Muhamedrahimov, R. J., Palmov, O. I., & Nikiforova, N. V. (2019). Early caregiver-child interaction and children's development: Lessons from the St. Petersburg-USA orphanage intervention research project. *Clinical Child and Family Psychology Review, 22*(2), 208–224. https://doi.org/10.1007/s10567-018-0270-9.

11. Mooney, C. G. (2000). *Theories of Childhood: An Introduction to Dewey, Montessori, Erikson, Piaget & Vygotsky*. Redleaf Press.

12. Onigbanjo, M. T., & Feigelman, S. (2020). The first year. In R. M. Kliegman, J. W. St. Geme, N. J. Blum, S. S. Shah, R. C. Tasker, & K. M. Wilson (Eds.), *Nelson Textbook of Pediatrics* (21st ed., chap. 22). Elsevier.

13. Parks, E. P., Shaikhkhalil, A., Sainath, N. N., Mitchell, J. A., Brownell, J. N., & Stallings, V. A. (2020). Feeding healthy infants, children, and adolescents. In R. M. Kliegman, J. W. St. Geme, N. J. Blum, S. S. Shah, R. C. Tasker, & K. M. Wilson (Eds.), *Nelson Textbook of Pediatrics* (21st ed., Chap. 56). Elsevier.

14. Poulin-Dubois, D., Brooker, I., & Chow, V. (2009). The developmental origins of naïve psychology in infancy. In *Advances in Child Development and Behavior* (Vol. 37, pp. 55–104). https://doi.org/10.1016/S0065-2407(09)03702-1.

15. Ridley, M. (2011). *Nature Via Nurture: Genes, Experience and What Makes Us Human*. Harper Perennial.

16. Roggman, L. A., Boyce, L. K., & Innocenti, M. S. (2008). *Developmental Parenting: A Guide for Early Childhood Practitioners*. Brookes Publishing Co.

17. Sharma, A., Cockerill, H., & Sanctuary, L. (2021). *Mary Sheridan's from Birth to Five Years: Children's Developmental Progress* (5th ed.). Routledge.

18. Shonkoff, J. P., & Phillips, D. A. (2000). *From Neurons to Neighborhoods: The Science of Early Childhood Development.* National Academies Press.

19. Stiles, J., & Jernigan, T. L. (2010). The basics of brain development. *Neuropsychology Review, 20*(4), 327–348. https://doi.org/10.1007/s11065-010-9148-4.

20. Tau, G. Z., & Peterson, B. S. (2010). Normal development of brain circuits. *Neuropsychopharmacology, 35*(1), 147–168. https://doi.org/10.1038/npp.2009.115.

21. Vannest, J., Karunanayaka, P. R., Schmithorst, V. J., Szaflarski, J. P., & Holland, S. K. (2009). Language networks in children: Evidence from functional MRI studies. *AJR. American Journal of Roentgenology, 192*(5), 1190–1196. https://doi.org/10.2214/AJR.08.2246.

22. Villar, J., Fernandes, M., Purwar, M., Staines-Urias, E., Di Nicola, P., Ismail, L. C., Ochieng, R., Barros, F., Albernaz, E., Victora, C., Kunnawar, N., Temple, S., Giuliani, F., Sandells, T., Carvalho, M., Ohuma, E., Jaffer, Y., Noble, A., Gravett, M., & Kennedy, S. (2019). Neurodevelopmental milestones and associated behaviors are similar among healthy children across diverse geographical locations. *Nature Communications, 10*(1), 511. https://doi.org/10.1038/s41467-018-07983-4.

Chapter 5

NUTRITION

Contents

INTRODUCTION

A nutrient is an element that the body needs for growth and maintenance and that gives it nourishment. There are seven categories of nutrients: water, minerals, vitamins, carbs, protein, fat, and fiber. Every group is necessary for the body to function as it should. While micronutrients are essential for biochemical processes, macronutrients are used as a source of energy. Water is one of the most vital nutrients because it is a solvent, a means of transportation, and a substrate for many important metabolic processes.

Orientation and Directional Terms

Term	Definition	Illustration
Carbohydrates	Carbohydrates, or carbs, are sugar molecules. Along with proteins and fats, carbohydrates are one of the three main nutrients found in foods and drinks.	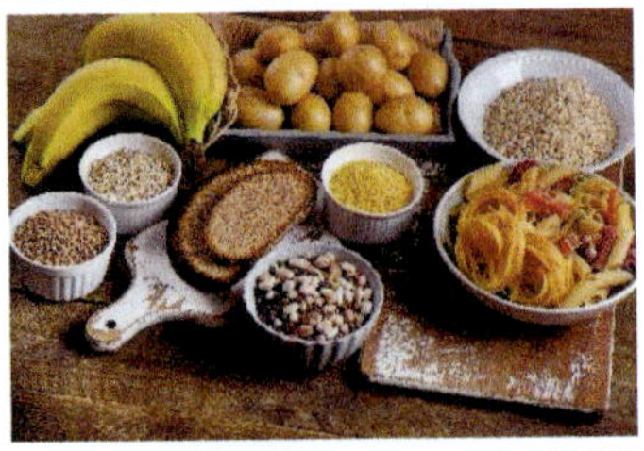
Proteins	Provide energy as well as repair and build body tissues like skin, hair, bone and muscle. It is present in food items like fish, eggs, nuts (almonds, cashew, etc.,), beans, peas and many more.	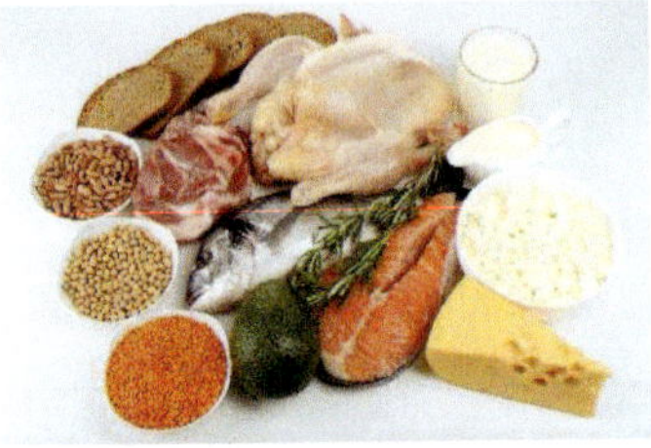
Fats	Provides energy in the absence of carbohydrates, insulates the body (keeps the body warm) and also protects the internal organs. It is present in different types of oils, fish, nuts, and avocados.	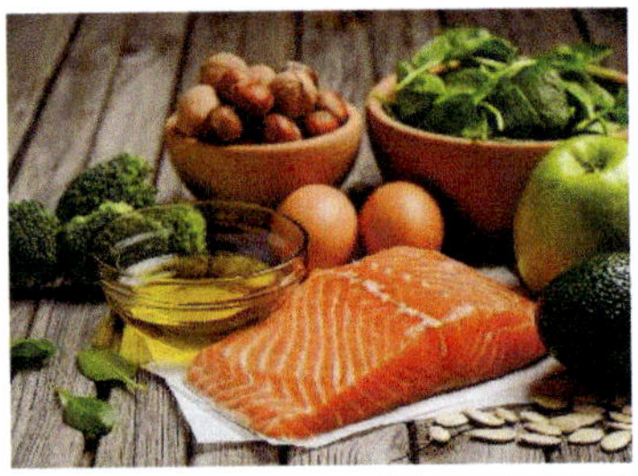
Colostrum	The first thick, yellow milk secreted by the breasts in the first few days after childbirth.	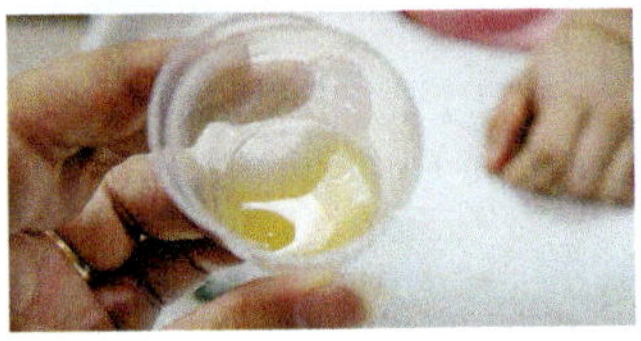
Infant formula	Infant formulas come in powder, liquid concentrate, and ready-to-feed forms. They are designed to be prepared by the parent or caregiver in small batches and fed to the infant, usually with either a cup or a baby bottle.	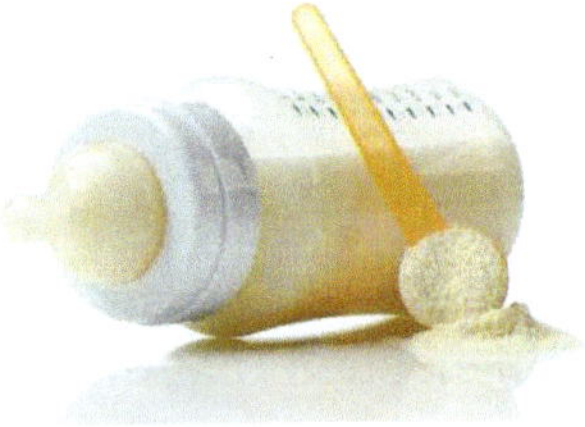
Kwashiorkor	Kwashiorkor is a serious form of malnutrition caused by a lack of protein.	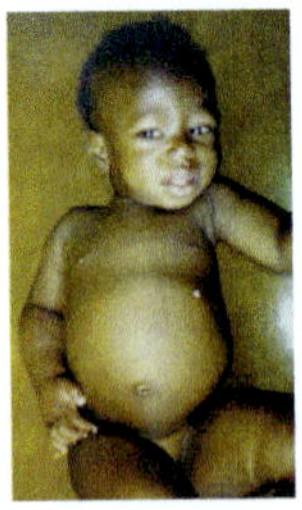

5.1. NUTRIENT-GENE INTERACTION

To define the critical elements in nutrient-gene interaction at the cell, individual, and population levels, a plethora of recently developed novel genomic, proteomic, and metabolomic techniques—with high throughput capacities in nutrition research—promise to facilitate the study of food nutrients and other diet constituents. Recent studies on nutrition have highlighted the impact of nutrients on the regulation and expression of genes. One of the well-established phenomena in prokaryotes is the response of gene expression to modifications in nutritional status. The regulation of gene expression in multicellular organisms is different from that in single-celled organisms in many ways and entails intricate interactions between hormonal, neurological, and nutritional factors. Notwithstanding their less widespread recognition, nutrients influence mammal gene expression as well. Every dietary component has an impact on the regulation of gene expression, and each genotype has a unique expression.

The study of how naturally occurring substances in food affect an individual's genetic information's molecular expression is known as nutrigenomics. A protein is created when a gene is expressed, or activated. By using molecular biology and genomics techniques, researchers have pinpointed the genes that produce vital proteins for proper nutrition, like digestive enzymes and transport molecules that deliver nutrients and cofactors to their intended locations. A phenotype, which is a representation of an organism's physical attributes or observable traits, such as weight, hair color, or the presence or absence of a disease, is created by gene expression patterns. Phenotypic traits are not invariably produced by genes alone. Nutrition has an impact on phenotypic expression. Dietary modifications affect homocysteine levels, obesity, and cholesterol levels and types (LDL, HDL, and their ratios); these responses vary among individuals (genetic component) (Hendricks, 2000; Holden, 2000; Baker and Robert, 2001; Suskind et al, 2011; Marotz, 2012; Koletzko, 2015; Kliegman, 2020).

5.1.1. Nutrition and Gene Regulation

Nutritional factors influence every stage of the metabolic process from gene to protein or metabolic product, including signal transduction and posttranslational modifications of proteins, so the effects on gene expression are just the tip of the iceberg. The relationship between diet and cancer or other diseases is well-established, and new genomic technologies have made it possible to investigate how nutrients, micronutrients, and phytochemicals can modulate the carcinogenesis pathway nutritionally. These technologies include transcriptomics, metabolomics, epigenomics, and nutrigenomics. Transcriptomics examines the expression level of mRNAs in a given cell population. Metabolomics studies the distinct chemical fingerprints left behind by specific cellular processes. Investigating how nutrients affect DNA damage and repair mechanisms, DNA methylation—which affects gene expression and cellular phenotypes—antioxidant rearranging and oxidative stress, target receptors and signal transduction pathways, cell cycle controls and checkpoints, apoptosis, and antiangiogenic processes are all part of the study of nutrient-modulated carcinogenesis. By utilizing nutritional genomics, proteomics, and metabolomics, researchers can concurrently clarify the biological impacts of food components on gene expression and cell function.

Transcription factors are the primary mechanisms by which nutrients affect the expression of genes. With 48 members in the human genome, the nuclear receptor superfamily of transcription factors is one of the most significant groups of nutrient sensors. This superfamily contains many receptors that bind nutrients and their metabolites. For instance, nuclear receptors bind as heterodimers with retinoid X receptor to particular nucleotide sequences (response elements) in the promoter regions of a large number of genes. These receptors include peroxisome proliferators activator receptor (PPAR), which binds fatty acids, and liver X receptor, which binds cholesterol metabolites. Nuclear receptors experience a conformational shift in response to ligand binding, which coordinates the dissociation of co-repressors and the recruitment of co-activator proteins to facilitate transcriptional activation. These transcription factors function as nutrient sensors in metabolically active organs like the liver, intestine, and adipose tissue by adjusting the level of DNA transcription of particular genes in response to nutrient fluctuations. Numerous processes, such as nutrition metabolism, embryonic development, cell proliferation, and cellular differentiation, are regulated by nuclear receptors.

5.1.2. Effects of Nutrients on Gene Expression

5.1.2.1. Nutrient-Gene Interactions

The three main kinds of nutrient gene interactions that take place are as follows.

- Direct interactions: Sometimes nutrients act as transcription factors that can bind to DNA and quickly induce the expression of a gene after interacting with a receptor.
- Epigenetic interactions: The structure of DNA or the histone proteins that make up chromatin can be changed by nutrients, changing gene expression over time.
- Genetic variations: Single nucleotide polymorphisms (SNPs), a common genetic variation, can change how a gene expresses or functions.

These mechanisms can all lead to changes in metabolism and dietary needs for specific nutrients.

5.1.2.2. Acute Effects of Nutrients on Gene Transcription

Nutrients can function as transcription factors to change the expression of genes in a variety of ways. When vitamin A or its retinoid derivatives interact with retinoic acid receptor proteins, they form complexes that either activate or repress transcription depending on which motif in the gene promoter region they bind to (such as retinoic acid response elements). Peroxisome proliferator-activated receptors, which bind to DNA and alter gene expression, can be influenced by dietary fatty acids. Additional instances of nutrient-response element interactions that alter gene expression are those between zinc and metal responsive transcription factor 1, calcium and calcineurin, and vitamin D and the vitamin D receptor. In each of these cases, a nutrient serves as a transient signal that acutely modifies gene transcription; the effect usually ends when the nutrient is no longer exposed. These kinds of examples are not the subject of this discussion because most nutrition scientists are familiar with them.

5.1.2.3. Epigenetics and Nutrition

DNA methylation, histone acetylation, biotinylation, or a combination of these processes can mediate epigenetic effects. Changes in gene expression brought about by such epigenetic modifications may endure a lifetime and even pass down through generations. DNA methylation affects gene transcription and genomic stability and typically happens at cytosine bases that are followed by guanosine (5′ CpG 3′ islands). 60–90% of the 5′ CpG 3′

islands in mammals are methylated. Expression is changed when this modification takes place in gene promoter regions. Because methylated 5′ CpG 3′ islands attract capping proteins that prevent transcription factors that normally induce gene expression from accessing the gene, increased methylation is typically linked to reduced or silenced gene expression. There are a few rare exceptions where gene methylation blocks the binding of inhibitory factors, causing the gene to be derepressed. Every time a gene is copied, the methylation that has already occurred on the 5′ CpG 3′ islands of the gene is replicated. Therefore, methylation's effects may last. Histone proteins, which encircle DNA, block access to gene promoter sequences when they are densely arranged. These histones can be uncoiled by methylation, acetylation, and possibly biotinylation, which opens up channels for transcription factors to pass through and activate gene promoters. Histone alterations are frequently brought about by the methylation of 5′ CpG 3′ islands in gene DNA. Gene expression and the ensuing phenotype can be modified by stable changes in gene methylation brought about by variations in the methyl groups that are available in the diet.

5.1.2.4. Genetic Variation

The human genome contains roughly 50,000 SNPs and is heterozygous. A portion of these SNPs either modify the expression of the gene or the gene product itself, changing the structure and function of proteins. Although it seems impossible to fully understand how millions of SNPs could affect nutrient requirements, recent developments have made this endeavor more doable. The amount of markers available for each gene now makes it expensive to genotype every marker, even though genotyping costs have significantly decreased. As a result, researchers must choose a set of markers for genotyping that would remove the need to measure every single single SNP. Haplotype blocks are short segments of a gene that contain combinations of related SNPs that are shared by several unrelated individuals. These SNPs are inherited over numerous generations and remain connected to one another. It is known that several SNPs that are rather common have an impact on nutrient requirements. For instance, the metabolism of folate involves the enzyme 5, 10-methylenetetrahydrofolate reductase (MTHFR). The C677T allele, a common SNP in the MTHFR gene, causes decreased enzymatic activity. Unless they consume large amounts of folate, homozygous individuals have elevated plasma homocysteine concentrations. Between 15–30% of people carry this SNP. Research on SNPs that altered the likelihood of organ damage or dysfunction in humans given diets low in choline provides another example. While some people did not experience muscle and liver damage or fatty liver, others did. On a low-choline diet, premenopausal women [carriers of a very common SNP (MTHFD1-G1958A)] were 15 times more likely than non-carriers to exhibit symptoms of choline deficiency.

Interestingly, mothers carrying this SNP had a four-fold higher risk of having a child with a neural tube defect when compared to women consuming diets in the upper quartile of choline intake. It would be interesting to find out if the highest-risk individuals carry the G1958A SNP in MTHFD1. The protein that the PEMT gene encodes is in charge of the liver's endogenous choline synthesis, which is stimulated by estrogen. An SNP in the PEMT gene's promoter region (rs12325817) was linked, but not in men, to a markedly increased susceptibility to choline deficiency in studies of organ dysfunction following choline deficiency in humans. This common allele, known as the "variant" one because the wild type was established by the codon found in lower mammals, had a frequency of 0.74. Research is being conducted to find additional genetic variations that may account for the variation in choline requirements among individuals from their diets.

To put it simply, gene expression refers to the sequential processes of transcription, translation, and post-transcriptional and translational modifications that result in the synthesis of particular proteins, which may be hormones, enzymes, or other active proteins. Protein is the final result of gene expression and may have particular physiological or biochemical functions in the body of an animal. Numerous factors, including transcriptional, translational, posttranscriptional, and translational modification factors as well as their regulators and environmental influences, affect the expression of genes. Nutrients are among the major environmental factors that can have a significant impact on gene expression in the ways listed below.

5.1.3. Effect of Carbohydrate on Gene Expression

Feeding high-energy diets causes obesity and metabolic syndrome to develop early in life, presumably because the body is unable to handle the diet's high energy density. A decrease in the mRNA levels of Ag RP (Agouti Related Peptide), NPY (neuropeptides Y), and oxygenic neuropeptides in the ARC (Arcuate nucleus) was linked to obesity even in the presence of decreased overall weight gain. The effects of hyperglycemia on the expression of the angiotensinogen (AGT) gene in the liver were observed to increase the expression of the AGT gene in the liver by about three times.

It has been demonstrated that eating different carbohydrates, such as sucrose, fructose, galactose, and glycerol, increases lactase activity and LPH (lactase/phlorizin hydrolase) mRNA level in the jejunum in a coordinated manner. LPH mRNA levels were elevated and lactase activity was slightly elevated after feeding the glucose diet.

5.1.4. Glucose Regulated Gene Expression

The most prevalent monosaccharide in nature, glucose, offers a prime illustration of how organisms have evolved regulatory systems to deal with varying nutrient availability. Glucose helps yeast use itself by promoting the expression of genes related to its metabolism and suppressing the expression of genes related to the uptake of other carbon sources. It is now well-known how glucose influences the expression of genes in yeast. Mammals have a more complex response to dietary glucose because it combines effects secondary to glucose-dependent hormonal modifications with effects related to glucose metabolism itself, primarily pancreatic stimulation of insulin secretion and inhibition of glucagon secretion. Glucose serves as the main physiological signal for controlling insulin synthesis and secretion in the pancreatic β-cells. Genes encoding glucose transporters, glycolytic and lipogenic enzymes, such as fatty acid synthase, acetyl-CoA carboxylase (ACC), and L-type pyruvate kinase (L-PK), are expressed in the liver in response to insulin and glucose. Conversely, genes of the gluconeogenic pathway, such as the phosphoenolpyruvate carboxykinase gene, are repressed. It has only recently been discovered that carbohydrates play a significant role in transcriptional regulation, although insulin and glucagon have long been recognized as essential for controlling gene expression. Recent studies have characterized DNA sequences and DNA binding complexes involved in glucose-regulated gene expression in β-cells and the liver.

5.1.4.1. Glucose-6-Phosphate Dehydrogenase (G6PD)

Understanding how a cell responds to dietary energy in the form of carbohydrates versus energy in the form of triacylglycerol can be gained by studying the family of enzymes involved in lipogenesis. Among this class of enzymes, glucose-6-phosphate dehydrogenase (G6PD) is special because it takes part in several metabolic pathways, including lipogenesis, reductive biosynthesis, oxidative stress defense, and cellular proliferation. Dietary carbs increase G6PD activity, whereas dietary polyunsaturated fats inhibit it. Variations in the G6PD gene's expression lead to these variations in G6PD activity. In response to dietary modifications, the majority of lipogenic enzymes experience significant changes in the rate of gene transcription; G6PD, on the other hand, is regulated at a step after transcription. This step regulates the efficiency of splicing the nascent G6PD transcript, which in turn affects the rate at which mature mRNA is synthesized in the nucleus.

5.1.5. Effect of Dietary Fat on Gene Expression

A crucial macronutrient for the growth and development of all living things is dietary fat. Apart from its function as a source of energy and its impact on the composition of lipids in membranes, dietary fat also significantly alters gene expression, resulting in modifications to cell differentiation, growth, and metabolism. An adaptive response to variations in the amount and kind of fat consumed is reflected in the effects of dietary fat on gene expression. It has been determined that certain transcription factors in bacteria, amphibians, and mammals are regulated by specific fatty acids. These factors include HNF4a (hepatocyte nuclear factor 4a), NFkB (nuclear factor kappa B), SREBP1c (sterol regulatory element binding protein 1c), and peroxisome proliferator–activated receptors (PPARa, -b, and -g) in mammals. A direct binding of fatty acids, fatty acyl–coenzyme A, or oxidized fatty acids can control these factors. Alternatively, oxidized fatty acid (eicosanoid) regulation of G-protein–linked cell surface receptors can control these factors and activate signaling cascades that target the nucleus. Lastly, oxidized fatty acid regulation of intracellular calcium levels can control nucleus-targeting cell signaling cascades.

The physiological reaction of cells to fatty acids is determined by the following factors: (a) amount, composition, and length of fat consumed; (b) fatty acid metabolism specific to each cell (oxidative pathways, kinetics, and competing reactions); (c) abundance of particular nuclear and membrane receptors within the cell; and (d) participation of particular transcription factors in gene expression. These systems regulate the synthesis of cytokines, adhesion molecules, and eicosanoid compounds, as well as the metabolism of fats and carbohydrates, cell differentiation, and growth. Fresh perspectives on the potential involvement of dietary fat in health and disease are offered by the effects of fatty acids on the genome.

Polyunsaturated fatty acids, or PUFAs, control SREBP-1 post-transcriptionally and inhibit its expression. SREBP-1 mRNA levels were altered in BeWo cells by PUFA. By raising the intracellular regulatory pools of cholesterol, PUFA may also reduce the transcription of SRE-regulated genes and the amount of mature SREBP-1 protein. Enzymatic cleavage is triggered when cells in LPDS media are starved of cholesterol, leading to an increase in the amount of mature SREBP-1 in the nucleus. We hypothesize that the PUFA-induced effect on leptin expression may involve a reduction in mature SREBP-1 because n-3 fatty acid (FA) did not lower the leptin mRNA level in conjunction with increased mature SREBP-1. Additionally, it has been demonstrated that dietary FA composition may affect human plasma leptin concentration. Furthermore, it has been demonstrated that PUFA lower leptin gene expression *in vitro* and *in vivo* through pathways linked to decreased SREBP-1 and PPARg gene expression (Hendricks, 2000; Holden, 2000; Baker and Robert, 2001; Suskind et al, 2011; Marotz, 2012; Koletzko, 2015; Kliegman, 2020).

5.1.5.1. Role of PUFA on Gene Expression

PUFA regulates gene expression in tissues that are lipogenic as well as those that are not. Feeding a diet high in 60% linoleic acid resulted in a decrease in lipogenic enzymes in the liver. Numerous genes related to the liver include fatty acid synthase, acetyl-CoA carboxylase, L-pyruvic kinase, malic enzyme, and S14 protein. While the majority of initial research indicated that the PUFA response was unique to the liver, more recent studies have shed light on the impact of PUFAs on adipose tissues as well. Gene specific to adipocytes was regulated by N-3 fatty acids linoleate (18:3). Arachidonic acid (n-6) and linoleic and eicosapentaenoic acid both reduced SCD1 m RNA stability in the 3T3-L1 adipocyte cell line in a dose-dependent manner (80% maximum repression). In skeletal muscle, as well as possibly in cardiomyocytes and β-cells, dietary n-6 and n-3 polyunsaturated fats decrease the build-up of triglycerides.

5.1.5.2. PUFA-mediated Suppression of Lipogenesis

Through SREBP1, nuclear factor Y, and hepatic nuclear factor-4 (HNF-4), PUFAs influence lipogenesis. Many hepatic enzymes involved in glucose metabolism and fatty acid biosynthesis, including acetyl CoA carboxylase, fatty acid synthase, steroyl CoA desaturase, glucose 6-phosphate dehydrogenase, glucokinase, and pyruvate kinase, are suppressed by PUFA. The transcription of the PPAR-a master switch mediates the aforementioned action. This intriguing theory was bolstered by findings that strong PPARa pharmacological activities somewhat decreased lipogenic transcription, PUFA decreased liver SREBP-1's nuclear content, and both of these effects were linked to a reduction in the rate at which fatty acid synthase and the S14 gene transcript.

Finally, gene expression in mouse liver is acutely influenced by dietary unsaturated fatty acids, particularly docosahexaenoic acid and other PUFAs. This effect is almost entirely mediated by PPARa, despite the presence of numerous other putative fatty acid-dependent transcription factors. Therefore, in terms of the regulation of particular target genes and the molecular mechanism, which includes coregulator interactions, dietary PUFAs closely resemble the effect of synthetic PPARa agonists on hepatic gene expression. However, they are obviously less potent PPARa agonists than WY14643 ([[4-chloro-6-[2,3-dimethylphenyl amino]-2-pyrimidinyl] thio]-acetic acid) and fenofibrate.

5.1.6. Effect of Protein on Gene Expression

The majority of genes carry the instructions required to assemble the useful molecules known as proteins. Some genes generate regulatory molecules that facilitate the assembly of proteins within the cell. Within every cell, the process from gene to protein is intricate and strictly regulated. Translation and transcription are the two main processes. Gene expression is the combined term for transcription and translation.

The information contained in a gene's DNA is transferred to a molecule called RNA (ribonucleic acid) in the cell nucleus during the transcription process. Although a chain of building blocks known as nucleotides is shared by both RNA and DNA, their chemical makeup is slightly different. Because messenger RNA (mRNA) transports the information, or message, from the DNA outside of the nucleus and into the cytoplasm, it is the type of RNA that carries the instructions needed to make a protein.

The cytoplasm is where translation, the second stage from a gene to a protein, happens. The ribosome, a specialized complex that reads the sequence of mRNA nucleotides, interacts with the mRNA. A codon is a group of three nucleotides that typically codes for a single amino acid. The building blocks of proteins are amino acids. The protein is put together one amino acid at a time by a sort of RNA known as transfer RNA (tRNA). Up until the ribosome comes across a stop codon—a string of three nucleotides that do not code for an amino acid—protein assembly continues. One of the main ideas of molecular biology is the information flow from DNA to RNA to proteins. It is sometimes referred to as the "central dogma" because of how crucial it is.

5.1.7. Protein Under-Nutrition

The majority of the essential amino acids have their plasma levels reduced after feeding a low-protein diet for an extended period of time. Leucine and methionine, for instance, can have concentrations dropped from 100–150 mM and 18–30 mM to 20 and 5 mM, respectively, in the plasma of kids afflicted with kwashiorkor. As a result, people need to modify many physiological processes to cope with this amino acid shortage. The primary effect of feeding a low-protein diet is a marked inhibition of growth in both young animals and children. Insulin-like growth factor binding protein-1 (IGFBP-1)3, which binds to insulin-like growth factors-1 and -2 and modifies their mitogenic and metabolic properties, is thought to be dramatically overexpressed in this case, which is responsible for growth inhibition. Expression of IGFBP-1 is controlled by insulin, glucose, or growth hormone. Nevertheless, these three explanations alone are insufficient to account for the elevated IGFBP-1 levels linked to feeding a diet low in protein. Here, the induction of IGFBP-1 is directly caused by a decrease in the concentration of amino acids. Thus, through the induction of IGFBP-1 expression, amino acid limitation, such as that which results from dietary protein deficiency, contributes to the downregulation of growth.

5.1.7.1. Effect of Minerals on Gene Expression

Like other nutrients, the majority of minerals are expressed in multiple genes. Zinc is a necessary trace element that acts as a cofactor in many proteins involved in hormone secretion pathways, immune defense mechanisms, and intermediary metabolism. Zinc also regulates gene expression in the thymus, small intestine, and hepatocytes. Mettallothionin I and II are regulated by MTF-I (Metal Responsive element Factor-I), a Zn-dependent transcriptional activator, via MRE (metal responsive element). Using oligonucleotide array analysis, the transcriptome of HT-29 cells grown for 16 hours under low or normal Zn conditions was examined. Of the 10,000 genes examined, 309 had changes in their mRNA levels; 231 genes showed downregulation upon intracellular zinc depletion, while 78 genes showed upregulation. The transcription factor KLF4 (Kruppel-like factor 4) depleted zinc is involved in the HT-29 cell protein synthesis. Zn is a constituent of the other proteins, including cytochrome c, ATP synthase, and Zn-regulated NADP dehydrogenase I and II. Increased DNA oxidation, DNA breaks, and an increased rate of chromosome damage occur in zinc deficiency.

Collagenases, elastases, and other extracellular matrix metalloproteases (MMP) along with their endogenous inhibitors (tissue inhibitor of metalloproteinase) have been identified in relatively large numbers and are a rapidly expanding field of study, particularly with regard to their roles in immunology, development, cancer, and wound healing. Because these enzymes need zinc for catalytic activity, they most likely get it during translation from intracellular sources. When zinc levels are low, the holoenzyme's secretion may be reduced. However, the enzyme's affinity for zinc may be such that, following secretion, zinc exchanges with the surrounding environment, leading to a reduction in enzymatic activity. There are undoubtedly large fluctuations in zinc levels, particularly when there is a deficiency, which may directly impact the activity of some of these enzymes and, consequently, their metabolic feedback pathways, if serum zinc levels can be extrapolated to be a measure of extra-cellular zinc levels. Feedback pathways can include a decrease in stimulus to a signal transduction pathway that triggers a compensatory response or an increase in the apoenzyme's protein degradation.

A rise in the zinc-deficient state is indicated by changes in mRNA levels seen in the majority of differential displays. This is a little surprising considering how many transcriptional enzymes require zinc; however, since these enzymes are intracellular, intracellular zinc pools may provide them with greater protection. If this were the case, the preponderance of mRNA increases over decreases may be explained by the induction of genes involved in zinc-sensitive enzyme activities caused by metabolic feedback.

In a juxtaglomerular cell line, thapsigargin downregulates renin gene expression, suggesting that an increase in cytosolic calcium concentration can inhibit renin gene expression. Thapsigargin inhibits endoplasmic Ca^{2+}-ATPase, which raises the cytosolic calcium concentration. The inhibition of renin gene expression also occurred as a result of cyclopiazonic acid's inhibition of endoplasmic Ca^{2+}-ATPase and the intracellular Ca^{2+}-chelator BAPTA-AM(1, 2-bis (2-aminophenoxy) ethane-N, N, N,' N'-tetra acetic acid-acetoxymethyl ester), which blocked the effects of both pharmacological agents on renin gene expression.

Ribonucleotide reductase and mitochondrial cytochromes both require iron. Its absence results in a decreased ability to repair DNA and a heightened susceptibility to oxidative damage to mitochondrial DNA. A mutation in a recently discovered major histocompatibility complex (MHC) class I-like gene causes hemochromatosis (HFE) protein level, which is elevated in human intestinal cells when cellular iron status rises. The idea that enterocyte HFE levels are involved in iron homeostasis and the observation that iron regulates HFE protein are congruent with the changes in HFE mRNA that are seen after iron treatment in Caco-2 cells. Furthermore, the idea that a protein with a short half-life may typically act to repress HFE gene transcription is consistent with the noticeable effect of inhibition of protein synthesis on HFE mRNA levels. It is currently unknown who this putative transient repressor protein is that controls the expression of HFE mRNA. Furthermore, it is unknown whether iron affects this protein's activity. However, other MHC class I genes have previously been shown to have a precedent for a repressor transcriptional control mechanism. By reducing silencer factors and concurrently increasing enhancer factors of MHC class I transcription, inhibition of protein synthesis leads to the super-induction of MHC class I mRNA. Magnesium is also necessary for microtubule polymerization and chromosome segregation, as well as a cofactor for several DNA polymerases, nucleotide excision repair, base excision repair, and mismatch repair. Its absence results in decreased DNA replication fidelity and DNA repair ability (Hendricks, 2000; Holden, 2000; Baker and Robert, 2001; Suskind et al, 2011; Marotz, 2012; Koletzko, 2015; Kliegman, 2020).

5.1.8. Effect of Vitamins on Gene Expression

Vitamins are micronutrients that the human diet requires in extremely small amounts. Vitamins mostly affect how genes are expressed. While deficiencies in these vitamins are linked to higher baseline levels of DNA strand breaks, chromosome breaks, oxidative DNA lesions, and lipid peroxide adducts on DNA, vitamins

C and E are useful in preventing oxidation to DNA and lipid oxidation. The synthesis of dTMP from dUMP, methylation of DNA, and effective folate recycling are all aided by folate and vitamin B12. However, when these nutrients are deficient, chromosome breaks, DNA hypomethylation, and uracil misincorporation occur. Poly (ADP-ribose) polymerase (PARP), which is involved in DNA cleavage and rejoining as well as telomere length maintenance, needs niacin as a substrate. Lack of it increases the number of unrepaired nicks in DNA, more chromosome rearrangements and breaks, and increased susceptibility to mutagens. Insulin-like growth factor (IGF) and PEPCK (phosphoenol pyruvate kinase) gene expression are influenced by vitamin A. At the gene level, biotin is involved in the synthesis of several important proteins (enzymes). Vitamin C has a role in the expression of genes in the liver. The impact of vitamin A on PEPCK and the function of biotin on the gene expression of OTC (ornithine transcarbomaylase) are discussed below.

5.1.9. Vitamin A and Gene Expression

The enzyme phosphoenolpyruvate carboxykinase (PEPCK) is dependent on vitamin A. One of the critical processes in gluconeogenesis, the conversion of oxaloacetate to phosphoenol pyruvate, is facilitated by PEPCK. The chromosomal structure of RARE (retinoic acid responsive element) is altered in vitamin A deficiency, and this in turn alters co-regulatory binding and activity. The interaction between PEPCK-RARE and the pre-initiation complex reduces the amount of RNA polymerase II that associates with the PEPCK promoter. This, in turn, improves gluconeogenesis when PEPCK levels are low or absent. When blood glucose levels are lowered during a food-deprived state, PEPCK gene expression is significantly increased in mice receiving adequate amounts of vitamin A. Nonetheless, PEPCK gene expression is either barely expressed or not expressed at all in their vitamin A-deficient counterparts. Serum IGF-I concentrations and the gene expression of IGF-I, IGF-IR, and IR in a variety of tissues are all influenced by dietary vitamin A levels. Vitamin A deficiency led to a downregulation of serum IGF-I concentrations and tissue IGF-I mRNA, while there was an overall upregulation of IGF-IR and IR mRNA expression. The growth retardation observed in animals deficient in vitamin A could potentially be explained by the significant decrease in serum IGF-I concentrations and IGF-I mRNA levels.

5.1.10. Role of Biotin on OTC Gene Expression

As a component of acetyl coenzyme carboxylase, propionyl CoA carboxylase, and b-methyl crotonyl CoA carboxylase, as well as gluconeogenesis, fatty acid synthesis, and amino acid catabolism (via pyruvate carboxylase), biotin plays a direct role in these vital metabolic processes. Furthermore, it plays a crucial role in the expression of the ornithine trans carbamylase (OTC) gene. In addition to clinical symptoms like coma, seizures, skin rashes, alopecia, and pica, deficiencies in the utilization of biotin in humans result in hyperammonemia and acidosis. Mammals remove ammonia primarily through two mechanisms: glutamine synthesis, which is catabolized by glutamine synthetase, and urea synthesis, which is facilitated by the urea cycle enzyme. The gene expression and activity of the urea cycle enzymes can be changed by biotin. The process at play is that OTC changes ornithine into citrulline, a crucial urea cycle step. Since biotin is a prosthetic group of OTC, a deficiency in biotin results in a reduction in OTC enzyme, which affects the body's normal urea cycle and urea synthesis (Hendricks, 2000; Holden, 2000; Baker and Robert, 2001; Suskind et al, 2011; Marotz, 2012; Koletzko, 2015; Kliegman, 2020).

5.2. FEEDING THE INFANT

The greatest source of nourishment for babies is thought to be their mothers' milk. Numerous bioactive substances found in breast milk alter how the immune system, the gastrointestinal tract, and the developing brain function. As a result, breast milk is widely acknowledged as a biological fluid necessary for the best possible development and growth of infants. Recent research has also revealed that breast milk may protect against type 2 diabetes and obesity in particular, as well as mitigate the programming of late metabolic diseases in infants.

For the first six months of their lives, infants should only be breastfed, according to recommendations from the World Health Organization. Breastfeeding for a minimum of 12 months is also advised by the American Academy of Pediatrics. The Academy of Nutrition and Dietetics recently updated and reaffirmed its mission statement, which states that the best feeding pattern for infants is to breastfeed with complementary foods from six months of age until at least 12 months of age, and that exclusive breastfeeding provides optimal nutrition and health protection for the first six months of life. Apart from its nutritional benefits, breastfeeding is affordable, practical, and a bonding experience for both the mother and the child.

The choice to breastfeed is very private and frequently impacted by a variety of factors. Breastfeeding may need to be interrupted or stopped in certain circumstances if it is not appropriate, feasible, or sufficient. Just 38% of babies worldwide receive only breast milk. Just 75% of babies in the US begin breastfeeding from birth, but by the time they are three months old, 27% of them, or 2 million babies, depend on infant formula for some portion of their diet. The six-month "any breastfeeding" rate for all new mothers in the U.S. is 43% of the population, only 13% of whom adhere to the six-month breastfeeding recommendation.

The purpose of infant formula is to serve as a practical replacement for breastfeeding. All attempts have been made to replicate the nutritional profile of human breast milk for healthy infant growth and development, even though it is not possible to produce a product that is exactly like breast milk. The most popular bases are cow milk or soymilk, to which additional ingredients such as iron, nucleotides, and fat blend compositions are added to improve the resemblance of the base to human breast milk and to achieve health benefits. Docosahexenoic acid (DHA) and arachidonic acid (AA) are added fatty acids. Probiotics and genetically engineered compounds are either already included in formulas or are being explored for inclusion. Giving babies the best nutrition possible during their first six months of life is essential because undernutrition can have serious consequences (Figure 5.1).

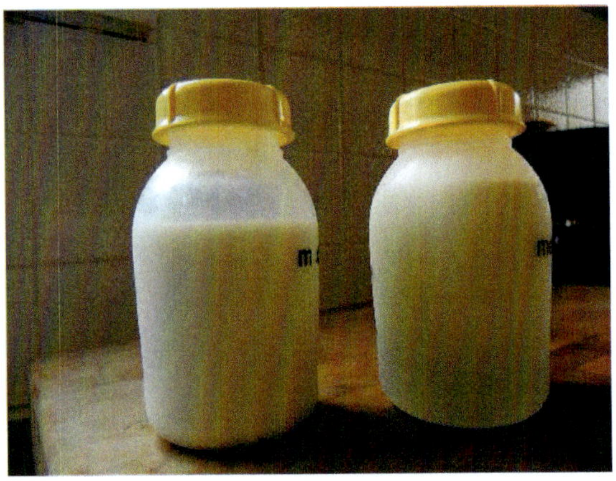

Figure 5.1. *Formula (left bottle) and pumped breastmilk (right bottle).*

Source: By Jengod - Own work, CC BY-SA 3.0, https://commons.wikimedia.org/w/index.php?curid=86780183.

5.2.1. Human Breast Milk

Carbs, protein, fat, vitamins, minerals, hormones, and digestive enzymes are all present in human breast milk. It is abundant in immune cells, such as macrophages and stem cells, in addition to these nutrients and a host of other bioactive substances. Certain bioactive molecules, like oligosaccharides, are derived from proteins and lipids, while others are derived from proteins and cannot be digested. By overflowing the infant gastrointestinal tract with decoys that bind pathogens and keep them off the intestinal wall, human milk oligosaccharides (HMOs) have anti-infective properties against pathogens like *Salmonella*, *Listeria*, and *Campylobacter*. Additionally, oligosaccharides help colonize up to 90% of the infant biome and are crucial for the development of a balanced and diverse microbiota, which is necessary for appropriate innate and adaptive immune responses.

5.2.1.1. Composition of Human Breast Milk

A complex matrix, human breast milk is primarily composed of 87% water, 3.88% fat, 1.0% protein, and 0.7% lactose. The milk's total energy content is made up of 50% fat and 40% lactose, respectively. However, the makeup of human breast milk is dynamic and ever-changing, molding itself to the changing requirements of the developing infant. For example, during a nursing session, the milk expressed first (called foremilk) is thinner and contains more lactose, which quenches a baby's thirst; the milk expressed later (called hindmilk) is creamier and contains much more fat for the baby's needs. There are also differences in the nursing stage (baby age), nutrition, health, and exposure to the environment for mothers. During early lactation, the protein content in human milk ranges from 1.4–1.6 g/100 mL, to 0.8–1.0 g/100 mL after three to four months of lactation, to 0.7–0.8 g/100 mL after six months. The amount of fat varies greatly depending on the mother's diet and is positively correlated with weight gain during pregnancy. Surprisingly, even in cases where a mother's nutrition is inadequate, her breast milk is nearly always sufficient in the vital nutrients required for the growth and development of her term infant. Specific nutritional supplementation is necessary for mother's milk given to preterm infants, even though the mean concentrations of protein, sodium, chloride, and potassium in early preterm milk are sufficient to meet the estimated requirements for preterm infants.

Mature milk (after 21 days postpartum) has a relatively constant lactose content, in contrast to protein and fat. To keep the osmotic pressure in human milk constant, lactose concentration must remain stable. Calcium and mineral absorption are also facilitated by lactose. Numerous bioactive carbohydrates, including oligosaccharides, are linked to lactose in breast milk. Lactose malabsorption and intolerance syndromes can occur if the small intestine does not produce enough of the enzyme lactase to break down these sugar complexes. Malabsorption and diseases caused by lactase deficiency are very uncommon in infants who are exclusively breastfed.

5.2.1.2. Protein in Human Breast Milk

Breast milk contains two types of protein: Casein and whey. Casein forms clots in the stomach, while whey remains in liquid form and is easier to digest. The ratio of whey to casein in breast milk varies depending on the stage of lactation, ranging from 80/20 to 50/50. This ratio is higher than that of other mammals, such as cows, where whey proteins make up only 18% of the total protein. Infant formulas traditionally have higher levels of casein, making them harder to digest compared to breast milk. The amino acid profiles of casein and whey proteins in breast milk also vary depending on the stage of lactation. Glutamine, the most abundant free amino acid, is significantly higher in mature milk compared to colostrum. Glutamine plays an important role in providing energy for the body, including acting as a neurotransmitter in the brain and fueling intestinal cells (Figure 5.2).

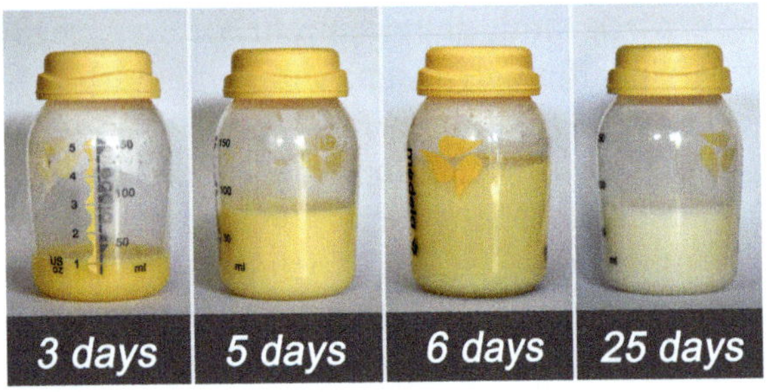

Figure 5.2. *From colostrum to breastmilk. (days after birth).*

Source: By Amada44 – Own work, CC BY-SA 3.0, https://commons.wikimedia.org/w/index.php?curid=73729325.

The primary whey proteins, including alpha-lactalbumin, lactoferrin, and secretory IgA, are essential components. Additional proteins like lysozyme, folate-binding protein, bifidus factor, casein, lipase, amylase, alpha1-antitrypsin, anti-chymotrypsin, and haptocorrin play important roles as well. Upon consumption, these proteins are quickly broken down into amino acids for absorption and use. Many of these proteins also have functions beyond nutrition, such as alpha-lactalbumin's role in lactose synthesis and mineral binding. Casein helps with calcium and phosphorus binding, while lactoferrin and lysozyme protect against harmful bacteria, particularly in infants. The IgA antibody destroys bacteria and maintains the gut's mucosal surface.

5.2.1.3. Fats in Human Breast Milk

The most significant component of breast milk is fat, which gives the baby energy and aids in the development of the central nervous system. Additionally, milk fat transports flavor and fragrance. Generally speaking, during lactation, the fat content of human breast milk varies between 3.5% to 4.5%. At roughly 95% of total lipids, triglycerides make up the majority of the lipid fraction. Saturated fatty acids make up nearly half of the fat in milk, while palmitic acid (C16:0) makes up 23% of the total fat. Milk contains the largest amount (36%) of oleic acid (18:1w9), a monounsaturated fatty acid. Two other essential fatty acids found in human breast milk are alpha-linolenic acid (C18:3w3) at 0.35% and linoleic acid (C18:2w6) at 15%. Arachidonic acid (AA, C20:4w6) and eicosapentaenoic acid (EPA, C20:5w3) are the products of the conversion of these two essential fatty acids, respectively. The latter is then transformed into docosahexaenoic acid (DHA, 22:6w3). The development of a newborn's immune system, growth, inflammatory responses, vision, cognitive function, and motor systems are all influenced by AA, EPA, and DHA.

Long-chain polyunsaturated fatty acids are passed from mother to fetus through the placenta during the third trimester, and, after birth, to infants through breast milk. Brain tissue is rapidly synthesized in the final trimester and during the neonatal period. Certain requirements of DHA and AA are necessary for cell differentiation and the development of active synapses in the brain. From the 26th week of pregnancy to delivery, 80% of the brain's DHA is acquired. Notably, due to premature enzyme activity, the synthesis of AA and DHA from linoleic acid (18:2w6) and alpha-linolenic acid (18:3w3) is limited in the fetus and neonate. Therefore, the mother must provide the necessary amounts of AA and DHA during pregnancy or as breast milk after the baby is born. According to one study, between the sixth week and the sixth month of lactation, there is a significant increase in the fat content and percentage of all polyunsaturated fatty acids in breast milk. There is proof that the main source of AA in milk is the gradually rotating maternal body pools. The amount of AA present in breast milk is correlated, dose-dependently, with the intake of foods high in AA by nursing mothers.

The amounts of EPA and DHA in breast milk are also directly correlated with the amount of these nutrients in the mother's diet. Human milk from nursing mothers who follow vegan or vegetarian diets contains less than 0.1% DHA, while mean DHA intakes in the US and China are between 0.2%–0.4% and ≥0.8%, respectively, depending on DHA intake from fish or other sources. It has been suggested that to reach human milk levels of 0.3%–0.35% DHA, intakes of less than 300 mg DHA daily are required. The effects of fatty acids found in human milk, however, are complicated, especially since neurodevelopment is evaluated after the first six months of exclusively feeding an individual human milk.

The transfer of these fatty acids from the placenta to the fetus is disrupted during the crucial final trimester of premature birth. Research has also demonstrated a link between neonatal morbidities and lower postnatal blood levels of arachidonic and docosahexaenoic acid in premature infants. Therefore, the preterm infant's ability to get enough fatty acid levels after birth depends on having a healthy diet. When compared to an infant receiving no supplementation, preterm infant formulas containing DHA and AA initially had positive effects on visual acuity, visual attention, and cognitive development.

5.2.1.4. Vitamins, Minerals and Other Bioactive Components in Breast Milk

Except for vitamins D and K, human breast milk provides sufficient levels of most vitamins to support a newborn's normal growth. Exclusively breastfeeding infants get far less vitamin D than is advised for their diet and far less than the minimum recommended intake. These babies run the risk of developing rickets, insufficient bone mineralization, and vitamin D deficiency. However, total sun exposure is also associated with the risk of vitamin D deficiency in breastfed infants, with the risk rising in regions with lower sun indices. Addition of 400–2000 IU (International Unit) to the mother. vitamin D/day can raise the amount of vitamin D in breast milk, but the infant needs a higher dose (2000 IU) to receive adequate levels of 25-OH-D. Within eight weeks, the normal vitamin D stores that are present at birth are depleted. It is advised to expose breastfed infants to sunlight and to take supplements of vitamin D. Compared to breastfed babies, formula-fed infants frequently have serum concentrations of vitamin D metabolites that are higher. The protein involved in blood coagulation depends on vitamin K. But the amount of vitamin K that crosses the placenta and enters the fetus is limited. Thus, a newborn baby is susceptible to hemorrhagic disease due to their frequently abnormally low vitamin K concentration. Supplementing with vitamin K is advised after delivery.

Minerals found in human breast milk support a range of physiological processes, serving as vital components of numerous enzymes and having biological significance for molecules and structures. Human and cow's milk are similar in terms of their mineral content. Numerous other bioactive substances, such as growth factors, hormones, and immunological components, have been found in human milk over the years.

5.2.2. Human Milk Options—Milk Donors and Milk Banks

When a mother's milk is not available, the World Health Organization and the American Academy of Pediatrics advise preterm infants to be fed pasteurized human donor milk. When donor milk is pasteurized, many of the normal commensal microbes are eliminated. Additionally, live immune cells, bioactive proteins, and enzymes are either greatly reduced or completely destroyed, which limits the milk's potential health benefits when compared to that of a mother's milk. There is continuous research being done to maximize donor breast milk. It is recommended that mothers speak with their child's healthcare providers prior to using donor breast milk.

5.2.3. Infant Formulas

Formulated to closely resemble the nutritional makeup of breast milk, infant formula serves as an efficient replacement for breast milk. Formulas meet the requirements for adequate biological quality of protein components (enough protein in a form that infants can use) and normal physical growth. Only healthy infants without uncommon medical or dietary issues should use infant formula. For the manufacturing process to satisfy both domestic and global quality standards, strict regulations and oversight are in place.

5.2.3.1. The Infant Formula Market

According to UN estimates, the current population of 7.2 billion people will increase by one billion during the next 12 years, reaching 9.6 billion people by the year 2050. The demand for infant milk formula will rise as a result, particularly for cutting-edge brands that incorporate components like prebiotics and particular milk protein fractions. The $50 billion infant formula market is predicted to grow at the fastest rate among packaged food categories over the next five years, with annual gains expected to exceed 7%. A few industry analysts anticipate a yearly growth rate of 8%–9%, which is considerably higher. A study indicates that the demand for infant formulas will be driven by Asia, specifically China and that the industry will continue to grow at a compound annual growth rate of 11%.

Three forms of infant formula are available: (1) powder, which is the least expensive and needs to be mixed with water before feeding; (2) liquid, which is a concentrated liquid that needs to be mixed with an equal amount of water; and (3) ready-to-feed, which is the most expensive and doesn't need to be mixed.

5.2.3.2. Guidelines for Manufacturing of Infant Formula

The right proportions of water, carbohydrates, protein, fat, vitamins, and minerals must be included in infant formulas. Government agencies have established strict regulations regarding the composition of infant formula, and manufacturers are required to adhere to these guidelines. For example, the effectiveness of each of the main ingredients added to the formula (protein, fats, and carbohydrates) has a range of minimum and maximum values. These parts need to have a track record of safe usage. Every nutrient's necessary range needs to be preserved for the duration of the product's shelf life. Only L forms of amino acids may be added; D forms must be avoided as they have the potential to cause D-lactic acidosis. Because of fructose intolerance, fructose should be avoided. Hydrogenated oils and fats are likewise prohibited. The formula product cannot be exposed to ionizing radiation since it could deteriorate the product. When infant formula is prepared and ready to be consumed, its energy content should be between 60 and 70 kcal (250 and 295 kJ) per 100 mL. Moreover, medical and nutritional research results must serve as the foundation for product reformulation. "Manufacturers must demonstrate that the formula containing the new ingredient is capable of sustaining physical growth and development over 120 days when the formula is likely to be the sole source of infant nutrition," according to the committee's recommendation regarding the "Evaluation of the addition of Ingredients New to Infant Formula."

According to the Food and Drug Administration (FDA) in the US, the safety criterion for introducing new ingredients to baby formula is "reasonable certainty of no harm." Under no circumstances should infants be given unmodified cow's milk or unmodified goat's milk, according to the World Health Organization (WHO). The WHO guidelines are used by federal and local agencies worldwide to oversee and manage infant formula regulations, which include national standards for quality and manufacturing procedures. It is in the best interests of manufacturers to keep refining their products so that they resemble human breast milk as closely as possible.

5.2.3.3. Classes of Infant Formula Products

Infant formulas fall into three main categories: soy-based formula, cow-milk-based formula, and specialty formula. Their cost, digestion, taste, nutrition, and caloric content vary. There are different types of formulas available to suit different needs. Certain alternatives to cow's milk are made from amino acids or include casein or whey proteins that have been thoroughly hydrolyzed. Some formulas are based on rice.

5.2.3.4. Cow Milk-Based Formula

The majority of baby formula is made with cow's milk. But in comparison to human breast milk, bovine milk has higher levels of fat, minerals, and protein. To make cow milk more like human breast milk, it must be skimmed and diluted. Most healthy full-term infants can consume additional vegetable oils, vitamins, minerals, and iron from cow-milk-based infant formula.

The study concludes that human milk or infant formula should not be substituted with raw, unprocessed, or unpasteurized cow's milk for children under one year of age. Furthermore, unadulterated milk is deficient in iron, vitamin E, and important fatty acids. Moreover, the high protein, sodium, and potassium content of raw cow's milk is too much for an infant's system to handle. For normal infants, formulas with a protein content of 2–3.5 g/100 mL and a protein/energy ratio of less than 3 g/100 kcal are utilized; higher protein contents (2.9 g/100 mL) and higher protein/energy ratios (3.05 g/100 kcal) are reserved for infants with extremely low birth weights or preterm babies. According to recent research, infant formula with a high protein content is linked to excess weight gain during infancy, which increases the risk of obesity by 20% in later life.

One of the first foods given to a baby is cow's milk, which is also one of the main causes of food allergies. Clinical reactions typically begin very early in life, following the cessation of breastfeeding and the introduction of cow's milk into the diet; lactation is rarely the time for symptoms to manifest. The kind and intensity of cow milk allergy symptoms vary greatly. It can be characterized as a repeatable negative response mediated by at least one immune mechanism to one or more milk proteins (typically caseins or whey beta-lactoglobulin). Research on the prevalence of cow milk allergy varies, as do diagnostic standards and baby food regimens. Its estimated population prevalence ranges from 2 – 3%, or as high as 7%, and it manifests in the first year of life. Nonetheless, the incidence of IgE-mediated cow milk allergy may be as low as 0.5%, according to data from recent cohort studies and a randomized trial of early introduction of allergenic foods in the diet of breastfed infants. It is possible that, at the very least, some non-IgE-mediated allergy cases may have been included in IgE-mediated cow milk allergy cases in previous reports because there is no definition for distinguishing between IgE-mediated and non-IgE-mediated cow milk allergy, and the clinical symptoms of both overlap significantly.

An allergy to cow's milk can manifest symptoms right away or later. Roughly 60% of adverse reactions induced by cow milk are caused by mechanisms associated with IgE. These usually affect the skin, respiratory system, and gastrointestinal tract and manifest immediately or within 1 to 2 hours of ingestion. A severe cow milk allergy may also result in anaphylactic reactions throughout the body. The delayed onset of non-IgE-associated symptoms can occur anywhere from two hours to several days following the consumption of cow milk. Two hours is useful in ruling out non-IgE-associated or non-allergic reactions. The gastrointestinal tract is primarily affected by the non-lgE-associated clinical symptoms, which include eosinophilic esophagitis, proctocolitis, enteropathy, and enterocolitis. The majority of symptoms for non-lgE-mediated gastrointestinal food-induced allergic disorders go away in one to five years, and the prognosis is favorable.

5.2.3.5. Soy-Based Formulas

For babies with congenital lactase deficiency or galactosemia, soy protein formulas are a good option. They alleviate colic and milk allergies; however, on rare occasions, infants with cow milk allergies may also have soymilk allergies. Infants with food allergies younger than six months should not use soy products. The use of soy-based formulas is restricted due to the possibility of harm to the infant due to the presence of phytoestrogens, albeit this is still debatable.

5.2.3.6. Hypoallergenic Formulas

Formulas containing protein hydrolysate are designed for infants and babies who cannot tolerate formulas containing cow's milk or soy. They have protein that has been hydrolyzed, either completely or partially, into smaller-sized pieces than what is found in products made from cow or soy. Formulas with extensive hydrolyzation provide a good substitute for babies with protein allergies.

5.2.3.7. Amino Acid Formulas

For infants with severe cow milk allergies who react to or refuse to eat appropriate amounts of extensively hydrolyzed formula, amino acid formulas represent an additional option. They supply protein as free amino acids only—no peptides (Hendricks, 2000; Holden, 2000; Baker and Robert, 2001; Suskind et al, 2011; Marotz, 2012; Koletzko, 2015; Kliegman, 2020).

5.2.4. Non-Bovine Milk Sources

During a time when infants and children are developing, the complete elimination of cow milk products without the use of appropriately modified and fortified substitutes may result in malnutrition and/or specific nutrient deficiencies. To manage cow milk allergy in infants and children, infant milk formulas derived from other animals (such as goats, ewes, mares, donkeys, or camels) or formulas based on lamb or chicken have been widely marketed as alternatives to cow milk. However, due to a lack of reliable randomized clinical trials, several animal-milk-based formulas are currently not approved in many areas.

5.2.5. Probiotics and Prebiotics

Human milk oligosaccharides are distinct from other milk proteins due to their high concentration and structural diversity. When probiotics and prebiotics are not supplemented, Bifidobacterium species do not typically dominate the gut microbiota of formula-fed infants. Research indicates that compared to formula-fed newborns, breastfed newborns have a more consistent and homogenous population of oligosaccharides. One important tactic for lowering the incidence and severity of diarrhea is to incorporate probiotics into infant formula. There are many different types of complex oligosaccharides found in domestic animal milk. Roughly 80–90% of the total pool of milk from all domestic animals is made up of sialylated oligosaccharides. Grazing cows' milk has higher sialic acid concentrations than non-grazing cows' milk. A variety of sialylated oligosaccharides that can be added to infant formula may be found in cow's milk. Additionally, synthetic oligosaccharides that are chemically identical to those found in human milk can now be added to commercial infant formula.

The probiotic strains added to the formula are mostly derived from food or the microbiota found in the feces of infants. Even though probiotics are increasingly being used for therapeutic and preventive purposes, more research is still needed to confirm which strains have the potential to be antiallergenic.

94 infants (gestational age 32 to 36 weeks and birth weight >1,500 g) were randomly assigned to receive prebiotics (a mixture of galacto-oligosaccharide and polydextrose 1:1), probiotics (*Lactobacillus rhamnosus* GG), or a placebo during the first two months of life. A one-year follow-up period was used to assess the effects of early pre- and probiotic intervention on the well-being, crying, growth, and microbiological programming of the infants. According to the findings, the prebiotic and probiotic groups experienced significantly less crying than the placebo group (19% *vs.* 19% *vs.* 47%, respectively; $p = 0.02$). The placebo group had a higher percentage of *Clostridium histolyticum* bacteria in their stools than the probiotic group did (13.9% *vs.* 8.9%, respectively; $p = 0.05$). Another study on safe and simple strategies to prevent viral respiratory tract infections between 3 and 60 days of life has demonstrated that prebiotics or probiotics had significantly less ($p < 0.001$ and $p = 0.022$) viral respiratory tract infections compared with those receiving placebo. Additionally, the incidence of rhinovirus-induced episodes, which comprised 80% of all respiratory tract infections, was significantly lower in the prebiotic ($p = 0.003$) and probiotic ($p = 0.051$) groups than in the placebo group.

5.2.6. Fatty Acids and Milk Fats from Different Mammalian Species

For developing infants, the lipid component of human milk constitutes the primary energy source, accounting for 45% to 55% of total energy. Mammalian milk (cow, buffalo, donkey, sheep, and camel) and human milk were compared for their lipid compositions in terms of phospholipid, triacylglycerol (TAG), fatty acid compositions, melting and crystallization profiles, and fatty acid profiles. The findings demonstrated that the overall fatty acid composition of these milk fats, particularly sheep milk fat, was very similar to that of human milk fat. Other chemical characteristics, however, differed less. The results show that these commercialized mammalian milk fats do not meet the standards for human milk fat substitutes, but they make good starting materials for the manufacturing of baby formula in large quantities. Although milk fat globule membranes were previously not included in baby formulas, their constituents are active and help to prevent infection. Supplementing infant formula with milk fat globule membrane also reduces the cognitive development gap between breastfed and formula-fed infants (Hendricks, 2000; Holden, 2000; Baker and Robert, 2001; Suskind et al, 2011; Marotz, 2012; Koletzko, 2015; Kliegman, 2020).

5.2.7. Bioactive Proteins

After being isolated, novel dairy fractions from bovine milk are now offered for sale. Proteins, including α-lactalbumin, lactoferrin, osteopontin, and milk fat globule membrane proteins, make up a large number of these constituents. It's crucial to lower the formula's overall protein content when incorporating bioactive proteins. It's crucial to consider the amino acid composition of formula; an infant's serum concentration of essential amino acids shouldn't be any less than that of a breastfed baby. For instance, α-Lactalbumin, which is frequently the first amino acid to become limited in baby formulas, breaks down into smaller peptides that possess prebiotic and antimicrobial properties as well as immunostimulatory properties. It also improves the absorption of minerals. Osteopontin is a highly glycosylated and phosphorylated protein that induces Th1/Th2 switching and regulates immune response. It may also influence bone growth and mineralization and support lactoferrin's physiological role.

The best food for a baby's growth and development is breast milk, which is also high in antibodies that give a newborn's digestive tract its initial supply of adaptive immunity. The best source of breast milk for preterm or low birth weight babies is the mother's own milk; if it is not available, donor breast milk is thought to be the next best option. Formula is currently the preferred option for healthy newborns whose mothers are unable to provide enough breast milk (Hendricks, 2000; Holden, 2000; Baker and Robert, 2001; Suskind et al, 2011; Marotz, 2012; Koletzko, 2015; Kliegman, 2020).

5.3. FEEDING THE CHILD AND ADOLESCENT

Adolescence and childhood are times of ongoing development and growth. An infant's weight doubles at five months of age and triples at one year of age due to rapid growth. In the second year, the child grows four times its birth weight in addition to an additional 7–8 cm of height. The pre-adolescent stage is characterized by an average annual growth in height of 6–7 cm and weight gain of 1.5–3 kg, along with the development and maturation of various tissues and organs.

Adolescent (or teenage) years span nearly 10 years. Rapid weight and height gain, hormonal changes, sexual maturation, and extreme mood swings are its defining characteristics. For girls, the teenage growth spurt begins around age 10–12, and for boys, it begins two years later. The highest annual rates of weight and height are 8–10 kg and 9–10 cm, respectively. During this time, critical bone mass must develop because it lays the foundation for preserving the mineral integrity of the bone later in life. Throughout childhood and adolescence, the pattern and proportion of different body components, such as body water, muscle mass, bone, and fat, increase until they reach adult values by the time a person is 18 years old. Due to menstruation, teenage girls experience higher levels of physiological stress than boys. Their dietary requirements are especially crucial because they must get ready to become mothers. Because of all these quick anabolic changes, more nutrients are needed per unit of body weight.

Older kids and teenagers should drink a lot of milk to meet their high calcium needs. Cooking oils (25–50g) ought to be eaten. Excessive consumption of fats can be prevented. Consuming too much salt is not recommended, especially for kids whose families have a history of high blood pressure. Adolescence is a time when unhealthy eating habits and unhealthy behaviors like chewing tobacco, smoking, and alcohol consumption are most likely to develop. These ought to be stayed away from. Children and adolescents should be encouraged to engage in appropriate lifestyle practices, physical activity, such as games and sports, and the consumption of a nutritious, well-balanced diet.

5.3.1. Nutrition in the Toddler Years

Children have progressed from infancy to becoming school-age by the time they are two years old. In comparison to their early development, their physical growth and motor skills slow down. Toddlers, however, go through significant cognitive, emotional, and social development. Naturally, food and nutrition still have a significant impact on a child's development. The diet entirely changes at this point from breast milk or bottle milk to solid foods plus wholesome juices and other liquids. A toddler's appetite declines because their metabolism slows down in comparison to an infant's. Toddler parents should also be aware of some nutrition-related concerns that may arise at this developmental stage of the human lifecycle. For instance, because children are more likely than adults to become dehydrated, toddlers have higher fluid requirements relative to body size. It is recommended that toddlers consume approximately 1.3 liters of fluids daily, with a preference for low-sugar beverages. Toddlers require less fluid, energy, and protein per kilogram than babies do.

To ascertain whether the child is the right size for their age, many evaluations will be performed. These comprise weight and height charts: weight for age and height for age. A child would be classified as stunted or underweight if their weight falls below the fifth percentile. As an additional screening method, BMI can be used to estimate body fatness indirectly. Should the child's weight fall below the fifth percentile, they would be classified as underweight. The child is overweight if it exceeds the 95th percentile. We'll also measure the circumference of the head.

5.3.1.1. The Toddler Years (Ages Two to Three)

Children are mobile and grow more slowly than infants during this stage of human development, but they are also far more active. Their dietary requirements rise with age but fall with each kilogram of body weight. As toddlers learn to eat independently and start to form personal preferences, the toddler years present interesting challenges for parents or other caregivers. Toddlers can, however, continue to develop and grow at a healthy rate if they are given the right food and supervision.

5.3.1.2. Nutritional Requirements

The toddler's diet can be guided by MyPlate (www.choosemyplate.gov/preschoolers.html). Serving sizes for toddlers should be about 1/4 of those for adults. For young children, a good rule of thumb is one tablespoon per year of life. At a meal, a child who is two years old would receive two tablespoons of fruits or vegetables, whereas a child who is four years old would receive four tablespoons or a quarter cup. An illustration of a toddler-sized meal is this one:

- 1 ounce of meat or chicken, or 2 to 3 tablespoons of beans
- One-quarter slice of whole-grain bread
- 1 to 2 tablespoons of cooked vegetable
- 1 to 2 tablespoons of fruit

5.3.1.3. Energy

Two to three-year-olds need between 1,000 and 1,400 calories per day in energy. Energy requirements can also be computed using the formula kcal/d = ((89*weight in kg)-100_+20. A toddler needs to eat roughly 40 calories for every inch of height, on average. A young child measuring 32 inches, for instance, needs to consume 1,300 calories on average per day. However, the amount of calories that are advised depends on how active a child is. Toddlers need small, frequent meals and snacks that are high in nutrients to meet their energy needs. A toddler's daily calorie needs determine how much food they require from each food group (Table 5.1).

Table 5.1. Guideline Values

Elements	Guideline Values	
Ca	AI	280 mg/day
Cu		0.4 mg/day
K		750 mg/day
Mg		80/mg/day
Mn		0.02–0.05 mg/day
Mo		10 µg/day
Na		0.2 g/day
Zn	PRI	2.9 mg/day
Fe		11 mg/day
Al	TWI	1 mg/kg body weight/week
B	UL	0.16 mg/kg body weight/day
Ba	TDI	0.2 mg/kg body weight/week
Cd	TWI	2.5 µg/kg body weight/week
Ni	TDI	2.8 µg/kg body weight/day
Pb	BMDL	0.5 µg/kg body weight/day
Sr	UL	0.13 µg/kg body weight/day
V		1.8 mg/day

AI = Adequate intake; PRI = Population reference intake; TWI = Tolerable weekly intake; RDI = Reference daily intake; TDI = Tolerable daily intake; BMDL= Benchmark dose (lower confident unit); UL= Tolerable upper intake level.

Source: González-Suárez S, Paz-Montelongo S, Niebla-Canelo D, Alejandro-Vega S, González-Weller D, Rubio-Armendáriz C, Hardisson A, Gutiérrez-Fernández ÁJ. Baby Food Jars as a Dietary Source of Essential (K, Na, Ca, Mg, Fe, Zn, Cu, Co, Mo, Mn) and Toxic Elements (Al, Cd, Pb, B, Ba, V, Sr, Li, Ni). Applied Sciences. 2022; 12(16):8044. https://doi.org/10.3390/app12168044.

5.3.1.4. Macronutrients

The Acceptable Macronutrient Distribution Range (AMDR) for the consumption of carbohydrates is 45 to 65% of daily calories (113 to 163 grams for 1,000 daily calories). Toddlers require more in order to support the development of their bodies and minds. Nutrient-dense and visually appealing to young children, brightly colored, unrefined complex carbohydrates like peas, orange slices, tomatoes, and bananas also add visual appeal to a plate. Emphasize low-sugar snacks over those with added sugar. The recommended daily allowance (RDA) for protein is 5–20% of total calories (13–50 grams for 1,000 calories). Toddlers' daily fat consumption should not exceed 30 -40% of calories (33 to 44 grams for 1,000 calories). Essential fatty acids are necessary for nerve and other tissue types as well as the development of the eyes. Nonetheless, foods high in trans and saturated fats should not be given to toddlers. Rather, young children need the daily equivalent of three teaspoons of healthy oils, like canola oil.

5.3.1.5. Micronutrients

A child's needs for micronutrients rise as they get older. With a few notable exceptions, children who eat a balanced diet can meet their needs for vitamins and minerals, including fluoride, iron, and vitamin D. In general, well-nourished children do not require supplements. As per the American Academy of Pediatrics, children and toddlers require 600 international units of vitamin D daily, regardless of their age. Cereals and milk with added vitamin D can assist in meeting this requirement. Toddlers who do not obtain enough of this micronutrient, however, ought to take an additional supplement. Toddlers who live in areas with low fluoride water quality may also be prescribed a fluoride supplement by their pediatricians. A significant worry for kids between the ages of two and three is iron deficiency. The child may not be getting enough vitamins A and C if they are not eating enough fruits and vegetables. Their calcium intake may be low if they don't eat or drink enough dairy products or if they avoid it.

5.3.1.6. Learning How to Handle Food

As kids get bigger, they like taking care of themselves, which includes feeding themselves. Offering kids foods that they can manage on their own and that protect them from choking and other risks is crucial during this stage. Examples include sections of orange or grapefruit, sliced fresh fruit, mashed potatoes or peas for safety, a cup of yogurt, and bagels or whole-grain bread that has been divided into pieces. Learning can be chaotic, even with thorough planning and instruction. Therefore, by offering the following, parents and other caregivers can assist kids in learning how to feed themselves.

- small utensils that fit a young child's hand
- small cups that are difficult to overturn.
- plates with edges to prevent food from falling off
- small servings on a plate
- cushions, high chairs, or booster seats to get to a table.

5.3.1.7. Feeding Problems in the Toddler Years

Parents may experience a variety of food- and nutrition-related issues when their child is a toddler. Challenges could include fighting over messy eating habits at the dinner table or having a hard time helping a small child overcome their fear of unfamiliar foods. Parents and other caregivers must make sure their preschooler has wholesome options at every meal, even in the face of issues and conflicts. For instance, parents ought to keep serving veggies to their children even if they adamantly refuse to eat them. The child might eventually have a change of heart and take a liking to foods they had previously detested. It's crucial to keep in mind that now is the perfect moment to create or strengthen healthy habits.

Parent and child share the duty of feeding one another. Infants are in charge of how much they eat, but parents are in charge of what their children eat. Children are in charge of how much food they eat and whether they eat, but parents are in charge of what their toddler-aged children eat, when they eat, and where they eat. A parent or other caregiver's responsibilities when it comes to feeding include the following:

- choosing and cooking meals (it can be enjoyable to include the toddler).
- supplying meals and snacks on a regular basis.
- enhancing the fun and interaction of mealtimes.
- teaching kids the lessons they need to learn about proper dining manners.
- When the child is hungry at the start of the meal, introduce new foods to them.
- keeping kids from eating between meal or snack times.

5.3.1.8. High-Risk Choking Foods

Some foods can be dangerous for toddlers and increase the risk of choking. It is important to avoid giving children under the age of four big chunks of food, large amounts of peanut butter, popcorn, nuts, and certain raw vegetables like baby carrots, cherry tomatoes, green beans, and celery. Instead, offer toddlers well-cooked vegetables cut into manageable bite-size pieces for safe eating.

5.3.1.9. Picky Eaters

Toddler parents may observe a sudden decrease in their child's appetite. At this age, kids are frequently very particular about the foods they eat. Even after taking only a few bites, they might look away. Or, during mealtimes, they might object to sitting at the table. Additionally, they may have erratic tastes in food when it comes to certain meals and times of the day. Toddlers' picky eating has a valid reason, despite the apparent suggestion that their food intake should increase to correspond with their activity level. After infancy, a child's growth rate slows, and toddlers between the ages of two and three don't need as much food.

5.3.1.10. Food Jags

Toddlers may go through phases where they only want to eat one or two preferred foods for weeks at a time. It's normal for young children to have inconsistent food preferences as they develop their eating habits. This is a way for them to assert their independence and individuality. However, if a child continues to only eat the same foods for several months, it's important to address the issue. Some options to help include offering a variety of foods, staying calm to avoid making the situation worse, and talking to a pediatrician. Children should not be forced to eat foods they don't like. It's important to remember that food jags usually do not have long-lasting effects on a toddler's health and will typically resolve on their own.

5.3.1.11. Toddler Obesity

Toddler obesity is another possible issue in the early childhood years. The US Department of Health and Human Services reports that during the last three decades, the percentage of obese children—including infants and toddlers—has more than doubled. A little over 20% of kids between the ages of two and five are overweight or obese, and nearly 10% of babies and toddlers weigh more than is appropriate for their length.

There are several factors leading to this increasing issue. One of them is the scarcity of time. Busy parents and caregivers are constantly on the move and struggle to squeeze in homemade meals, turning to fast food and other quick but unhealthy options instead. Additionally, limited access to fresh fruits and vegetables plays a role, especially in low-income areas where stores may not offer a variety of produce. Sedentary lifestyles also contribute, as inactive toddlers are more prone to becoming overweight or obese. Lack of support for breastfeeding is another key factor, as breastfed children tend to have lower obesity rates compared to those who were bottle-fed.

Parents and other caregivers can take the following actions to prevent or address toddler obesity:

- Eat at the kitchen table rather than in front of the TV so you can keep an eye on your child's portion sizes.
- Give a child a wholesome serving. A toddler's fist size serves as a suitable serving size.
- Schedule time each day for at least 60 minutes of physical activity. Toddlers shouldn't engage in sedentary activities like watching television for longer than 60 minutes every day.

5.3.1.12. Early Childhood Caries

Toddler years are still a potential time for early childhood caries. The increased consumption of foods high in sugar by children increases their risk of developing caries during their early years. Children between the ages of two and five consume approximately 200 calories of added sugar per day, according to the National Health and Nutrition Examination Survey. As a result, parents of young children ought to stay away from processed foods like vending machine snacks and sugary drinks like soda. At this age, parents should also teach their children how to brush their teeth to prevent tooth decay and help the toddler form healthy habits.

5.3.1.13. Iron-Deficiency Anemia

Iron-deficiency anemia can occur in an infant who transitions to solid foods but does not consume enough foods high in iron. This disorder develops when the body does not produce enough hemoglobin, a red blood cell protein that carries oxygen throughout the body, due to an iron deficiency. Anemia is caused by insufficient hemoglobin production for new blood cells. Many issues are brought on by iron-deficiency anemia, such as irritability, weakness, pale skin, and shortness of breath. Additionally, it may cause behavioral, intellectual, or motor issues. Iron-deficiency anemia can develop in infants and toddlers as they wean themselves off of foods high in iron, like breast milk and formula with added iron. They start eating solid foods, which might not contain enough of this particular nutrient. Consequently, at a time when iron is essential for brain development and growth, their iron stores are depleted.

Parents and caregivers can take steps to prevent iron-deficiency anemia in children by incorporating more iron-rich foods into their diet, such as lean meats, fish, poultry, eggs, legumes, and iron-enriched whole-grain breads and cereals. Toddlers should aim to consume 7 to 10 milligrams of iron daily. While milk is important for calcium intake, it should not be overconsumed to avoid displacing iron-rich foods. Children may also benefit from a daily supplement, such as infant vitamin drops with iron or ferrous sulfate drops. If iron-deficiency anemia occurs, treatment typically involves a daily dosage of 3 milligrams per kilogram before breakfast, often in the form of ferrous sulfate syrup. Additionally, consuming vitamin C, such as orange juice, can aid in improving iron absorption.

5.3.1.14. Toddler Diarrhea

Just like adults, toddlers can experience diarrhea for a variety of reasons. Some possible causes include bacterial or viral infections, food allergies, or lactose intolerance. Additionally, consuming too much fruit juice (more than one 6-ounce cup per day) can also result in diarrhea.

Young children's diarrhea is especially concerning because of their small stature, which puts them at risk for dehydration. If a toddler has had diarrhea for longer than 24 hours, is vomiting, or shows symptoms of dehydration (such as sunken eyes, cheeks, or abdomen, or a dry mouth or tongue), parents should take them to the pediatrician. Replacing lost fluids and electrolytes—sodium and potassium—is part of preventing or treating dehydration in toddlers. The best course of action is to give specific fluids orally or administer oral rehydration therapy.

5.3.1.15. Developing Habits

Early life experiences shape eating habits. They usually form in the first few years of life and are thought to last for years, if not forever. Therefore, parents and other adults who care for children must assist them in developing good habits and avoiding bad ones. Early on, kids start to express their preferences. Parents have to strike a balance between giving their children a chance to express themselves, assisting them in forming healthy habits, and seeing to it that their nutritional needs are met. Poor diet and bad habits compound each other. Your health will be impacted by the foods you eat when you're younger, from childhood into later life. Therefore, eating well now will result in optimal health later on.

5.3.1.16. Lead Poisoning

Ingesting lead paint is typically the cause of lead poisoning, which is one of the most common forms of poisoning at this age. Lead is a heavy metal that builds up in the kidneys, teeth, brain, and bones. Iron deficiency, learning impairments, altered behavior, paralysis, nerve damage, and severe toxicity are all consequences of lead poisoning.

5.3.1.17. Effect of Food on Behavior

Food additives and sugar have been linked to hyperactivity. These assertions are unsupported by scientific data. Consuming foods high in sugar will make you more active for a short while, but that will pass quickly. Once the initial stimulation wears off, a high sugar dose may have sedative properties. Not just coffee contains caffeine; other foods also contain this stimulant. Caffeine can be found in chocolate and sodas, so check the ingredient list to see if it's included. As a stimulant, caffeine can make some kids hyperactive. Some kids are caffeine sensitive. Research has indicated that eating breakfast enhances academic achievement. Kids who miss breakfast tend to be less focused and have shorter attention spans. During the toddler years, young children gain the ability to feed themselves and start forming eating habits and preferences. Toddlers typically need between 1,000 to 1,400 calories per day, with a general guideline of consuming about 40 calories for every inch of height. Growth tends to slow down during this stage, but toddlers are more physically active and experience significant cognitive, emotional, and social growth. Common food and nutrition issues that may arise during the toddler years include choking, selective eating, food obsessions, tooth decay, low iron levels, and digestive problems.

5.3.2. Childhood and Nutrition

As children grow out of the toddler stage, their nutritional needs change. School-aged children grow steadily between the ages of four and eight, albeit more slowly than babies and toddlers. They also go through the process of losing their deciduous, or "baby," teeth and getting their permanent teeth, which usually starts around age six or seven. Many children experience some malocclusion, or tooth malposition, as new teeth erupt, which may impair their ability to chew food. Other factors that impact nutrition include the foods that schools and after-school programs offer, which can account for a significant portion of a child's diet, and the impact that peers have on dietary decisions. For young children, food allergies, malnourishment, and tooth decay are all possible food-related issues. Furthermore, gaining too much weight at a young age can cause obesity in adolescence and adulthood.

5.3.2.1. Childhood (Ages Four to Eight): "Growing Pains"

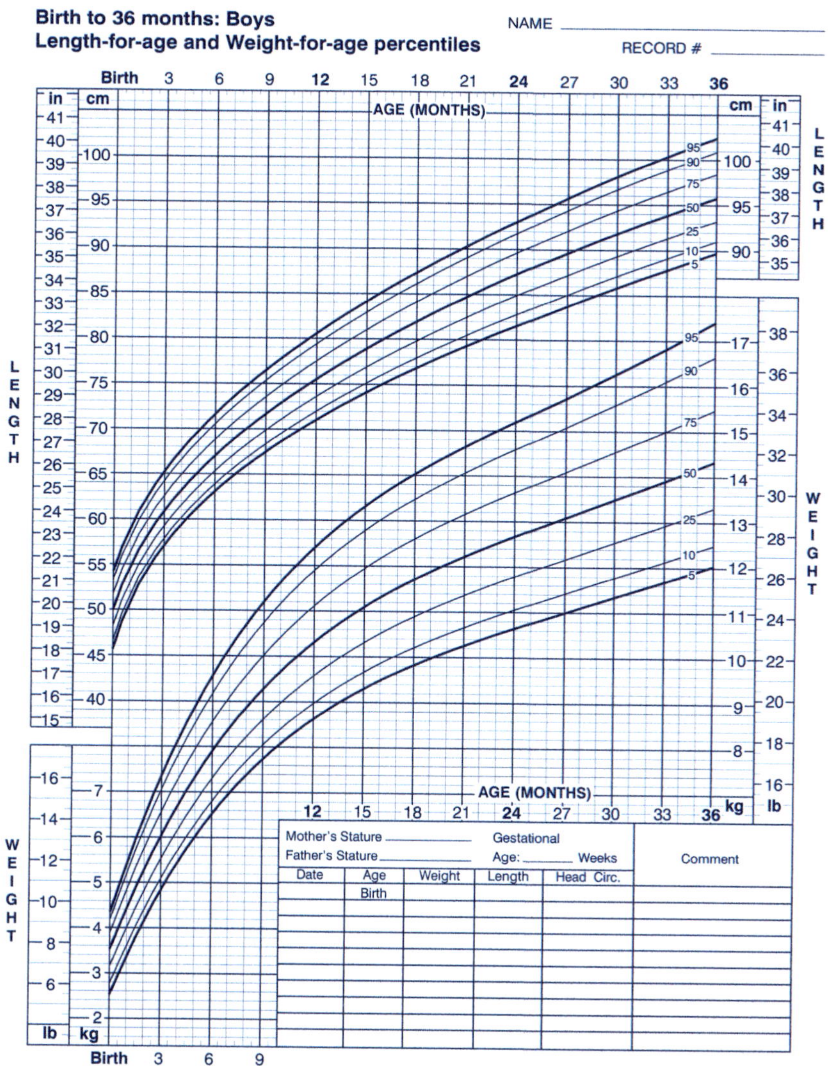

Figure 5.3. *In school-aged children, muscle mass and strength increase and motor skills show improvement.*

Source: https://med https://en.wikipedia.org/wiki/File:CDC_growth_chart_boys_birth_to_36_mths_cj41c017.pdf.

A nutritious diet promotes both physical and mental development at this stage of life and aids in preserving overall health and well-being. Children in school grow at a steady, consistent rate, gaining 2–3 inches (5–7 centimeters) in height and 4–6 pounds (2–2 kg) in weight annually on average. Furthermore, the growth rate of the extremities is higher than that of the trunk, leading to more adult-like proportions. Muscles and ligaments are stretched during long-bone growth, which is why many kids get "growing pains," especially at night (Figure 5.3).

5.3.2.1.1. Energy

Children's energy needs vary based on their growth and physical activity levels, as well as their gender. Girls between the ages of four and eight typically require 1,200 to 1,800 calories per day, while boys need 1,200 to 2,000 calories daily, potentially more depending on their activity level. In addition, children require higher intakes of macronutrients and most micronutrients relative to their body size compared to adults. It is important to provide children with nutrient-dense foods at meals and snacks, but overfeeding should be avoided to prevent childhood obesity, which will be discussed in the following section.

5.3.2.1.2. Macronutrients

The Acceptable Macronutrient Distribution Range (AMDR) for carbohydrates is 45–65% of daily calories (135–195 grams per day for 1,200 daily calories). The majority of intake should consist of high-fiber carbohydrates. For protein, the AMDR ranges from 10 – 30% of daily calories (30 to 90 grams for 1,200 calories). For the development and growth of their muscles, children have a high protein requirement. To support growth, high levels of essential fatty acids are required, albeit not as high as in infancy and the toddler years. For fat, this means that the AMDR is 25–35% of daily calories (33–47 grams for 1,200 calories). Youngsters need to consume 17–25 grams of fiber daily.

5.3.2.1.3. Micronutrients

Foods should fulfill needs for micronutrients first. To make sure that dietary needs are satisfied, parents and other caregivers should choose a range of foods from each food group. Children need high-iron foods like lean meats, legumes, fish, poultry, and iron-enriched cereals because they grow so quickly. Sufficient fluoride is essential for strong teeth. Getting enough calcium and vitamin D in childhood is one of the most crucial micronutrient requirements. To create strong, dense bones, both are required. 10 micrograms (400 international units) of vitamin D should be given as a supplement to children who do not get enough of it each day. (Note that the recommendations are the same for boys and girls. As we progress through the different stages of the human life cycle, there will be some differences between males and females regarding micronutrient needs) (Table 5.2).

Table 5.2. Estimated Daily Intake (mg/day) and Percentages of Contribution to the AI of the Studied Essential Elements Considering a Consumption of 130 g/day and 250 g/day of Baby Food from Jars

Guideline Values [20,27,46,47,48,49, 50,51, 52]		Fruits				Vegetables				Meat				Mixed			
	EDI (mg/Day)		% AI		EDI (mg/Day)		% AI		EDI (mg/Day)		% AI		EDI (mg/Day)		% AI		
	130 g/Day	250 g/Day	130 g/Day	250 g/Day	130 g/Day	250 g/Day	130 g/Day	250 g/Day	130 g/Day	250 g/Day	130 g/Day	250 g/Day	130 g/Day	250 g/Day	130 g/Day	250 g/Day	
Ca	280 mg/day	28.7	55.3	10.3	19.8	59.3	114	21.2	40.7	104	200	37.1	71.4	120	230	42.9	82.1
Cu	0.4 mg/day	0.35	0.68	87.5	170	0.22	0.43	55.0	108	0.23	0.44	57.5	110	0.18	0.35	45.0	87.5
Fe	11 mg/day	0.71	1.36	6.45	12.4	1.09	2.10	9.91	19.1	1.02	1.96	9.27	17.8	1.37	2.63	12.5	23.9
K	750 mg/day	505	971	67.3	130	479	922	63.9	123	548	1053	73.1	140	529	1017	70.5	136
Mg	80 mg/day	40.0	76.8	50.0	96.0	41.5	79.8	51.9	99.8	39.3	75.5	49.1	94.4	41.1	79.0	51.4	98.8
Mn	0.02–0.5 mg/day	0.42	0.80	2100–84.0	4000–160	0.38	0.73	1900–76	3650–146	0.30	0.57	1500–60	2850–114	0.30	0.57	1500–60	2850–114
Mo	10 µg/day	0.008	0.02	80	200	0.02	0.05	230	500	0.02	0.04	200	400	0.02	0.03	200	300
Na	Not established	-															
Zn	2.9 mg/day	0.38	0.73	13.1	25.0	0.80	1.54	27.6	53.1	1.63	3.13	56.2	108	2.42	4.65	83.4	160

Source: *González-Suárez S, Paz-Montelongo S, Niebla-Canelo D, Alejandro-Vega S, González-Weller D, Rubio-Armendáriz C, Hardisson A, Gutiérrez-Fernández ÁJ. Baby Food Jars as a Dietary Source of Essential (K, Na, Ca, Mg, Fe, Zn, Cu, Co, Mo, Mn) and Toxic Elements (Al, Cd, Pb, B, Ba, V, Sr, Li, Ni).* Applied Sciences. *2022; 12(16):8044. https://doi.org/10.3390/app12168044.*

5.3.2.1.4. Factors Influencing Intake

Children's eating patterns and attitudes toward food can be influenced by a multitude of factors. The family environment, media messages, taste preferences, and societal trends all influence how children feel about their diet. Children may be persuaded to eat refined carbohydrates, sugary goods, fatty fast food, excess calories, and sodium by watching television commercials. Parents and other adults must guide kids toward healthy decisions as a result. Adding excitement and fun to meal and snack times is one way to motivate kids to eat well. Children should be involved in the planning and preparation of meals. This can involve helping to make a salad or choosing items during a grocery shop. Parents can also teach their kids about kitchen safety at this time. Cutting meats, sandwiches, or pancakes into unique or tiny shapes could be useful. Furthermore, parents ought to serve wholesome desserts like fresh fruit rather than calorie-dense cakes, cookies, ice cream, and salty snacks. Additionally, research indicates that kids who regularly attend family meals eat a diet higher in nutrients (Hendricks, 2000; Holden, 2000; Baker and Robert, 2001; Suskind et al, 2011; Marotz, 2012; Koletzko, 2015; Kliegman, 2020).

5.3.2.2. Children and Malnutrition

Many children suffer from malnutrition, both in developed and developing countries. Despite North America's abundance of food, a large number of kids suffer from malnourishment or go without food. The following categories represent how the US Census Bureau classifies households:

- food secure
- food insecure without hunger
- food insecure with moderate hunger
- food insecure with severe hunger

Both the quantity and quality of food that is readily available cause millions of children to grow up in homes where there is food insecurity and inadequate nutrition. Approximately 20% of American households with children experience some level of food insecurity. In half of those, food insecurity affects only adults, while in the other half, it affects both adults and children, meaning that children occasionally lack access to sufficient, nourishing meals.

Being raised in a home where there is insufficient access to food can cause many issues. Limited development, sickness, and stunted growth can arise from iron, zinc, protein, and vitamin A deficiencies. The risk of hunger and malnutrition in school-aged children is addressed by federal programs like the Summer Feeding Program, the School Breakfast Program, and the National School Lunch Program. They fill in the gaps and increase the availability of wholesome meals for kids from households experiencing food insecurity.

5.3.2.2.1. The National School Lunch Program

Children eat at least one meal in a school setting starting in preschool. A lot of kids eat breakfast and lunch somewhere other than at home. For this reason, schools must serve nutrient-dense food. Over 31.1 million children from economically disadvantaged households receive meals from the National School Lunch Program in the United States. This federally funded program provides free or inexpensive lunches for schools as well as snacks for after-school programs. The US Department of Agriculture (USDA) provides funding to participating school districts for each meal they serve.

The Healthy School Lunch Campaign educates parents, food service personnel, government officials, and school administrators about how to better the food that kids eat at school and how to support their short- and long-term health. This organization, which is sponsored by the Physicians Committee for Responsible Medicine, pushes schools to stock more low-fat and cholesterol-free options in their cafeterias and vending machines.

5.3.2.3. Children and Vegetarianism

Making the decision to support a child's transition to a vegetarian or vegan diet is another challenge that some parents have with school-age children. For reasons related to health, culture, or other factors, some parents and other caregivers choose to raise their kids as vegetarians. Concerns for the environment or animals may lead preteens and teens to choose vegetarianism on their own. For whatever reason, parents of vegetarian children need to be careful to make sure their kids eat wholesome, nutrient-dense foods that meet all their needs.

5.3.2.3.1. Types of Vegetarian Diets

Vegetarians come in different varieties, each with their own dietary restrictions.

- **Ovo-Vegetarians:** Eggs are consumed by ovo-vegetarians, but no other animal products are.
- **Lacto-Ovo-Vegetarians:** Those who follow a lacto-ovo-vegetarian diet consume dairy products and eggs but not meat.
- **Lacto-Vegetarians:** Dairy products are consumed by lacto-vegetarians, who abstain from all other animal products.
- **Vegans:** Vegans consume only plant-based foods—no animal products at all.

Some animal products, like cheese, eggs, and other dairy products, can help children meet their nutritional needs. Planning is necessary to ensure that a child eating a strict vegan diet gets enough protein, iron, calcium, vitamin B12, and vitamin D. Meat can be replaced with legumes and nuts, and cow's milk can be substituted with soy milk fortified with calcium and vitamins D and B12.

5.3.2.4. Food Allergies and Food Intolerance

It is concerning when food allergies start to develop in toddlers. Children who are in school still have this problem. Three million children under the age of 18 are allergic to at least one type of food, according to recent studies. The most popular foods that cause allergies are shellfish, peanuts, milk, eggs, soy, and wheat. An allergy develops when a food protein sets off an immunological reaction that releases histamine, antibodies, and other defense mechanisms against foreign substances. Itchy skin, hives, stomach pain, vomiting, diarrhea, and nausea are examples of possible symptoms. Usually, minutes to hours after ingesting a food allergen, symptoms appear. Food allergies, particularly those to wheat, milk, eggs, or soy, can outgrow a child.

A potentially fatal reaction known as anaphylaxis causes breathing difficulties, edema in the mouth and throat, low blood pressure, shock, or even death. It is most likely to be caused by milk, eggs, wheat, soybeans, fish, shellfish, peanuts, and tree nuts. An injection of the medication epinephrine is frequently given via a "pen" to treat an individual experiencing anaphylactic shock. A food intolerance that some kids have doesn't result from an immunological reaction. The telltale signs of a food intolerance are unpleasant symptoms that appear after eating a particular food. One example is lactose intolerance, which is uncommon in very young children. Children with this illness react negatively to lactose, which is present in milk products. It is brought about by the small intestine's incapacity to generate adequate amounts of the lactase enzyme. Lactose intolerance symptoms can include bloating, abdominal pain, gas, nausea, and diarrhea; they typically affect the GI tract. The best way to manage an intolerance is to alter your diet and stay away from anything that makes you react.

5.3.2.5. The Threat of Lead Toxicity

Children in school age are susceptible to lead toxicity, also known as lead poisoning. Lead can occasionally be found in the soil, lead-based paint, and the plumbing in older homes. Lead poisoning can occur from contaminated food and water, increasing exposure and raising dangerous blood lead levels. Youngsters younger than six are particularly at risk. They might eat things that are contaminated with lead, like paint that has chips in it. Lead dust in carpets is another frequent source of exposure; the dust flakes off wall paint. Children are at risk when they play or roll around on lead-coated carpets. Lead is unbreakable, and the human body finds it difficult to change or eliminate it once it has been consumed. Before symptoms appear, it can subtly accumulate in the body for months or even years. Lead poisoning can harm the brain and central nervous system, impairing perception, reasoning, and thought processes.

Removing the child from the contaminated area and removing lead from the body are part of the treatment for lead poisoning. Chelation therapy, which binds with lead to allow its excretion in urine, may be used in extraction. If a patient's blood lead level is more than 45 mcg/dL, another treatment protocol called EDTA therapy involves giving them a medication called ethylenediaminetetraacetic acid. Thankfully, lead poisoning is largely avoidable. It entails locating possible dangers and eliminating them before kids are exposed to them, such as lead paint and pipes. Compared to the nutrient requirements of adults, the recommended intakes of macronutrients and micronutrients for children are higher in relation to body size. Furthermore, a child's daily energy requirements differ based on their gender and degree of physical activity. Boys and girls between the ages of four and eight require 1,200 and 2,000 calories, respectively. Children in school may experience food and nutrition-related issues such as lead poisoning, food allergies, food intolerances, and malnourishment (Hendricks, 2000; Holden, 2000; Baker and Robert, 2001; Suskind et al, 2011; Marotz, 2012; Koletzko, 2015; Kliegman, 2020).

5.3.3. Puberty and Nutrition

Adolescence begins with puberty. The development of primary and secondary sex traits, growth spurts, an increase in body fat, and an increase in bone and muscle development are all brought on by the onset of puberty. Sufficient intake and dietary choices that promote health are necessary to support all of these changes.

5.3.3.1. The Onset of Puberty (Ages 9 to 13)

There are two stages to this physical development period. The first stage entails a 20–25% increase in height. When it comes to the fastest growth of the long bones stretching to their final, adult size, puberty is second only to the prenatal stage. Boys are taller by 4–12 inches (10–30 centimeters), while girls are taller by 2–8 inches (5–20 centimeters). Weight gain associated with the growth of bone, muscle, and fat tissue characterizes the second phase. The development of secondary sexual traits like pubic hair and reproductive organs is triggered by sex hormones during puberty. Girls grow "curves" as well, but boys get bigger and stronger.

5.3.3.2. Energy

Preteens have varying energy needs based on their activity level, growth, and gender. Based on daily needs rather than body weight, the highest energy requirements occur during this time. Girls should consume roughly 1,400 to 2,200 calories per day and boys should consume 1,600 to 2,600 calories per day between the ages of 9 and 13. Preteens who engage in regular physical activity, such as sports or exercise, require a higher caloric intake to meet their increased energy needs.

5.3.3.3. Macronutrients

The recommended daily intake for carbohydrates is 45–65% of daily calories, which equates to 158–228 grams for 1,400–1,600 daily calories. It is recommended that carbohydrates high in fiber be the main source of intake. Protein is essential for growth, with the recommended daily intake being 10 to 30%of daily calories, or 35–105 grams for 1,400 daily calories for girls and 40–120 grams for 1,600 daily calories for boys. The recommended daily intake for fat is 25 to 35% of daily calories, or 39–54 grams for 1,400 daily calories for girls and 44–62 grams for 1,600 daily calories for boys. These recommendations vary based on caloric intake and activity level.

5.3.3.4. Micronutrients

During puberty, vitamins D, K, and B_{12} are essential. Consuming enough calcium is crucial for promoting bone growth and averting osteoporosis in later life. Young males require extra iron for the development of lean body mass, while young females require more iron at the onset of menstruation. Except for iron, almost all of these requirements should be satisfied by dietary choices rather than supplements. Protein metabolism and energy production require the B vitamins. DNA and cell growth require folate and vitamin B_{12}. Teenagers who abstain from milk are at risk of becoming deficient in calcium, vitamin D, and riboflavin. Given that the bones are growing longer and that this is a crucial period for laying down bone mass, vitamin D and calcium are particularly concerning. A shortage of iron is also possible in women because it coincides with the onset of menstruation, while in men it helps build muscle (Table 5.3).

Table 5.3. The Role of Diet in Early Life and During Childhood on Timing of Puberty

Period	Dietary Source	Mechanism of Action	BMI Dependent and/or Independent Action	Effect on Puberty
Early-life nutrition	Breastfeeding	Overweight prevention through normal hormonal and microbiome balance and positive psychosocial influence	Both	Precocious puberty prevention
	Formula feeding	Overweight development and predisposition to childhood obesity through increased IGF-1 and consequent enhanced sex steroid production	BMI dependent	Increased risk for precocius puberty

	Soy-based formulas	Weak estrogenic effects of soy isoflavones	BMI independent	Uncertain increased risk for precocius puberty
	Complementary feeding	Overweight development in case of age-inappropriate feeding and high protein consumption	BMI dependent	Increased risk for precocius puberty
	Soy-based foods	Weak estrogenic effects of soy isoflavones	BMI independent	Uncertain increased risk for precocius puberty
Childhood nutrition	High-energy diet	Higher levels of leptin, IGF-1 activation, adrenal androgen overproduction, and increased conversion of androgens to estrogens	BMI dependent	Increased risk for precocius puberty
	Protein intake	Adiposity rebound before pubertal onset, IGF-1 secretion	Both	Increased risk for precocius puberty
	Fat intake	Direct effect on steroidogenesis and mammary gland development, indirect effect through induction of low-grade hypothalamic inflammation	BMI independent	Increased risk for precocius puberty (PUFAs). Uncertain increased risk for precocius puberty (MUFAs)
	Carbohydrate intake	Rapid increase in insulin concentration in high-glycemic-index diets resulting in increased availability of sex hormones and IGF-1	BMI independent	Uncertain increased risk for precocius puberty
		Further studies are needed to identify the possible mechanisms	BMI independent	Uncertain increased risk for precocius puberty
	Mediterranean diet	Reduction in circulating levels of estrogen, follicle-stimulating hormone, and luteinizing hormone. Increased excretion of estrogen. Stimulation of hepatic synthesis of SHBG, which reduces the biological availability of sex hormones	BMI independent	Precocious puberty prevention
	Vegetarian diet	Lower leptin levels	BMI dependent	Uncertain increased risk for later puberty

	New dietary patterns	A combination of the above mechanisms of high energy, fat, glycemic, and protein intake associated with unbalanced micronutrient supplies	Both	Increased risk for precocius puberty

Source: *Calcaterra V, Verduci E, Magenes VC, Pascuzzi MC, Rossi V, Sangiorgio A, Bosetti A, Zuccotti G, Mameli C. The Role of Pediatric Nutrition as a Modifiable Risk Factor for Precocious Puberty.* Life. *2021; 11(12):1353. https://doi.org/10.3390/life11121353.*

5.3.3.5. Childhood Obesity

For healthy growth, children require a sufficient amount of calories, so it's crucial to avoid imposing extremely restrictive diets. But regularly consuming more calories than needed can result in childhood obesity, a serious issue in North America. In the US, one in three kids and teenagers are overweight or obese. Approximately 26% of children and adolescents in Canada are obese or overweight (Figure 5.4).

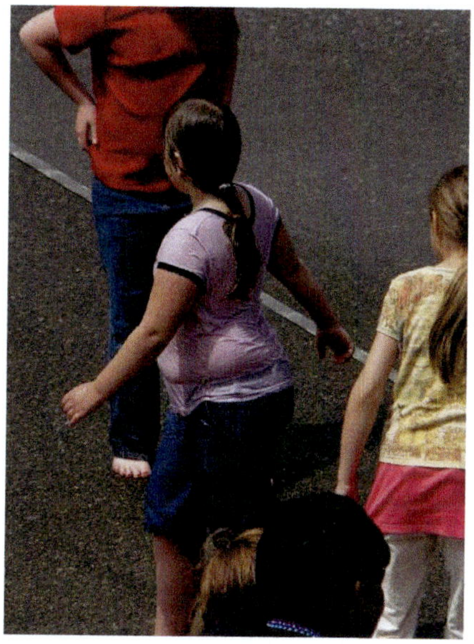

Figure 5.4. *Children with varying degrees of body fat.*

Source: By Walter Siegmund – Own work, CC BY 2.5, https://commons.wikimedia.org/w/index.php?curid=2165293.

The issue of childhood obesity is caused by several factors, such as:

- larger portion sizes
- restricted availability of nutrient-rich foods.
- improved availability of fast food options and vending machines
- inadequate assistance for breastfeeding.

- school physical education programs are deteriorating.
- a sedentary lifestyle and insufficient exercise.
- messages in the media that promote eating unhealthy foods.
- high fat, high energy snacks

Obese children have a higher likelihood of becoming overweight or obese adults. Obesity has a significant impact on energy, activity level, and self-esteem. More significantly, it poses a significant risk for several diseases that arise later in life, such as hypertension, stroke, Type 2 diabetes, cardiovascular disease, and some types of cancer. To assess whether a child is overweight or obese, a body mass index (BMI) percentile tailored to the child's age and gender is used. This is more appropriate than the adult BMI categories because children's body composition varies with development and is different for boys and girls. Limiting energy-dense, low-nutrient snack foods is advised for parents and caregivers of children who gain weight unsuitable for their growth. Additionally, kids three years old and up can adhere to the National Cholesterol Education Program's recommendations, which include consuming no more than 350 mg of cholesterol daily and no more than 35% of their calories from fat (10% or less from saturated fat). A child's physical activity should also be increased, and sedentary activities like watching TV, playing video games, and using the Internet should be minimized.

Behavior modification, exercise counseling, psychological support or therapy, family counseling, and meal-planning advice for the family are some of the programs available to address childhood obesity. For most, allowing height to catch up with weight as the child grows is more important than focusing on weight loss. For preteens and younger children, rapid weight loss is not advised due to the risk of deficiencies and stunted growth.

5.3.3.6. Avoiding Added Sugars

Consuming added sugars is one of the main causes of childhood obesity. In addition to being added to food at the table, added sugars can also be found in bread, cookies, cakes, pies, jams, soft drinks, and other baked goods. Store-bought products may contain added sugar under the names brown sugar, white sugar, honey, malt syrup, maple syrup, molasses, concentrated fruit juice, high-fructose corn syrup, and anhydrous dextrose. Natural sugars found in food, such as the fructose in fruits and the lactose in milk, are not included. Furthermore, sugars are frequently "hidden" in condiments like ketchup and salad dressing that are added to meals after they have been prepared. The National Center for Health Statistics estimates that added sugars account for 322 calories, or roughly 16% of daily calories, consumed by young children and adolescents.

Processed and packaged foods, as well as soda and other beverages, are the main culprits. These foods frequently replace healthier options because they are not only high in sugar but also low in nutrients. Limiting daily intake of added sugar to 100–150 calories can help deter unhealthy eating patterns.

5.3.3.7. Tools for Change

Preteens and teens should engage in moderate-to-intense physical activity for 60 minutes each day. This includes bone- and muscle-strengthening exercises in addition to aerobic activity. But a lot of young people fail miserably to achieve this aim. To prevent or treat childhood obesity, preteens need to be encouraged to lead more active lifestyles. Kids are encouraged to start exercising by the Let's Move! campaign in the United States. First Lady Michelle Obama started this initiative in 2010 to address the growing issue of childhood, preteen, and teen obesity. It helps kids get more active, provides information to parents and teachers, and advocates for better food options in classrooms and after-school programs. The program encourages preteens and teens to find something they love to do as one way to promote physical activity. Kids are more likely to get moving and maintain their health when they find an activity they enjoy, whether it's riding a bike, playing football, joining a soccer team, or dancing in a crew.

Preteens go through growth spurts and develop the traits of primary and secondary sex during puberty. Preteens' daily energy needs vary depending on their activity level, growth, and gender. Boys and girls between the ages of 9 and 13 should consume 1,600 and 2,600 calories daily, respectively. Obesity and malnutrition are two nutritional issues that older children should be aware of. It is important to support preteens in forming positive habits, such as eating a balanced diet and engaging in regular physical activity or sports.

5.3.4. Older Adolescence and Nutrition

We'll talk about the nutritional needs of teenagers between the ages of 14 and 18 in this section. Making food choices is one way that teenagers show their independence. They typically eat more meals away from home and have the means to buy food on their own. Additionally, older teenagers may be inquisitive and receptive to new concepts, which includes experimenting with their diet and trying out new foods. Teens, for instance, occasionally choose to snack in place of their main meal. That in and of itself is not troublesome. It matters more what they choose to eat than where or when they eat it.

However, young people may become nutritionally vulnerable if they make too many bad decisions. It is best to discourage teenagers from consuming fast food, which is high in fat and sugar, as well as from going to convenience stores and using vending machines, which usually have subpar food options. Adolescents may also struggle with eating disorders and obesity. Young people still require parental and other caregiver guidance regarding nutrition-related issues at this stage of life. Young people can benefit from hearing about how eating well can enhance their favorite activities, like skating or dancing, or link to their goals or interests, like having a trimmer body, performing better in sports, or having better cognitive abilities.

5.3.4.1. Adolescence (Ages 14 to 18): Transitioning into Adulthood

Males and females grow and develop differently during adolescence, just as they do during puberty. Teenage boys have greater increases in muscle and bone mass and a decrease in body fat, whereas fat makes up a larger portion of body weight in girls. With the end of puberty, both primary and secondary sex characteristics have fully developed and the rate of growth slows. Furthermore, an older adolescent's motor abilities are similar to those of an adult. Once more, this stage of growth and development is supported by a healthy diet and dietary choices. Adolescents who suffer from acne, substance abuse, obesity, and adolescent pregnancy are more likely to become malnourished, which can have long-term consequences.

5.3.4.2. Energy

The increased nutritional needs result in increased appetites. Except for pregnancy, adolescence has higher nutritional needs than any other stage of life. Depending on activity level, girls need 1,800–2,400 calories and boys need 2,000–3,200 calories per day between the ages of 14 and 18. The extra energy needed for adolescent physical development should come from nutrient-dense foods rather than "empty calories." Teens who play sports must also make sure they get the extra energy they require.

5.3.4.3. Macronutrients

While older teenagers are more in charge of their diet than younger kids, parents and other adults still need to make sure that teens are getting all the nutrients they need. The AMDR ranges from 45 -65% of daily calories for carbohydrates (203–293 grams for 1,800 daily calories). Compared to younger children, adolescents need greater servings of grains, and they should consume whole grains like brown rice, oats, wheat, and barley. Increased protein consumption is advised by the Institute of Medicine to support adolescent population growth. Lean proteins, such as meat, chicken, fish, beans, nuts, and seeds, are great sources of protein to help meet the AMDR of 10 -30% of daily calories (45–135 grams for 1,800 calories).

Depending on daily calories and activity level, the AMDR for fat is 25–35% of daily calories (50–70 grams for 1,800 daily calories), and the AMDR for fiber is 25–34 grams per day. Due to their increased risk of dehydration, young athletes and other physically active teens must ensure they consume adequate fluids.

5.3.4.4. Micronutrients

Although children at this age require more of some minerals to promote bone growth (such as calcium and phosphorus, along with iron and zinc for girls), the micronutrient recommendations for adolescents are largely the same as those for adults. Once more, food should be the primary source of vitamins and minerals, with supplements only needed for specific micronutrients (like iron).

The micronutrients iron, calcium, vitamin D, and vitamin A are the most crucial for teenagers. Getting enough calcium and vitamin D is crucial for increasing bone mass. For both boys and girls, 1,300 milligrams of calcium is advised. Low-fat dairy products, such as milk and cheeses, are great sources of calcium and can help young people avoid cholesterol and saturated fat. Adolescents who consume products fortified with calcium, like orange juice and breakfast cereals, may also benefit from doing so. Lean body mass and muscle growth are aided by iron. When they begin to menstruate, teenage girls must also make sure they are consuming enough iron. Girls between the ages of 12 and 18 need 15 milligrams of iron daily. Increased vitamin C intake, such as that found in orange juice and other foods, can help the body absorb iron. Additionally, consuming enough fruits and vegetables enables one to meet one's vitamin A needs.

5.3.4.5. Acne

Acne in teenagers can occur for reasons other than eating chocolate or other high-sugar or greasy foods. Rather, an infection of the skin's sebaceous gland is the cause. Clogged gland ducts cause skin oils to build up. This results in the gland becoming agitated and inflamed, as well as the related heads appearing. Stress exacerbates acne, which also tends to run in families (hereditary link). Reducing the stressors, topical ointments, antibiotics, and/or the medication Accutane are all part of the treatment. Since accutane and vitamin A are similar, the drug's toxicity will be closely watched.

5.3.4.6. Eating Disorders

An eating disorder affects many teenagers and can be harmful to diet and general health. 24 million Americans and 70 million people worldwide are affected by these conditions. Although adolescent boys have been more affected by these disorders recently, adolescent girls are still more likely to experience them. Adolescents with eating disorders are deprived of the vital nutrients their still developing bodies need because eating disorders frequently result in malnourishment. It is unknown what causes eating disorders, but it is most likely a result of a combination of factors. The condition may be brought on by a combination of biological, psychological, and/or social factors. Hormonal changes associated with puberty give rise to biological factors, which may also be hereditary. Puberty brings about changes in personality and behavior, which may hasten the emergence of an eating disorder. Lastly, the media shapes our ideas about what constitutes a desirable body weight and affects how we perceive our own weight. Adolescent athletes frequently believe that lighter weight equates to superior performance.

Extreme food and exercise-related behavior is a feature of eating disorders. They include a range of conditions characterized by undereating or overeating and are sometimes referred to as "starving or stuffing." Among these conditions are the following:

- **Anorexia Nervosa:** The potentially fatal symptoms of anorexia nervosa include excessive weight loss and undereating. Individuals suffering from this disorder exhibit unhealthy levels of obsession with food intake, calories, and dieting. Because of their negative body image, anorexics experience anxiety, food avoidance, strict exercise regimens, fasting, and hunger denial. Women are primarily affected by the illness. This eating disorder affects between 0.5 and 1% of women and girls in the United States. Men make up 5% of the population. Anorexia nervosa affects two to five percent of teenage girls.

Diagnostic guidelines for eating disorders are established by the American Psychiatric Association. Refusal to maintain body mass above a minimal weight for age and height (15% below expected body mass) is one of the DMS-IV criteria for anorexia nervosa. the following: (1) a distorted self-image and/or denial of the severity of low body mass (satisfied with certain body parts but critical of other areas); (2) an intense fear of gaining weight or becoming fat despite being underweight; and (3) the absence of at least three consecutive menstrual cycles. The person may appear physically malnourished, with hair loss, tooth loss, and rough, dry, and cold skin. They might have very high standards, be obsessive, and have competitive psychological traits. Their family might be conflictual, overly protective, rigid, and overly involved.

One prevalent nutritional consequence of anorexia nervosa is protein-energy malnutrition. Reduced white blood cell counts in the immune system; decreased body temperature, heart rate, and bone mass; anemia; constipation; amenorrhea; multiple organ failures; and an elevated risk of suicide are among the medical complications.

A medical team experienced in treating anorexia nervosa should be involved in therapy. The nutritional objective is to gain weight gradually, which is accomplished by increasing daily caloric intake by about 200 kcal. Supplements may be necessary to ensure that the diet meets nutritional requirements. It's critical to recognize the emotional triggers and develop behavioral control strategies to modify eating habits. Family, group/individual, and/or relapse therapy may be used to achieve this.

- **Disorder of Binge Eating (Also Known as Compulsive Overeating):** Individuals with binge-eating disorders frequently go through phases where they eat a lot of food in a short amount of time without purging. The most prevalent eating disorder, it is also prevalent in people who are extremely obese. Those who engage in compulsive binge eating often believe they have no control over the behavior. In addition to contributing to obesity, high blood pressure, high cholesterol, Type 2 diabetes, and other health issues, this behavior frequently results in feelings of embarrassment and shame. Males and females with binge-eating disorder are both affected. One to five percent of people are impacted.

Recurrent binges occurring at least twice a week for six months are necessary to diagnose binge eating disorder. The person overindulges in food even when they are not hungry because they feel like they are eating excessively. They frequently eat by themselves because they feel disgusted and guilty about overindulging in food and are embarrassed about how much they ate. The majority of sufferers of this eating disorder are obese or overweight. They may be depressed and have low self-esteem. Their excessive adipose stores are the cause of their medical issues, which can be treated by losing weight and altering their lifestyle to keep the weight off.

- **Nervous Bulimia:** With alternating cycles of overeating and undereating, bulimia nervosa is more common than anorexia nervosa. Individuals who experience it engage in compulsive exercise, self-induced vomiting, laxative use, diuretics, enemas, medication, fasting, and compulsive eating as compensatory behaviors. The majority of people lose control over how much they eat during a binge episode. Similar to anorexia, the majority of sufferers are female, single, highly educated, and close to their ideal body weight. This eating disorder affects between 1% and 2% of women and girls in the United States.

The DMS-IV criteria for bulimia nervosa include: (1) frequently occurring binge-eating episodes; (2) frequently occurring, inappropriate compensatory behavior to avoid gaining weight; (3) both compensatory behavior and binge eating occurring on average at least twice a week for three months; (4) dissatisfaction and/or distortion of body image; and (5) disturbance not occurring during anorexia nervosa episodes. Individuals suffering from this eating disorder may weigh normal or change their weight by 20% in a short period of time.

An unsuccessful diet may lead to the development of this eating disorder. The person could be depressed, passive, high-stress, perfectionist, low on self-esteem, or depressed. Usually, they are aware that the behavior is strange. Their family might be permissive and disengaged. Poor kidney function, weakened immunity, an increase in UTIs, low blood potassium (hypokalemia), and irregular heartbeats are examples of medical complications. If they vomit in an attempt to purge, they run the risk of developing infections in the salivary glands and esophagus, rupturing the stomach or esophagus, tooth erosion, and potassium loss. Creating regular eating routines, meal planning, keeping a food journal, and maintaining consistent body weight and food intake are all part of the treatment. They need to treat depression, break the purge cycle psychologically, improve their body image, increase their self-esteem, and adopt a positive outlook on food and their bodies.

Stress, low self-esteem, and other psychological and emotional problems are the root causes of eating disorders. Parents should be on the lookout for sudden weight loss, loose clothing, lethargy, a decline in grades, social isolation, eating alone, vomiting after meals, and appetite suppressant use, among other symptoms of these disorders. If treatment is not received, eating disorders may result in major complications or even death. Treatment involves nutritional, behavioral, and cognitive therapy, and a qualified practitioner is needed.

5.3.4.7. Muscle Dysmorphia (Adonis Complex)

Being preoccupied with not being slender and strong enough is known as an Adonis Complex. While there are many similarities between it and anorexia nervosa, the person's perception of their body is obviously distorted. Most sufferers of this eating disorder are big, strong individuals. Their obsession with being slender and strong is evident in their frequent self-weighing and/or mirror gazing (narcissistic behavior). They enjoy dressing in loose-fitting clothing or altering it to highlight their muscles. They follow a strict diet and engage in excessive exercise to gain muscularity. They also abuse dietary supplements. Surprisingly, they may spend more than three hours contemplating their muscularity, even though they do not perceive themselves as small and feeble.

Numerous physical changes occur in older adolescents, and in order to support these changes and meet their nutrient needs, they must increase their energy intake. Except for pregnancy, adolescence has higher nutrient requirements than any other stage of life. Depending on activity level, girls between the ages of 14 and 18 need 1,800 to 2,400 calories per day and boys between the ages of 2,000 and 3,200 calories per day. Eating disorders are among the nutritional concerns that older adolescents face (Hendricks, 2000; Holden, 2000; Baker and Robert, 2001; Suskind et al, 2011; Marotz, 2012; Koletzko, 2015; Kliegman, 2020).

5.4. NUTRITION IN PEDIATRIC INTENSIVE CARE

When a critical illness strikes, the body's first defensive response is based on basic phylogenetic targets that aim to deliver oxygen and energy (E) to the essential organs. While in the acute stage (e.g., shock), a number of immunological, endocrine, and metabolic responses are triggered in an effort to lessen the initial damage. This stage is typically linked to impaired protein and energy delivery; failure in energy utilization may also manifest. All substrates, including amino acids, are used in glycogenolysis and gluconeogenesis (with muscle breakdown) when maximal effort is made to ensure adequate delivery of E. Insulin resistance, stress hyperglycemia, and the shift to catabolism are all linked to these metabolic abnormalities during the acute phase of critical illness. Although these metabolic disturbances are initially life-saving, if they persist past the acute phase of illness, they can cause profound catabolism, severe malnutrition, and an increase in morbidity and mortality. Pediatric critical care therefore includes early nutritional support and initial nutritional assessment within 48 hours of admission (after initial stabilization). Given the potential for up to 25% malnutrition rate at pediatric intensive care unit (PICU) admission, nutritional support should be tailored case-by-case. Target E and protein delivery should be closely monitored during the PICU stay.

In critical illness, muscle breakdown and protein wasting occur in the initial state, making it important for nutritional support to aim at minimizing negative protein balance. Delivering excessive nutrition (overfeeding) can be harmful during this acute phase due to ineffective substrate utilization. Protocol-based nutritional support in the Pediatric Intensive Care Unit (PICU) is recommended, with guidelines developed by organizations such as the European Society of Pediatric and Neonatal Intensive Care (ESPNIC), European Society for Clinical Nutrition and Metabolism (ESPEN), American Society for Clinical Nutrition and Metabolism (ASPEN), and Society of Critical Care Medicine (SCCM) being widely adopted and cited. Proper nutritional support has been shown to impact infection rates, length of stay, and mortality. When considering nutritional support for critically ill pediatric patients, key principles remain similar to adults, such as early nutritional status assessment and preferring enteral feeding over parenteral feeding. However, differences in nutritional status assessment and energy targets for different age groups should be taken into account. This review outlines a step-by-step approach for providing nutritional support to critically ill pediatric patients in the general population in the PICU, with a focus on excluding very small infants and neonates.

5.4.1. Nutritional Status Assessment

As was previously mentioned, PICU admission can be used to diagnose a high prevalence of malnutrition. Given the strong correlation between malnutrition (including obesity) and unfavorable clinical outcomes, a thorough evaluation of nutritional status should be conducted as soon as a patient is admitted to the intensive care unit. Nutritional risk screening and nutritional risk in critically ill patients (NUTRIC) have been approved and implemented for adult patients. Weight, height/length (in children under 2 years old), and the z score for body mass index (BMI) for age, mid upper-arm circumference, or weight for age can all be used with pediatric patients. The head circumference of infants younger than 36 months should also be observed. To assess the impact of nutritional interventions indirectly, anthropometric measurements should be taken frequently throughout the PICU stay (following the nutrition protocol). In addition to a thorough physical examination, the functional status and entire dietary history should be evaluated before PICU admission. In general, nutritional assessments take longer to complete, require specialized training, and require clinical expertise. Usually, a dietitian, nutrition specialist, or other licensed healthcare professional is needed to conduct such a formal nutritional assessment. Conversely, nutrition screening tools offer a rapid means of evaluating nutritional status and are designed to be easily administered (i.e., less than 15 minutes) and don't call for the caregiver to have any specialized training. Later on, the entire assessment can be completed, particularly for high-risk patients. There are several screening instruments in the literature, but none of them have PICU validation.

Although it cannot assess children with abnormal anthropometrics, the Screening Tool for Risk of Impaired Nutritional Status and Growth (STRONGKids) seems to be a good admission screening test for malnutrition in PICUs. Three of these more widely used screening tools showed some variability in the classification of malnutrition risk, and none of them were able to identify a proportion of children with subnormal anthropometric measures, according to a recent multicenter study of inpatients in 14 hospitals across 12 European countries. Thus, it makes sense to integrate screening instruments with anthropometric measurements and to periodically reevaluate them while the patient is in the intensive care unit. Other potential malnutrition screening techniques, like computed tomography (CT), bioelectrical impedance, and ultrasound, are presently primarily employed for research purposes and have not been proven to be accurate. Ultrasound muscle mass and density screening, on the other hand, appear to be promising techniques for the future because of their widespread accessibility, low-cost needs, and low experience requirements for staff.

5.4.2. Nutritional Support Initiation

It is best to start nutritional (enteral) support as soon as possible. Enteral feeding should begin within the first 24 hours of admission, unless there is a contraindication. Gastritis is the recommended delivery method; oral is ideal. A gastric tube should be used if a person is unable to eat naturally due to swallowing problems or a risk of aspiration. Under all circumstances, breastfeeding or tube feeding with breast milk should be encouraged for small infants (i.e., less than six months of age). Breast milk can serve as the only nutritional source for very small, critically ill infants. Tight bowel stenosis, severe diarrhea, severe malabsorption, gut ischemia, decompensated shock, severe acidosis and/or hypoxemia, uncontrolled upper gastrointestinal (GI) bleeding, bowel obstruction, abdominal compartment syndrome, and high-output fistula are the traditional list of contraindications for enteral feeding.

5.4.3. Optimal Energy and Protein Delivery for a Critically Ill Child

Throughout the PICU stay, there are significant differences in the optimal energy delivery (higher in the recovery state, lower in the acute state). Since newborns and infants have higher E demands per kilogram, a simple formula (such as 20–25 kcal/kg during the acute stage and 30–35 kcal/kg during recovery in adults) will not work for all age groups. The indirect calorimetry (IC) approach is thought to be the best one for estimating each person's E demand specifically. Nevertheless, IC is still not widely available in PICUs. The Schofield, Food Agriculture Organization, World Health Organization (WHO), or United Nations University equations without additional risk factors can be used in the absence of IC to calculate the optimal energy delivery; the ESPNIC prefers the Schofield equation, which combines age, gender, height, and weight. Volumetric measurement of VO_2 and/or VCO_2 is another suggested technique for optimal/individualized E-target estimation. In both adult and pediatric critical care, the Harris-Benedict equation—which has been in use for several decades—is no longer advised. In the acute phase of adult critical illness, a hypocaloric target of 70% energy expenditure should be used, though this is not well defined for the pediatric population (Table 5.4).

Table 5.4. Energy Delivery Calculation Equations with Model Examples

Schofield Equation (kcal/Day)			
males	<3 years	REE = 0.167 × W + 15.174 × H − 617.6	598.59
	3–10 years	REE = 19.59 × W + 1.303 × H + 414.9	950.03
	10–18 years	REE = 16.25 × W + 1.372 × H + 705.8	1865.29
females	<3 years	REE = 16.252 × W + 10.232 × H − 413.5	567.58
	3–10 years	REE = 16.969 × W + 1.618 × H + 371.2	888.56
	10–18 years	REE = 8.365 × W + 4.65 × H + 200	1467.31

Food Agriculture Organization (MJ/D)			
males	<3 years	REE = 0.255 × W – 0.226	545.89
	3–10 years	REE = 0.0949 × W + 2.07	948.37
	10–18 years	REE = 0.0732 × W + 2.72	1647.32
females	<3 years	REE = 0.255 × W – 0.214	558.32
	3–10 years	REE = 0.0941 × W + 2.09	949.33
	10–18 years	REE = 0.051 × W + 3.12	1440.49
World Health Organization (WHO)			
males	<3 years	60.9 × W – 54	555
	3–10 years	22.7 × W + 495	949
	10–18 years	17.5 × W + 651	1648.5
females	<3 years	61 × W – 51	559
	3–10 years	22.5 × W + 499	949
	10–18 years	22.2 × W + 746	2011.4

REE—resting energy expenditure, kcal—kilocalorie, MJ—megajoule, 1 kcal = 4184 × 103 MJ, W—weight in kilograms, H—height in centimeters. Examples of REE in kcal of three model patients can be seen in the third column: 10 kg 80 cm, 20 kg 110 cm, 57 kg 170 cm, respectively.

Source: Kratochvíl M, Klučka J, Klabusayová E, Musilová T, Vafek V, Skříšovská T, Djakow J, Havránková P, Osinová D, Štourač P. Nutrition in pediatric intensive care: A narrative review. Children (Basel). 2022, 9(7):1031. doi: 10.3390/children9071031. PMID: 35884015; PMCID: PMC9318205.

Preventing a negative protein balance is the goal of protein delivery (high risk in the early phase). Protein delivery for pediatric patients should be at least 1.5 g/kg/day (and possibly more in cases of burns and respiratory failure). Nevertheless, there is currently no data supporting the beneficial effects of increased protein delivery (above 1.5 mg/kg/day) on overall clinical outcomes during the acute phase of critical illness. Deliveries of protein (or amino acids) should not surpass 3 g/kg/day or 2 g/kg/day for stable teenagers. Adult patients receive hypocaloric nutrition (not more than 70% of energy target) during the acute phase of critical illness, with a progressive increase of up to 100% of the E target in the case of indirect calorimetry over a period of three days, despite the lack of data for pediatric patients. Conversely, if predictive equations are used to estimate energy needs, hypocaloric nutrition—which does not exceed 70% of calculated energy need—is advised during the initial week of a critical illness. When compared to the late phase, when the anabolic process predominates (ration 1 gN:130 or higher), the protein E to nonprotein E ratio (defined by grams of nitrogen to nonprotein kcal ratio) should be higher in the acute phase (e.g., 1 gN:80 nonprotein kcal).

In the first seven days following PICU admission, the E and protein delivery attempts to meet 66% (up to 100%) of the calculated targets, preferably by enteral route, if at all possible. During the first week of their PICU stay, patients who are severely malnourished or who are not able to tolerate enteral nutrition at all may receive parenteral nutrition or supplemental parenteral nutrition. Parenteral nutrition, however, can be securely postponed until the eighth day, particularly in previously healthy, well-fed children. In light of the findings of the multicentric observational trial PEPaNIC, which showed that delayed parenteral nutrition was linked to better clinical outcomes and a lower frequency of related complications in pediatric intensive care unit patients, the ESPEN guidelines advise delaying parenteral nutrition during the first week of a patient's stay in the intensive care unit, regardless of nutritional status.

5.4.4. Macronutrients

5.4.4.1. Proteins

Proteolysis, low protein delivery, and a negative protein balance continue to be prevalent issues in PICU settings. Several guidelines recommend a daily minimum protein dose of 1.5 mg/kg; however, a much higher dose may be required to maintain a neutral or even positive protein balance. However, the dose of protein and amino acids in newborns and infants should not exceed 3 g/kg/d, and in stable adolescents, it should not exceed 2 g/kg/d. Amino acid polymers make up proteins. Three categories can be used to categorize amino acids: nonessential, semi-essential, and essential. Since the essential amino acids cannot be produced in the body, they must be taken orally, enterally, or parenterally. Many clinical situations, including infancy, critical illness, trauma, burns, and others, can make semi-essential (conditionally essential) amino acids necessary. The amino acid classification is listed in Table 5.5. The so-called pharmaconutrition (e.g., glutamine, arginine supplementation) is not currently recommended for PICU settings. However, supplementing with arginine (to prevent necrotizing enterocolitis), tyrosine and cysteine has been linked to better outcomes in preterm newborns. One gram of protein has approximately 4 kcal (17 kJ) of energy, which is the same as one gram of carbohydrates. Between 15 and 30% of the mixed enteral or parenteral formula should contain proteins or amino acids as part of the E delivery system.

Table 5.5. Amino Acid Classification by the Possibility of Synthesis In Vivo

Essential	Semi-Essential (Conditionally Essential)	Nonessential
Arginine	Cysteine	Alanine
Histidine	Glutamine	Asparagine
Isoleucine	Hydroxyproline	Aspartate
Leucine	Proline	Glutamate
Lysine	Taurine	Glycine
Methionine	–	Serine
Phenylalanine	–	Tyrosine
Threonine	–	
Tryptophan	–	
Valine		

Source: Kratochvíl M, Klučka J, Klabusayová E, Musilová T, Vafek V, Skříšovská T, Djakow J, Havránková P, Osinová D, Štourač P. Nutrition in Pediatric Intensive Care: A Narrative Review. Children (Basel). 2022 Jul 11;9(7):1031. doi: 10.3390/children9071031. PMID: 35884015; PMCID: PMC9318205.

5.4.4.2. Carbohydrates

With 4 calories per gram, carbohydrates should make up 40–60% of an E diet. Enteral feeding allows for the delivery of carbohydrates as polysaccharides (starch), oligosaccharides (lactose, mannose, and dextrins), and monosaccharides (glucose and fructose). Following the delivery of carbohydrates, oligomers and polymers are broken down into monomers by rapid glycolysis, with glucose serving as the primary final carbohydrate E substrate to be transported to the tissues. In parenteral nutrition, the carbohydrates are administered as glucose (dextrose) solutions at concentrations of 5, 10, 20, 30%, 40%, or even 50%. The optimal glucose concentration is determined by the fluid intake (higher concentration preferred in patients with limited daily fluid intake) and the delivery route (a peripheral intravenous line can be used up to 850 mosmol/L ≈ 12% glucose solution or lower). The delivery of carbohydrates and glucose should satisfy metabolic and energy requirements, but it shouldn't result in overfeeding, which could result in hyperglycemia and excessive CO_2 generation. Aiming to meet the basal E needs, glucose/carbohydrate delivery should range from 0.5 to 10 mg/kg/min (0.7–14 g/kg/day), with a lower threshold in older children and during the acute phase of critical illness, a higher threshold in younger patients, and a later (recovery) stage during the ICU stay. Although it is not advised, the so-called tight glucose control, which aims to maintain the laboratory glycemia reference levels, is linked to worse outcomes; nonetheless, hypoglycemia (<2.5 mmol/L) and/or hyperglycemia (>10 mmol/L) should all patients receive intensive treatment. Validated point-of-care (POCT) glucometers can measure blood glucose at the bedside using peripheral or capillary blood samples; however, arterial or central venous blood samples are recommended for patients who require high vasopressor dosage or shock.

5.4.4.3. Lipids

Complex enteral and/or parenteral nutrition cannot exist without lipids. Since 1 g of lipid contains 9 kcal of E, lipids constitute a significant E substrate that is over two times denser than proteins or carbohydrates. Additionally essential to cell membranes, lipids (phospholipids) are involved in hormone synthesis, vitamin metabolism (particularly the lipid-soluble vitamins A, D, E, and K), signaling, and other critical biochemical processes. Like amino acids, fatty acids, which make up the majority of fat tissue, can also be classified as essential or nonessential depending on whether or not the patient's body can synthesize them *in vivo*. Polyunsaturated omega-3 (ω–3) and omega-6 (ω–6) acids (linoleic acid) are essential fatty acids (EFAs) that need to be supplemented in diet. Because of their limited capacity for conversion, some fatty acids, including docosahexaenoic acid (DHA) and eicosatetraenoic acid (EPA), can be regarded as conditionally essential. As such, intake of these fatty acids needs to be closely monitored. Fish oil, vegetable-based oil, soybean oil, or a combination of these can be the basis of lipid formulas containing essential fatty acids. Lipid emulsion with a 10% or, ideally, 20% concentration is sold for parenteral nutrition. Between 25 and 50% of nonprotein calories (or about 20 to 30% of total E delivery) is the ideal range for lipid E delivery percentage. The recommended dose of composite 20% lipid emulsion in parenteral form is between 1.0 and 3.0 g/kg/day (or up to 4.0 g/kg/day in preterm and term infants). When administering lipids, nutrition markers—particularly serum triglyceride levels and liver biomarkers—should be watched closely. Lipid intake should be reduced when plasmatic triglyceride levels are elevated above 3 mmol/L in infants or 4 ± mmol/L in older children.

5.4.5. Fluid—Electrolytes

Infusion therapy, a crucial aspect of intensive care management, is used to address dehydration, hypovolemia, and hemodynamic optimization. Fluids are also prescribed as part of nutritional support to maintain hydration and replenish daily fluid losses. It is important to individualize fluid and electrolyte intake based on the patient's clinical condition, with isotonic-balanced crystalloid solutions being the preferred choice. Age-based guidelines for fluid intake exist: <1 year (120–150 mL/kg/day), 1–5 years (80–120 mL/kg/day), 6–18 years (50–80 mL/kg/day). In cases where balanced crystalloid solutions are not appropriate, electrolyte supplementation may be necessary. When administering fluids to critically ill children, careful consideration should be given to the patient's current volume status and avoid hyperhydration. Be mindful of the use of "junk fluids," such as those used for medication administration, to prevent unnecessary fluid overload.

5.4.6. Micronutrients

Numerous metabolic cycles and biochemical processes depend on vitamins and trace elements. Complex enteral feeding formulas, or even mixed hospital nutrition (best prescribed in collaboration with nutrition support professionals), contain sufficient amounts of water- and fat-soluble vitamins as well as trace elements (e.g., Cu, Fe, Zn, Se, and others) for patients on an oral diet or enteral nutrition. Outside of clinical trials, routine supplementation is not currently advised, despite recent widespread research on vitamin C supplementation in critical illness showing some encouraging results. Conversely, essential vitamins and trace elements are necessary for healthy metabolism in patients receiving parenteral nutrition. There are complex multivitamins on the market, but their availability varies by region. The manufacturer's recommendation should be followed for dosage and administration, ideally through a prolonged infusion lasting up to 24 hours. Table 5.6 lists the suggested vitamin and trace element dosages based on ESPEN (the level of expert opinion).

Table 5.6. Recommended Dosing of Vitamins and Trace Elements by the European Society of Clinical Nutrition and Metabolism (ESPEN)

Fat-Soluble Vitamins (Vitamin A, D, E, K)	
Vitamin A	150–300 μg/kg/d
Vitamin D	40–150 IU/kg/d up to 400–600 IU/d
Vitamin E	2.8–3.5 mg/kg/d or 2.8–3.5 IU/kg/d 11 mg/d or 11 IU/d
Vitamin K	10 μg/kg/d (or 200 μg/d
Water-Soluble Vitamins (Vitamin C, B Vitamins)	
Vitamin C	15–25 mg/kg/d up to 80 mg/d
Vitamin B1 (Thiamine)	0.35–0.50 mg/kg/d up to 1.2 mg/d
Vitamin B2 (Riboflavin)	0.15–0.2 mg/kg/d up to 1.4 mg/d
Vitamin B3 (Niacin)	4–6.8 mg/kg/d up to 17 mg/d
Vitamin B5 (Pantothenic acid)	2.5 mg/kg/d up to 5 mg/d
Vitamin B6 (Pyridoxine)	0.15–0.2 mg/kg/d up to 1.0 mg/kg/d
Vitamin B7 (Biotin)	5–8 μg/kg/d up to 20 μg/d
Vitamin B9 (Folic acid)	56 mg/kg/d up to 140 mg/d
Vitamin B12 (Cyanocobalamin)	0.3 μg/kg/d up to 1 μg/d
Trace Minerals/Elements	
Iron	50–250 μg/kg/d up to 5 mg/d
Zinc	50–500 μg/kg/d up to 5 mg/d
Copper	20–40 μg/kg/d up to 0.5 mg/d
Iodine	1–10 μg/kg/d
Selenium	2–7 μg/kg/d up to 100 mg/d
Manganese	≤1 μg/kg/d up to 50 mg/d
Molybdenum	0.25–1 μg/kg/d up to 5 mg/d

Source: Kratochvíl M, Klučka J, Klabusayová E, Musilová T, Vafek V, Skříšovská T, Djakow J, Havránková P, Osinová D, Štourač P. Nutrition in Pediatric Intensive Care: A Narrative Review. Children (Basel). 2022 Jul 11;9(7):1031. doi: 10.3390/children9071031. PMID: 35884015; PMCID: PMC9318205.

5.4.7. Enteral Nutrition

Unless it is contraindicated, enteral nutrition is the recommended method of nutrition support for pediatric patients in critical condition. The integrity of the gastrointestinal mucosa is positively impacted by enteral feeding, even at low dosages, and enterocytes are trophically affected. Oral intake is the most natural method, if it is feasible. As a result, it is important to evaluate PICU patients every day and to promote oral intake and early breastfeeding support. For the delivery of certain enteral nutrition formula or (fortified) breast milk, a gastric tube—preferably nasogastric—can be utilized in cases of consciousness disorders, profound sedation, or the incapacity to swallow or drink. Post-pyloric feeding—a feeding tube placed and floated further in the jejunum or inserted by an endoscopist—is a viable option in cases of severe aspiration risk or gastric feeding intolerance. One option for enteral feeding in chronic intensive care (a stay of six weeks or more) is a percutaneous gastrostomy (PEG) or jejunostomy (PEG-J or surgical jejunostomy).

Enteral nutrition can be administered in multiple ways: continuous feeding, which uses a feeding pump to administer EN over a 24-hour period; cyclic feeding, which uses a feeding pump to administer EN over a time of less than 24 hours; intermittent feeding, which uses a pump or gravity assist to administer EN over a 20–60 minute period every 4–6 hours; and bolus feeding, which uses a syringe to administer EN over a 4- to 10-minute period (5–6 times per day, up to 7–8 times in small infants). If there is insufficient enteral feeding tolerance, the application should be continuous or cyclical. The goal, as optimally outlined in an executed local-based nutrition/feeding protocol, is to attain the estimated E and protein delivery in a stepwise manner two to three days following PICU admission. See Figure 5.5 for a potential step-by-step enteral nutrition strategy.

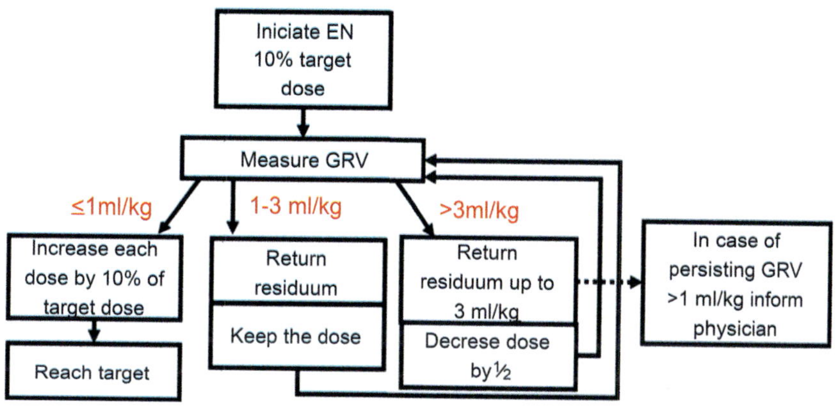

Figure 5.5. *Example of a stepwise approach to enteral nutrition.*

Source: Kratochvíl M, Klučka J, Klabusayová E, Musilová T, Vafek V, Skříšovská T, Djakow J, Havránková P, Osinová D, Štourač P. Nutrition in Pediatric Intensive Care: A Narrative Review. Children (Basel). 2022 Jul 11;9(7):1031. doi: 10.3390/children9071031. PMID: 35884015; PMCID: PMC9318205.

During the first seven days of enteral feeding, the goal is to achieve at least two-thirds of target E delivery. For most patients, the first formula can be the standard polymeric enteral one. An oligomeric or peptide-based formula can increase tolerance in patients who are not able to tolerate enteral feeding. Most nutrition formulas available in the market have an isocaloric value of 1 kcal/mL. One can use the dense/hypercaloric formulas (>1 kcal/mL) to set a daily maximum for enteral feeding volume. The best source of energy and nutrients for very small, critically ill infants should be breast milk. If breast milk is not available, certain infant formulas or formula milk with a low caloric content (approximately 0–0.75 kcal/mL) should be used. Although it is no longer advised for the evaluation of enteral feeding tolerance in critically ill enterally-fed children, routine gastric residual volume (GRV) assessment can still be used in regional feeding protocols. A clinical diagnosis of enteral feeding intolerance is made by an intensive care nurse, a clinician, or both based on the presence of diarrhea, abdominal distension, nausea/vomiting, or GRV > 3 mL/kg (if used, in ≥2 subsequent measurements). There are various approaches for managing enteral feeding intolerance, and healthcare professionals should adhere to their region's nutrition guidelines. Table 5.7 provides a list of strategies that can be used to mitigate possible enteral intolerance. For every patient receiving complete enteral nutrition, a daily minimum protein intake of ≥1.5 g/kg/d ought to be met. Add extra protein powders if the standard enteral formula does not accomplish this.

Table 5.7. Methods to Improve Enteral Feeding Intolerance

Prokinetics	Metoclopramide, Domperidone—agents for gastric motility improvement
Continuous enteral feeding via enteral feeding pump	Usually, 18–19 h of continuous administration via gastric tube with 5–6 h pause
Bowel stimulation	Erythromycin—stimulate the bowel motility Consider subcutaneous naltrexone in patients on opioids. Suppository rectally applied
Oligomeric formula	Oligomeric formula or peptide-based formula
Post-pyloric feeding	Jejunal tube placement and continuous enteral feeding without the night pause

Source: Kratochvíl M, Klučka J, Klabusayová E, Musilová T, Vafek V, Skříšovská T, Djakow J, Havránková P, Osinová D, Štourač P. Nutrition in Pediatric Intensive Care: A Narrative Review. Children (Basel). 2022 Jul 11;9(7):1031. doi: 10.3390/children9071031. PMID: 35884015; PMCID: PMC9318205.

5.4.8. Parenteral Nutrition

Compared to enteral nutrition, parenteral nutrition (PN) is linked to increased rates of morbidity, infectious complications, and mortality. For children who are not receiving any enteral nutrition, PN can be started individually during the first week of their PICU stay. Supplemental PN should be postponed for the first seven days (for patients receiving enteral nutrition). The daily content of supplemental PN should be customized based on the amount of enterally delivered feeding tolerance, protein and E targets, and other factors. In contrast, total parenteral nutrition should include trace minerals, vitamins, and electrolytes in addition to protein delivery based on an idealized mixed protein, carbohydrate, and lipids ratio (e.g., 25:50:25% of energy content). Osmolarity <850 mosmol allows for the administration of so-called peripheral parenteral nutrition through the peripheral venous cannula, reducing the risk of phlebitis and causing no irritation to the vein walls. Low osmolarity is caused by lower nutrient concentrations, a lack of lipid emulsion in the mixture, and glucose/dextrose concentrations below 10%. As a result, these types of PN cannot be used for total parenteral nutrition. Because of its high osmolarity, total PN should only be administered via a central vein catheter (CVC), peripherally inserted CVC (central venous catheter), tunneled CVC (central venous catheter), or central vein implanted port system. Total PN prescriptions can be made using either individually based nutrition (which includes all components of the system, including macronutrients and micronutrients recommended by the physician and primarily prepared by the hospital pharmacy) or commercially based/standard nutrition (made by pharmaceutical companies). To meet each patient's unique nutritional needs, the majority of patients (including newborns) should ideally use standard (commercially available default all-in-one preparations), with individually based PN serving as an additional option. Micronutrients should also be added using the prepared mixtures of water- and lipid-soluble vitamins and trace elements if standard parenteral nutrition is being used. Prematurely born babies have unique needs, and extra solutions may be required to meet those needs (such as higher calcium and phosphorus requirements).

5.4.9. Examples of Enteral and Parenteral Feeding Prescriptions in PICU

Example No. 1: a 6-year-old boy who was intubated and on mechanical ventilation after being admitted to the PICU due to septic shock and had no prior medical conditions.

- Anthropometric measurement and nutrition screening.—(e.g., Strong kids):
    - Low risk of malnutrition, weight = 25 kg, height 120 cm.
- Protein target calculation using indirect calorimetry, also known as Schofield equation E:
    - E Target: 1061 kcal/d, protein target at least: 37.5 g/d.

Within 24 hours of admission, gastric nutrition began following the insertion of a gastric tube and following the first stabilization measures (fluid resuscitation, antibiotics) following local protocol.

- In case of intolerance (GRV > 3 mL/kg, dose reduction and optimize to tolerance), the isocaloric enteral nutrition formula (1 kcal/1 mL, target 1061 mL/d) should be administered in bolus form five times a day. The initial bolus should be 10% of the estimated dose = 1061/5 times per day/10%≈ 20 mL of the first dose, 40 mL of the second dose, and 60 mL of the third dose.

Example No. 2. A female patient, 11 years old, was admitted to the PICU following a subtotal colectomy and had a low risk of refeeding syndrome. She had severe decompensated Crohn's disease.

- Anthropometric measurement and nutrition screening—(e.g., Strong kids):
    - High risk of malnutrition, weight = 35 kg, height 140 cm.
- Protein target calculation using indirect calorimetry, also known as Schofield equation E:
    - E target: 1276 kcal/d, protein target at least: 52.5 g/d.
- Enteral nutrition, severe abdominal distension, and gastric tube in

situ are currently contraindicated, according to the surgeon:

- Complete parenteral nutrition (including additional micronutrients) through a central line inserted centrally or peripherally, with regular evaluations of the potential for "trophic" enteral feeding.
- **If a Single Patient is Given the Following Dosage**: 53 g of 10% amino acids (525 mL) + 36 g of 20% lipid emulsion (180 mL) + 178 g of 40% glucose (445 mL) + 40 mL of 10% NaCl + 35 mL of 75% KCl + 5 mL of 10% $MgSO_4$ + 5 mL of Ca gluconicum + multivitamin + trace elements + 640 mL of Aqua Pro Injection (Holiday and Segar formula fluids 1875 mL/day).

5.4.10. Nutritional Status Evaluation During PICU Stay

Laboratory parameters (electrolytes, albumin, prealbumin, serum protein levels, serum transferrin, triglycerides, and other lipids) and nutritional status (anthropometric, weight gain/loss) should be closely monitored during the PICU stay. It is important to regularly assess the tolerance of patients receiving enteral feeding in order to quickly transition from gastric enteral feeding to a peroral diet. Because even a modest (so-called trophic) dose of enteral nutrition can have a positive effect on patients' overall morbidity and mortality (gut mucosa integrity, nutritional effect on enterocytes), it is important to regularly reevaluate enteral feeding in patients on PN.

One of the mainstays of intensive care for both adult and pediatric patients continues to be nutritional support. The accepted standard of care is the assessment of nutritional status and the provision of early nutritional support, preferably through enteral feeding, using a protocol-based approach. When possible, enteral nutrition is preferred over parenteral. Resuming oral intake should happen as soon as is practical. Breastfeeding and/or expressed breast milk consumption in infants should be encouraged; in fact, it may be the only source of nutrition (Hendricks, 2000; Holden, 2000; Baker and Robert, 2001; Suskind et al, 2011; Marotz, 2012; Koletzko, 2015; Kliegman, 2020).

5.5. PROTEIN-ENERGY MALNUTRITION

A type of malnutrition known as protein-energy undernutrition (PEU), formerly known as protein-energy malnutrition (PEM), is characterized by a variety of conditions resulting from an untimely shortage of dietary protein and/or energy (calories) in different amounts. There are three stages to the illness: mild, moderate, and severe.

5.5.1. Clinical Syndromes

The term "acute malnutrition" refers to a collection of related conditions that include marasmus, kwashiorkor, and intermediate stages of Marasmic kwashiorkor. Clinical findings are used to differentiate between them; edema is the main factor that sets kwashiorkor apart from marasmus. PEU is a relatively common condition that kills roughly 250,000 people a year worldwide in both adults and children. PEM is primarily seen in hospitals, is linked to illnesses, or is frequently observed in the elderly in the industrialized world. Keep in mind that PEU may develop as a side effect of other illnesses like cancer cachexia or chronic renal disease, which can also cause protein energy wasting (PEW).

Children are most affected by protein-energy undernutrition because they consume less protein. The few uncommon cases that do occur in the developed world almost exclusively affect young children due to fad diets or a lack of awareness of the nutritional needs of young people, especially in cases of milk allergy.

Types include:

- Kwashiorkor (predominant protein malnutrition).
- Marasmus (deficiency in calorie intake)
- Marasmic kwashiorkor, sometimes known as the most severe form of malnutrition, is characterized by a marked protein deficiency and a marked calorie insufficiency.

5.5.1.1. Marasmus

The word "marasmus" comes from the Greek word "marasmus," which means to wither or waste. The most common acute malnutrition syndrome is Marasmus. It results from consuming too little energy over several months to years. It is caused by a severe restriction in energy intake and is characterized by the wasting of body tissues, especially muscles and subcutaneous fat. It is the body's physiologic adaptive response to starvation in response to severe deprivation of energy and all nutrients. Due to their higher calorie needs and greater susceptibility to infections, children under the age of five are most frequently affected. These kids have bradycardia, hypotension, and hypothermia along with an emaciated, feeble, and listless appearance. Due to the loss of subcutaneous fat, their skin is xerotic, wrinkled, and loose; however, they do not exhibit any particular dermatosis. Because these areas of the body have lower metabolic activity, muscle wasting frequently begins in the axilla and groin (grade I), then moves to the thighs and buttocks (grade II), chest and abdomen (grade III), and lastly the face muscles (grade IV). In extreme situations, the children's faces appear older due to the loss of buccal fat pads. Children who are severely affected are often indifferent, but they can also get agitated and challenging to comfort.

5.5.5.2. Kwashiorkor

The word "kwashiorkor," which means "the sickness of the weaning," comes from the Kwa language of Ghana. In 1933, Cicely D. Williams coined the phrase. It is believed that eating too few calories but not enough protein causes kwashiorkor. It was initially discovered in kids whose diets consisted primarily of maize (these kids have been dubbed "sugar babies" because their meals are usually high in carbohydrates but low in protein). Kwashiorkor primarily affects older infants and young children and is common in developing nations. It mostly happens in places where there is famine or a shortage of food, especially in nations where the staple foods are beans, corn, and rice. Kwashiorkor is an example of an unsuitable starvation response. The hallmark of kwashiorkor—which is absent in marasmus—is edema, which is typically brought on by a confluence of factors including low serum albumin, elevated cortisol, and an incapacity to trigger the antidiuretic hormone. Grad I pedal edema is typically followed by grade II facial edema, grade III paraspinal and chest edema, and grade IV ascitis association. Clinical features include dermatoses, hypopigmented hair, distended abdomen, hepatomegaly, and nearly normal weight for age in addition to edema. Typically, hair is reddish yellow in color, dry, sparse, brittle, and depigmented. The typical cutaneous manifestations begin with dry, atrophic skin that confluences areas of hyperkeratosis and hyperpigmentation. When the skin is stretched, it splits, exposing underlying erythematous skin and causing erosions. These manifestations progress over several days. Children with kwashiorkor have a variety of skin abnormalities, such as dark erythematous pigmented macules (48%), shiny, varnish-like skin (64%), xerotic crazy paving skin (28%), residual hypopigmentation (18%), and hyperpigmentation and erythema (11%) (Figure 5.6).

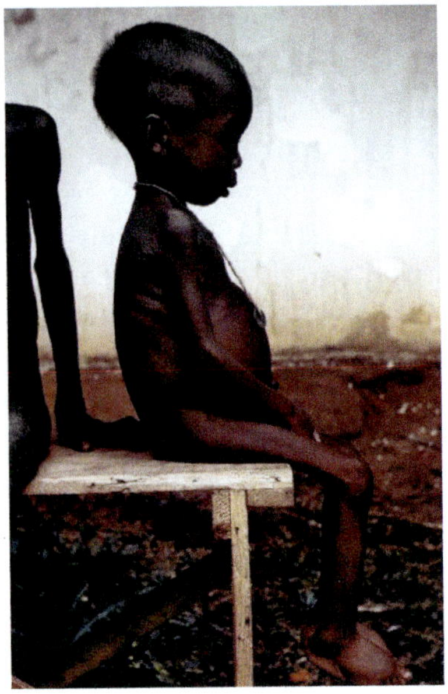

Figure 5.6. *A young girl with kwashiorkor in a relief camp during the Biafra War.*

Source: By Dr. Lyle Conrad – Centers for Disease Control and Prevention, Atlanta, Georgia, USAPublic Health Image Library (PHIL); ID: 6901http://phil.cdc.gov/, Public Domain, https://commons.wikimedia.org/w/index.php?curid=425975.

5.5.5.3. Marasmic Kwashiorkor

Marasmic kwashiorkor is a condition that combines characteristics of both marasmus and kwashiorkor. Children with this condition typically exhibit severe wasting and edema simultaneously. They may also experience mild skin and hair issues, as well as an enlarged, fatty liver that can be felt upon examination.

5.5.2. Epidemiology

Children from higher-income countries are also affected by protein energy malnutrition, including children from large urban areas in low socioeconomic neighborhoods, even though it is more common in low-income countries. Children who have chronic illnesses or who are hospitalized or institutionalized for a different diagnosis may also experience this. Intellectual disability as the primary diagnosis, cystic fibrosis, cancer, cardiovascular disease, end-stage renal disease, oncologic disease, genetic disease, neurological disease, multiple diagnoses, and extended hospital stays are examples of risk factors. Under these circumstances, the difficult nutritional management may be disregarded or undervalued, which could impair recovery prospects and exacerbate the condition.

Protein-energy malnutrition (PEM) is a prevalent issue globally, affecting both children and adults and leading to 250,000 deaths each year. In developed countries, PEM is most commonly observed in hospital settings, linked to various diseases, or prevalent among the elderly.

5.5.3. Co-Morbidity

A significant portion of kids with PEM also have other co-morbid illnesses. Of 66 subjects in the sample, diarrhea (72.2%) and malaria (43.3%) are the most common co-morbidities. Nonetheless, PEM has also been linked to a number of other illnesses, such as rickets, keratomalacia, HIV, TB, scabies, chronic suppurative otitis media, sepsis, severe anemia, and bronchopneumonia. These co-morbidities burden already malnourished children, lengthen their initial hospital stays for PEM, and raise their risk of death. Increased infectious comorbidity in malnourished individuals is generally explained by two factors: (1) malnutrition stresses and impairs immune function; and (2) the immune system keeps such diseases from spreading more widely in healthy, well-nourished individuals. Stated differently, malnutrition weakens the defenses against infectious diseases by causing (mild to moderate) immunodeficiency. For instance, this reversal is well known in relation to the fluctuating natural history of tuberculosis before the development of TB drugs. Epidemiological research has also shown links, through the shared underlying factor of poverty, between malnutrition and other health risks. For instance, condoms can stop the spread of HIV, but poor people frequently lack the funds or access to a store where they can purchase them. Furthermore, if an impoverished individual contracts a specific infection, they might not have access to the best care, which makes the illness worse, increases the risk of transmission, and so forth. Even in developing nations with universal health care and national health insurance, the poorest 25% of the populace may still have limited access to healthcare in practice.

5.6. THE ROLE OF NUTRITION IN MANAGING PEDIATRIC CHRONIC DISEASES

The health of their children is the top priority for all parents and physicians. Unfortunately, childhood chronic illnesses are becoming more and more common, leading to substantial morbidity and mortality. Childhood health and wellbeing are negatively impacted by many chronic conditions, including diabetes, obesity, and hypertension. More than 40% of children and adolescents in the US may have at least one chronic illness, according to a recent survey (e.g., obesity, asthma, etc.). The good news is that many disorders can be managed and prevented from starting with a proper diet.

5.6.1. Chronic Disease: Definition and Causes

Illnesses classified as chronic make worse with time. According to the World Health Organization (WHO), chronic illnesses account for 71% of all fatalities worldwide, making them the leading cause of mortality. Childhood obesity, diabetes, hypertension, and asthma are the most common chronic illnesses.

The following are a few of the frequently noted causes of pediatric chronic illnesses.

- **Genetics:** Genetic mutations that are inherited are the cause of some chronic illnesses, including sickle cell anemia and cystic fibrosis.
- Chronic illnesses like obesity and type 2 diabetes can be exacerbated by unhealthy lifestyle choices like poor eating, inactivity, and excessive screen time.
- Two conditions that increase the risk of chronic illnesses like asthma, heart problems, and type 2 diabetes are preterm delivery and low birth weight.
- **Exposure to Pollution:** Tobacco smoke, lead, and air pollution are examples of environmental contaminants that can increase a person's risk of developing chronic illnesses like allergies and asthma.

It is important to emphasize that many chronic illnesses have a complex and multifaceted etiology. Thus, early detection, prevention, and quality care are essential to improving outcomes for children with chronic illnesses.

5.6.2. Prevention of Chronic Disease with Nutrition

Prevention is key when it comes to treating chronic illnesses in children. Eating a healthy diet is one of the best ways to avoid chronic diseases. Children who eat a healthy, balanced diet are more likely to stay at a healthy weight, have stronger immune systems, and experience fewer chronic illnesses. Research indicates that children who consume a diet rich in fruits, vegetables, whole grains, and high-quality proteins are less likely to develop chronic illnesses. On the other hand, children who consume a diet high in processed foods, sugar, and saturated fats are more likely to develop chronic illnesses. Encouraging children to participate in meal planning and preparation, providing nutritious meals and snacks, and minimizing sugar-filled drinks and snacks can all contribute to healthy eating habits. Additionally, by offering nutrient-dense options in school meals and promoting physical activity, communities and schools can support the promotion of healthy eating practices.

5.6.3. Management of Chronic Disease with Nutrition

As was already mentioned, nutrition is crucial to preserving one's health. Therefore, a few dietary or nutrient-related adjustments can either prevent or manage the occurrence of chronic diseases in children. These actions are listed below:

- **Consultation with a Doctor or Qualified Dietitian:** Depending on the goals and health needs of the child, a registered dietitian or pediatrician can help create a customized nutrition plan.
- **Offer a Well-Balanced Diet:** Chronic condition management may benefit from a well-balanced diet high in fruits, vegetables, whole grains, lean meats, and healthy fats.
- **Regulated Portion Sizes:** To effectively manage chronic conditions like obesity, diabetes, and heart disease, portion sizes must be reduced. For assistance with portion control, consult a pediatrician or certified nutritionist.
- **Limit Your Intake of Harmful Fats and ADDED SUGARS:** CONSUMING added sugars, trans fats, and saturated and trans fats in excess may increase your risk of chronic illness. It's important to read food labels and steer clear of products that are high in added sugars and saturated fats.
- **Consume Enough Water and Fluids:** Diabetes and kidney disease are two chronic conditions that can be controlled by consuming more water and other fluids than necessary.
- **Consider Nutritional Supplementation:** Supplementing with nutrients may be necessary to maintain an adequate intake of vitamins and minerals in certain chronic conditions, such as inflammatory bowel disease or cystic fibrosis.

Lastly, maintaining a healthy diet is essential for managing and preventing childhood chronic illnesses. Children who eat a healthy, balanced diet are more likely to maintain a healthy weight, have stronger immune systems, and experience fewer chronic illnesses. Additionally, a healthy diet is essential for managing children's chronic illnesses because it reduces symptoms and improves overall health. To encourage healthy eating and prevent chronic illnesses, communities, schools, parents, and caregivers can all play a role (Hendricks, 2000; Holden, 2000; Baker and Robert, 2001; Suskind et al, 2011; Marotz, 2012; Koletzko, 2015; Kliegman, 2020).

A Closer Look

Marasmus

A severe form of malnutrition called marasmus is characterized by an energy deficit. Severe malnutrition can cause it in anyone, but children are typically the ones who experience it. Less than 62% of the typical (expected) body weight for the age is lost from the body. While the occurrence of kwashiorkor increases after 18 months, that of marasmus increases before the age of one. It differs from kwashiorkor in that whereas kwashiorkor is characterized by an adequate energy intake but a protein deficiency, marasmus is characterized by an inadequate energy intake in all forms, including protein. The clinical manifestation of marasmus and kwashiorkor cannot always be distinguished as kwashiorkor frequently occurs in the setting of inadequate caloric intake, leading to the possibility of mixed clinical presentations known as marasmic kwashiorkor. The main clinical signs of marasmus, which causes the ribs and joints to protrude, are muscular wasting and loss of subcutaneous fat. Protein wasting in kwashiorkor typically results in edema and ascites.

The outlook is more favorable than that of kwashiorkor. When children have co-morbid HIV and marasmus, which occurs in the latter stages of pediatric AIDS, their prognosis is extremely bad. Marasmus is the type of malnutrition most closely linked to HIV.

- **Signs and Symptoms:** A diminished, wasted appearance, loss of muscle mass, and subcutaneous fat mass are typical signs of marasmus. because of a lack of macronutrients and calories, particularly protein and adult survivors, which have an effect on development. The increased risk of pancreatic beta-cell dysfunction, which results in glucose intolerance and type 2 diabetes, is another long-term effect of marasmus. This could result in more visceral fat and less muscle mass. Additionally, there are metabolic ramifications such as decreased glucose metabolism and decreased insulin sensitivity. In addition, the risk of other non-communicable diseases (NCDs) and cardiovascular risk factors (CVRFs) is elevated. Not only are the survivors of mastitis affected, but also their progeny. There is a correlation between survivorship and low birth weight offspring. Long-term consequences of gene methylation also exist. Adult survivors of malaria may exhibit altered gene expression related to growth, immunity, and glucose metabolism.
- **Diagnosis:** Anthropometric measurements and a physical examination are the first steps in the diagnosis of marasmus. A physical examination can diagnose certain characteristics, such as severe wasting and stunting, as well as an abnormally thin appearance. Waste is computed by dividing weight by height. A child is deemed wasted if they deviate from the WHO standard by two standard deviations. The formula for stunting is the same, but for age ratios, it is based on height. The middle-upper arm circumference is another method used for measurement (MUAC). Blood

testing can be used to identify protein deficiencies as well as deficiencies in other important minerals and vitamins after a physical examination and measurements. This aids in assessing nutritional status and the presence of any marasmus indicators. Blood counts and stool samples are taken in severe infection cases. Some providers will check for edema to confirm that the patient has marasmus, as the nutritional condition is frequently linked to kwashiorkor. Edema is linked to kwashiorkor rather than marasmus.

- **Causes:** The following variables can lead to marasmus:
    - Maternal malnutrition
    - Maternal anemia
    - Poverty
    - Pathological conditions in a baby (e.g., diarrhea)
    - Pneumonia
    - Cyanotic heart diseases
    - Malaria
    - Necrotizing enterocolitis
    - Pyloric stenosis
    - Lactose intolerance
    - Intussusception
    - Meningitis
    - Anorexia nervosa
- **Treatment:** Treatment is required for the disorder's causes as well as its side effects, which include dehydration, infections, and circulation problems, all of which can be fatal if left untreated and result in a high death rate. First, the child is given boiled water mixed with dried skim milk. Refeeding must occur gradually in order to prevent refeeding syndrome. Children should have more nutritionally complete, balanced meals once they begin to heal. Children who have marasmus frequently get infections, which is why antibiotics or other drugs are used to treat them. Ultimately, when the body can no longer synthesize proteins, marasmus can advance to the point of no return. At this stage, feeding the patient food or protein won't cure the illness, and death is certain.
- **Prevent**ion: The most effective nutritional strategy to avoid marasmus is to eat a balanced, varied diet. Supplements containing protein and micronutrients, SAM treatment, and CTCs (comprehensive treatment centers) are additional interventions that specifically target nutrition. Education regarding nutrition, child development, and prenatal care is also crucial for moms and families. Supplementing with energy, protein, and micronutrients is essential to guaranteeing that the mother and child receive enough nourishment. To prevent marasmus and other forms of malnutrition in children under the age of two, it is also advised that children breastfeed exclusively for six months and 24 months to receive nutritional supplements.

Apart from proper nutrition, other preventive measures like access to clean water, sanitation, and hygiene play a crucial role in averting childhood illnesses and diarrheal disease, which can exacerbate severe acute malnutrition cases like marasmus. Additionally, a child with marasmus may become more susceptible to other diseases due to weakened immune systems. The child or anyone else who may be susceptible to malaria must have access to primary care in order to treat these conditions, prevent diarrheal illnesses that are frequently brought on by malnutrition, and track growth.

Summary

- The effects of nutrition on gene expression are only the beginning of the story because dietary components impact every step from gene to protein or metabolic product(s)—including signal transduction and posttranslational modifications of proteins.
- Feeding high-energy diet to rats leads to the early development of obesity and metabolic syndrome, apparently through an inability to cope with the energy density of the diet.
- Glucose, the most abundant monosaccharide in nature, provides a very good example of how organisms have developed regulatory mechanisms to cope with a fluctuating level of nutrient supply.
- Dietary fat is an important macronutrient for the growth and development of all organisms. In addition to its role as an energy source and its effects on membrane lipid composition, dietary fat has profound effects on gene expression leading to changes in metabolism, growth, and cell differentiation.
- Protein is essential for growth, to develop immunity, normal maintenance of body function and structure apart from reproduction and production (growth, milk, meat, egg, and wool).
- Prolonged feeding of a low-protein diet causes a decrease in the plasma level of most of the essential amino acids. For example, in the plasma of children affected by kwashiorkor, leucine and methionine concentrations can be reduced from; 100–150 mM and 18–30 mM to; 20 and 5 mM, respectively.
- Mothers' own milk is considered to be the best source of infant nutrition. Breast milk contains a variety of bioactive agents that modify the function of the gastrointestinal tract and the immune system, as well as in brain development.
- Human breast milk contains carbohydrates, protein, fat, vitamins, minerals, digestive enzymes and hormones. In addition to these nutrients, it is rich in immune cells, including macrophages, stem cells, and numerous other bioactive molecules.
- Infant formula is intended as an effective substitute for breast milk and is formulated to mimic the nutritional composition of breast milk. Formulas satisfy the quality factors of normal physical growth and a sufficient biological quality of protein components (adequate amounts of protein in a form that can be used by infants).
- Childhood and adolescence are periods of continuous growth and development. An infant grows rapidly, doubling its birth weight by 5 months and tripling it by 1 year of age. During the second year, the child increases not only in height by 7–8 cm but also gains 4 times its birth weight.
- Nutritional needs change as children leave the toddler years. From ages four to eight, school-aged children grow consistently, but at a slower rate than infants and toddlers. They also experience the loss of deciduous, or "baby," teeth and the arrival of permanent teeth, which typically begins at age six or seven.
- Puberty is the beginning of adolescence. The onset of puberty brings many changes, including the development of primary and secondary sex characteristics, growth spurts,

an increase in body fat, and an increase in bone and muscle development. All of these changes must be supported with adequate intake and healthy food choices.

- The initial protective body reaction to critical illness is based on simple phylogenetic targets aimed at oxygen and energy (E) delivery to the vital organs. During the acute phase (e.g., shock), multiple endocrine, immunology and metabolic reactions are initiated to minimize the initial insult. This stage is usually associated with compromised energy and protein delivery; moreover, energy utilization failure can also appear.
- Protein–energy undernutrition (PEU), once called protein-energy malnutrition (PEM), is a form of malnutrition that is defined as a range of conditions arising from a coincident lack of dietary protein and/or energy (calories) in varying proportions. The condition has mild, moderate, and severe degrees.
- Protein undernutrition is detrimental at any point in life, but protein undernutrition prenatally has been shown to have significant lifelong effects.
- Whether it involves managing chronic illnesses in children, prevention is everything. Proper eating is one of the most effective methods to prevent chronic illnesses. A nutritious and well-balanced diet can help youngsters maintain a healthy weight, strengthen their immune systems, and lower their risk of chronic illnesses.

References

1. Baker, R. D. Jr. (2001). *Pediatric Parental Nutrition* (1st ed.). Gaithersburg, MD: Aspen Publishers, Inc.
2. Beijers, R., Buitelaar, J. K., & de Weerth, C. (2014). Mechanisms underlying the effects of prenatal psychosocial stress on child outcomes: Beyond the HPA axis. *European Child & Adolescent Psychiatry, 23*(10), 943–956. https://doi.org/10.1007/s00787-014-0566-3.
3. Bhutta, Z. A. (2010). *Nutrition Interventions for Maternal and Child Health and Survival.* Karachi: Oxford University Press.
4. Collier, S., Fulhan, J., & Duggan, C. (2004). Nutrition for the pediatric office: Update on vitamins, infant feeding and food allergies. *Current Opinion in Pediatrics, 16*(3), 314–320. https://doi.org/10.1097/01.mop.0000131196.48763.d0.
5. Duggan, C., & Sonneville, K. (2014). *Manual of Pediatric Nutrition*. Shelton, Connecticut: People's Medical Publishing House-USA.
6. Durán Parada, K. (2012). Administration methods, infusion systems and necessary implements for home enteral nutrition. *Gastrohnup Journal, 14*(3), 129–130. Available at: https://revgastrohnup.univalle.edu.co/a12v14n3/a12v13n3art7.pdf (accessed on 11 September 2024).
7. Ferreyra, C. (2017). *Specialization in Critical Care Nursing*. Córdoba, Argentina: Faculty of Medical Sciences, pp. 16–20. Available at: http://lildbi.fcm.unc.edu.ar/lildbi/tesis/ferreyra-cynthia-soledad.pdf (accessed on 11 September 2024).
8. Hendricks, K. M., et al. (2000). *Manual of Pediatric Nutrition* (3rd ed.). Hamilton, Canada: B. C. Decker Inc.
9. Holden, C. (2000). *Nutrition and Child Health*. Edinburgh: Baillière Tindall, published in association with the RCN.

10. Kellams, A., Harrel, C., Omage, S., Gregory, C., & Rosen-Carole, C. (2017). ABM clinical protocol #3: Supplementary feedings in the healthy term breastfed neonate, revised 2017. *Breastfeeding Medicine, 12*(3), 188–198. https://doi.org/10.1089/bfm.2017.0036.
11. Kliegman, R. M., et al. (2020). Part V: Nutrition. In *Nelson Textbook of Pediatrics* (21st ed.). Elsevier.
12. Koletzko, B. (2015). *Pediatric Nutrition in Practice* (2nd ed.). Basel: Karger.
13. Laplante, D. P., Barr, R. G., Brunet, A., Du Fort, G. G., Meaney, M. L., & Saucier, J. F., et al. (2004). Stress during pregnancy affects general intellectual and language functioning in human toddlers. *Pediatric Research, 56*(3), 400–410. https://doi.org/10.1203/01.PDR.0000131780.95561.7F.
14. Letizia, A. G., Ge, Y., Vangeti, S., Goforth, C., Weir, D. L., Kuzmina, N. A., et al. (2021). SARS-CoV-2 seropositivity and subsequent infection risk in healthy young adults: A prospective cohort study. *The Lancet Respiratory Medicine, 9*(7), 712–720. https://doi.org/10.1016/S2213-2600(21)00134-6.
15. Lutz, C. A., & Przytulski, K. R. (2006). *Nutrition and Diet Therapy* (4th ed.). Philadelphia, PA: F. A. Davis Company.
16. Malawi. (2007). *Infant & Young Child Nutrition Policy*. Malawi: World Health Organization.
17. Marotz, L. R. (2012). *Health, Safety, and Nutrition for The Young Child* (8th ed.). Australia: Wadsworth Cengage Learning.
18. Morgan, R., Paul, S. M., & Fisher, M. F. (2004). Challenges and strategies for proper pediatric nutrition and weight control. *New Jersey Medicine: The Journal of the Medical Society of New Jersey, 101*(5), 33–36.
19. Pakistan. (2002). *Protection of Breastfeeding & Child Nutrition*. [Pakistan]: Dī Neṭvark, Ṣārifīn ke Taḥaffuẓ kā Idārah.
20. Rakers, F., Rupprecht, S., Dreiling, M., Bergmeier, C., Witte, O. W., & Schwab, M. (2020). Transfer of maternal psychosocial stress to the fetus. *Neuroscience & Biobehavioral Reviews, 117*, 185–197. https://doi.org/10.1016/j.neubiorev.2020.07.008.
21. Robertson, C. (2002). *Safety, Nutrition, and Health in Child Care*. Albany: Delmar Thomson Learning.
22. Salihagic-Kadic, A., Kurjak, A., Medić, M., Andonotopo, W., & Azumendi, G. (2005). New data about embryonic and fetal neurodevelopment and behavior obtained by 3D and 4D sonography. *Journal of Perinatal Medicine, 33*(6), 478–490.
23. Samour, P. Q. (2011). *Pediatric Nutrition* (4th ed.). Sudbury, MA: Jones & Bartlett Learning.
24. Samour, P. Q., & King, K. (2005). *Handbook of Pediatric Nutrition* (3rd ed.). Sudbury, MA: Jones and Bartlett Publishers, Inc.
25. Schetter, C. D., & Tanner, L. (2012). Anxiety, depression and stress in pregnancy: Implications for mothers, children, research, and practice. *Current Opinion in Psychiatry, 25*(2), 141–148. https://doi.org/10.1097/YCO.0b013e3283503680.
26. Suskind, D. L., & Lenssen, P. (2011). *Pediatric Nutrition Handbook*. West Sussex, UK: John Wiley & Sons, Ltd. https://doi.org/10.1002/9781118785034.
27. Temple, N. J., et al. (2006). *Nutritional Health: Strategies for Disease Prevention* (2nd ed.). Totowa, NJ: Humana.

Chapter

IMMUNIZATION AND INFECTIOUS DISEASES

6

Contents

INTRODUCTION

Immunizations are crucial for ensuring children have a healthy start in life and continue to be healthy as they age. The many vaccine-preventable diseases that were once common have not been seen by many parents today because immunization programs of the 20th and 21st centuries have been so successful. They might not be aware that those contagious illnesses might resurface. Certain diseases that are currently uncommon or nonexistent in the U.S. could arise if people decide not to vaccinate themselves or their children might come back. Infectious diseases that used to be common in children in the U.S. – including measles, polio, diphtheria, rubella (German measles) and chickenpox – are preventable with vaccines approved by the U.S. Food and Drug Administration. Vaccines have the power to stop infectious diseases that used to kill or seriously damage a lot of newborns, kids, and adults. The FDA makes sure that any vaccinations we approve or permit for use in emergencies within the U.S. satisfy our requirements for quality, safety, and effectiveness.

People require vaccinations throughout childhood to protect them from potentially dangerous infectious diseases, from babies to teenagers. Without vaccinations, kids would be more susceptible to diseases like measles, whooping cough, or meningitis caused by Haemophilus influenzae type b (Hib), which can cause serious illness, disability, or even death.

Orientation and Directional Terms

Term	Definition	Illustration
Tuberculosis	Tuberculosis (TB) is an infection that most often attacks the lungs, but in infants and young children, affects other organs like the brain. A severe case could cause serious complications or death.	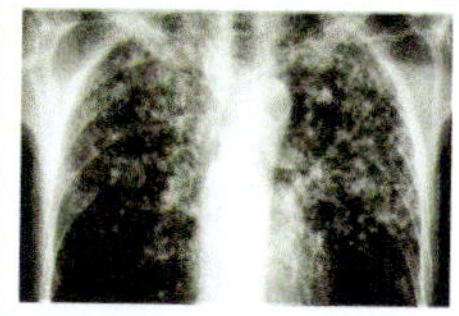
Hepatitis B	Hepatitis B virus is a dangerous liver infection that, when caught as an infant, often shows no symptoms for decades. It can develop into cirrhosis and liver cancer later in life.	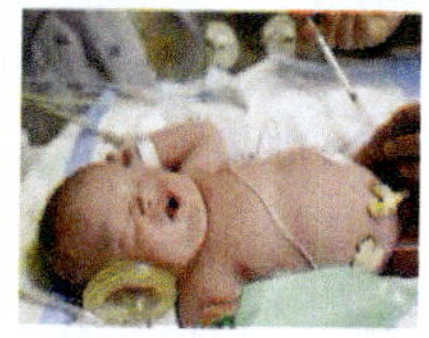
Polio	Polio is a virus that paralyzes 1 in 200 people who get infected. Among those cases, 5 to 10% die when their breathing muscles are paralyzed. There is no cure for polio once the paralysis sets in – only treatment to alleviate the symptoms.	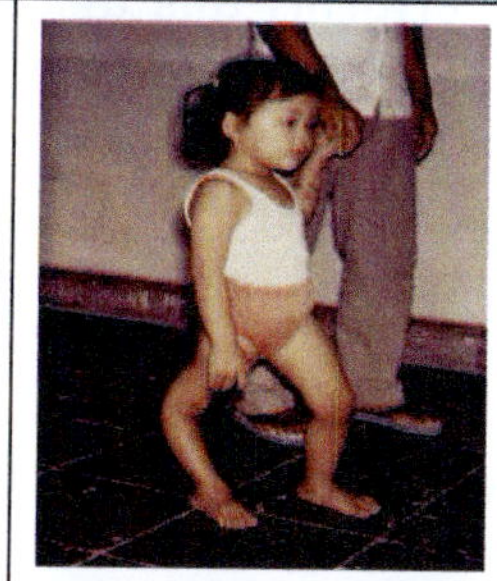
Diphtheria	Diphtheria infects the throat and tonsils, making it hard for children to breathe and swallow. Severe cases can cause heart, kidney and/or nerve damage.	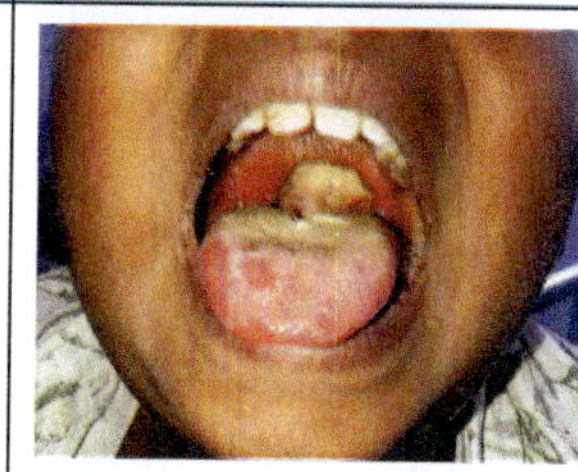
Tetanus	Tetanus causes very painful muscle contractions. It can cause children's neck and jaw muscles to lock (lockjaw), making it hard for them to open their mouths, swallow (breastfeed) or breathe. Even with treatment, tetanus is often fatal.	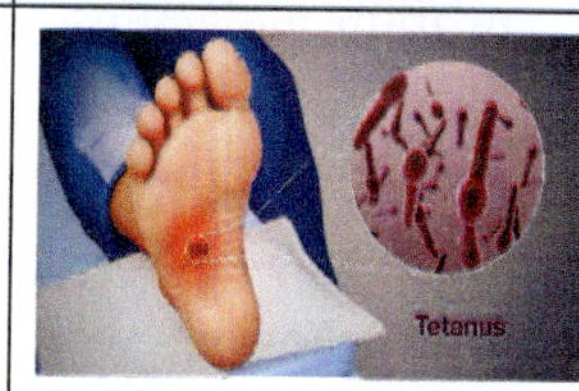
Pertussis	Pertussis (whooping cough) causes coughing spells that can last for weeks. In some cases, it can lead to trouble breathing, pneumonia, and death.	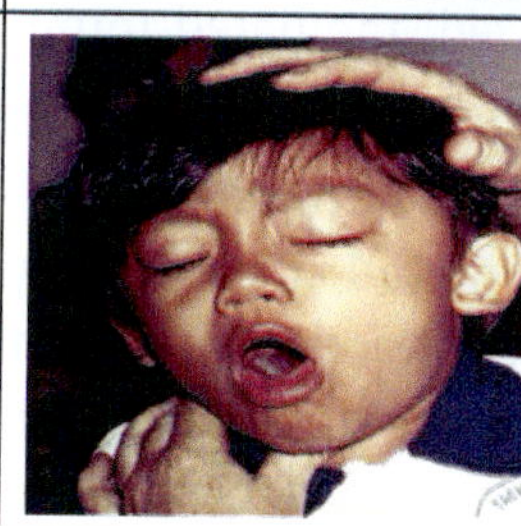

6.1. THE PRINCIPLES AND PRACTICE OF IMMUNIZATIONS

It helps to comprehend the fundamental operation of the human immune system to comprehend vaccinations and the basis of advice regarding their use. The human body's capacity to both eliminate foreign substances and tolerate the presence of materials that are native to it is known as immunity. The immune system is a complex network of interacting cells that performs this discriminatory ability to eliminate foreign substances. The majority of organisms, such as bacteria, viruses, and fungi, are considered foreign, so being able to recognize and get rid of them protects against infectious diseases. Generally speaking, immunity is restricted to a single organism or a small group of closely related organisms.

Antigens are chemicals that can activate the immune system, and the immune system builds a defense against them. The immune response, which is this defense, typically entails the production of:

- B-lymphocytes (B-cells) produce protein molecules (immunoglobulins or antibodies, the main component of humoral immunity).
- particular cells—such as T-lymphocytes, which are linked to cell-mediated immunity.

Immune responses are most successful when triggered by antigens found in live organisms. However, not all antigens need to come from live organisms to activate an immune response. For example, the hepatitis B surface antigen can still prompt a protective immune response even if not from a live virus. Some materials may not be as effective as antigens, potentially leading to a weaker immune response that offers less protection (Demirjian and Levy, 2009; Havelaar et al, 2010; Davis, 2011; Ginsburg et al, 2014; Rappuoli et al, 2017).

6.1.1. Anatomy and Physiology

Immune system modulation by vaccines is mainly mediated by B- and T-lymphocytes. The immune system is composed of B- and T-lymphocytes, each of which can react to a distinct antigen before exposure. Furthermore, a lot of antigens demand a joint response from T- and B-lymphocytes. We call this type of immunity T-cell-dependent immunity. It happens less frequently that an antigen stimulates B-lymphocytes and antibody production independently of T-lymphocyte assistance. It is known as T-cell-independent immunity.

The process that triggers the start of the immune response is initiated by the introduction of the antigen by the vaccine. First, macrophages phagocytize and degrade the foreign material. Subsequently, the breakdown of the protein material produces peptides that are transported to the surface of the macrophage cell, where they are visible. MHC-I and MHC-II, two different forms of Major Histocompatibility Complexes, are molecules that display these antigens. Several inflammatory mediators, such as cytokines and different interferons, are secreted in response to the antigen presentation, and this triggers an additional response.

T-helper cells identify the antigen and encourage corresponding B-lymphocytes to multiply and generate antibodies in T-cell-dependent immunity. B-lymphocytes divide into plasma cells that produce antibodies as they multiply. The production of antibodies serves a variety of purposes, the most significant of which are to neutralize pathogenic virus reproduction (neutralizing antibodies), facilitate intracellular bacterial digestion (lysins), inactivate soluble protein toxins (antitoxins), and inhibit bacterial adhesion to mucosal surfaces (antiadhesion). Following vaccination, the body gradually converts from producing mostly IgM antibodies to IgG antibodies over the course of several weeks. Vaccines can be categorized as subunits, toxoids (tetanus), killed or inactivated vaccines, or live attenuated vaccines.

6.1.2. Types of Immunity

Passive and active immunity acquisition are the two main methods.

6.1.2.1. Passive Immunity

Protection from antibodies or antitoxins produced by one animal or person and passed on to another is known as passive immunity. Although it offers momentary protection from infection, passive immunity does so. After a few weeks to months, the recipient will no longer be protected as the antibodies break down. The type of passive immunity that a newborn inherits from its mother is the most prevalent. During the final one to two months of pregnancy, antibodies—more especially, the IgG class of antibodies—are carried across the placenta. A full-term baby will therefore have the same kind of antibodies as the mother. During the first few months after birth, these antibodies can shield the baby from specific illnesses. Certain diseases (like measles, rubella, and tetanus) are better avoided by those with maternal antibodies than others (like polio and pertussis).

Transfusions of blood products can also result in the acquisition of passive immunity. Certain blood products, like reconstituted or cleansed red blood cells, have comparatively little antibody, whereas other blood products, like intravenous immune globulin and plasma products, have a lot. There are three main sources of antibodies used in human medicine, apart from blood products used in transfusions. These consist of heterologous hyperimmune serum, homologous human pooled antibody, and homologous human hyperimmune globulin.

Homologous pooled human antibody, also called immune globulin, is created by combining the antibody fraction—more especially, the IgG class of antibodies—from thousands of adult donors' blood. It has antibodies to a wide range of antigens since it comes from numerous donors. Its main uses are in the prevention of measles and hepatitis A, as well as in the treatment of specific congenital immunoglobulin deficiencies.

Homologous human hyperimmune globulins are antibody products with higher antibody titers directed toward more specialized antigens. These goods are created using high concentrations of the target antibody in donated human plasma. Hyperimmune globulins are mainly polyclonal, containing a wide variety of antibodies in smaller amounts, due to their human origin. For postexposure prophylaxis, hyperimmune globulins are used to prevent rabies, varicella, tetanus, and hepatitis B.

Heterologous hyperimmune serum, sometimes referred to as antitoxin, is made by animals—mostly horses—and is composed of antibodies that target a single antigen. Antitoxins can be used to treat diphtheria and botulism in the United States. Serum sickness is an immune response to the horse protein that can be brought on by these products.

Human immune globulin products are mainly made up of polyclonal antibodies, which consist of a variety of antibodies. Monoclonal antibody products are versatile and can be used for diagnosing specific cancers (such as colorectal, prostate, ovarian, and breast cancer), treating various types of cancer (like B-cell chronic lymphocytic leukemia and non-Hodgkin lymphoma), preventing transplant rejection, and treating autoimmune diseases (including Crohn's disease and rheumatoid arthritis) and infectious diseases.

Monoclonal antibody products, which are directed against a single antigen or a closely related group of antigens, do not interfere with the immune response to live-virus vaccines, in contrast to certain antibody products, such as immune globulins. Palivizumab (Synagis), a monoclonal antibody product, is available to prevent respiratory syncytial virus (RSV) infection. Synagis won't obstruct the body's reaction to a live vaccination because it only contains RSV antibodies.

6.1.2.2. Active Immunity

Protection generated by one's own immune system is known as active immunity. An antigen stimulates the immune system to produce both cell- and antibody-mediated immunity. Active immunity, in contrast to passive immunity, is often long-lasting—often lasting a lifetime. Surviving an infection with the disease-causing form of the organism is one way to develop active immunity. With a few exceptions, such as malaria, most people who recover from infectious diseases will have lifelong immunity to that illness. Immunologic memory is the capacity to retain protection for a considerable amount of time following an infection. Some memory B-cells stay in the bone marrow and circulate in the bloodstream for many years after the immune system is exposed to an antigen. When the antigen is encountered again, these memory cells quickly multiply and start to make antibodies in order to restore protection.

Vaccination is another method to create active immunity. Vaccines contain antigens that trigger the immune system to generate a response similar to that of a natural infection. Unlike natural infection, vaccination prevents the recipient from being infected by the disease and experiencing potential complications. Various factors can impact the immune response to vaccination, including the presence of maternal antibodies, the type and amount of antigen, the method of administration, and the use of adjuvants like aluminum-containing materials. Host factors like age, diet, genetics, and existing health conditions also play a role in affecting the immune response. Vaccines that closely resemble the disease-causing organism tend to produce a stronger immune response.

6.1.3. Classification of Vaccines

There are two basic types of vaccines:

- Live, attenuated, and
- Inactivated. The differences in their characteristics dictate the usage of each type.

6.1.3.1. Live, Attenuated Vaccines

Live vaccinations come from "wild" bacteria or viruses. In a lab setting, these wild viruses or bacteria are attenuated (weakened), usually through repeated culturing. For instance, the measles virus that is currently used in vaccinations was discovered in a child who had the illness in 1954. To convert the wild virus into the attenuated vaccine virus, a tissue culture medium had to be serially passed through for nearly 10 years.

Live, attenuated vaccines need to replicate in the recipient to elicit an immune response. When a virus or bacteria is given in relatively small doses, the body replicates the organism and produces enough of it to trigger an immune response. Live, attenuated vaccines do not always cause diseases similar to those caused by the organism in its wild form, although they do replicate.

When a live, attenuated vaccine does result in illness, it is typically far less severe than the underlying condition and is regarded as a vaccine adverse reaction.

Because the immune system cannot distinguish between an infection caused by a wild virus and an infection with a weakened vaccine virus, the immune response to a live, attenuated vaccine is essentially the same as that resulting from a natural infection. Most recipients of injected live, attenuated vaccines develop immunity after just one dose. A second dose of an injected live, attenuated vaccine (like the measles, mumps, and rubella [MMR]) is advised to provide an exceptionally high level of immunity in the population, as a small percentage of recipients do not respond to the first dose. Live, attenuated vaccinations given orally need multiple doses to induce immunity.

Due to unchecked vaccine virus or bacterial replication, a live, attenuated vaccination may result in serious or deadly infections. But only those with compromised immune systems—such as those afflicted with leukemia, certain medication side effects, or HIV infection—experience this. It is theoretically possible for a live, attenuated vaccine virus to revert to its pathogenic form. Only the live (oral) polio vaccine has been shown to cause this, and it is no longer accessible in the US.

A circulating antibody may interfere with the vaccine virus, preventing the development of active immunity from a live, attenuated vaccination. Any type of antibody can prevent the vaccine organism from replicating, which can result in a poor or nonexistent immune response—a condition known as vaccine failure. Examples of such immune sources include transplacental transfer to infants and blood product transfusions.

Vaccines that are live and attenuated are delicate and can be ruined by heat and light. They need to be handled and stored with caution. Currently available and regularly advised in the United States are live, attenuated viral vaccines against influenza (intranasal), varicella, rotavirus, and MMR. The adenovirus vaccine (used by the military), the typhoid vaccine (Ty21a), and the Bacille Calmette-Guerin (BCG) vaccine are additional live vaccines that are not frequently advised. In the US, BCG is administered as a bladder cancer treatment rather than as a vaccine.

6.1.3.2. Inactivated Vaccines

Vaccines that have been inactivated are not live and cannot spread. Even in those with compromised immune systems, these vaccinations cannot spread illness. Since inactivated antigens are less susceptible to circulating antibodies than live antigens, they can be administered when blood antibody levels are high (e.g., either during infancy or after receiving blood products containing antibodies).

Generally speaking, live, attenuated vaccinations produce immunity that lasts longer than inactivated vaccinations. It takes several doses spread over time to achieve sustained immunity. Generally speaking, the initial dosage "primes" the immune system rather than producing protective immunity. After the second or third dosage, an immune response that is protective arises. The immune response to an inactivated vaccine is primarily the production of antibodies, as opposed to live vaccines, which elicit an immune response that closely mimics a natural infection. There's little to no cellular immunity. Over time, antibody titers against inactivated antigens decrease. Therefore, to raise, or "boost," antibody titers, some inactivated vaccines might need to be administered infrequently at additional doses.

Whole-cell inactivated vaccines are among the inactivated vaccinations (e.g., hepatitis A, rabies, and polio vaccinations), subunit vaccinations (e.g., vaccinations against pneumococcal and influenza), toxoids (e.g., tetanus toxoid and diphtheria), as well as recombinant vaccines (e.g., flu [Flublok brand], hepatitis B, and human papillomavirus [HPV]).

Vaccines that are whole-cell inactivated contain viruses or bacteria that have been rendered inert via chemical or physical means. In the US, there are whole-cell inactivated viral vaccines against rabies, hepatitis A, and polio. Outside of the US, a vaccine against whooping cough (pertussis) is available. It is made from whole killed bacteria.

A subunit of the bacteria or virus is present in subunit vaccines. The organism's portion that is chosen is the portion required to trigger a defense immune response. In subunit vaccines, the antigens may be polysaccharides, proteins, or a mix of polysaccharides and proteins (i.e., conjugate vaccination, for example).

Subunit conjugate vaccine conjugation is the chemical process by which a polysaccharide from the surface of bacteria is joined to a protein molecule to create vaccines (such as pneumococcal conjugate and *Haemophilus influenzae* type B). Long-lasting protective immunity against a polysaccharide antigen is produced when the polysaccharide antigen is conjugated to a protein molecule.

Pure polysaccharide vaccines can stimulate B-cells without the aid of T-helper cells, as the immune response to these vaccines is generally T-cell-independent. Due to the immune system's immaturity, T-cell-independent antigens, such as polysaccharide vaccines, do not consistently elicit an immune response in children under the age of two. In populations where a polysaccharide vaccine is ineffective or only offers transient protection, bacterial infections can be prevented by attaching the polysaccharide antigen to a protein.

Toxins generated by bacteria are inactivated and used to make toxin vaccines. These toxins made of proteins are rendered inactive by heat, chemicals, or other means. Some bacteria (e.g., tetanus, and diphtheria) create toxins that lead to illness. The immune system's capacity to identify and get rid of these toxins shields the body from illness.

Recombinant DNA technology is used to create recombinant vaccines. Combining DNA from two or more sources is possible thanks to recombinant DNA technology. Vaccines against influenza (Flublok brand), hepatitis B, and human papillomavirus (HPV) are made by inserting a portion of the respective viral gene into the gene of a yeast cell or virus. When the modified yeast cell or virus multiplies, it produces pure influenza hemagglutinin, HPV capsid protein, or hepatitis B surface antigen. Using recombinant technology, proteins and outer membrane vesicles are produced as serogroup B meningococcal vaccines.

6.1.4. Indications

Vaccinations against various bacteria and viruses during childhood are recommended to prevent infections and their aftereffects. The recommended childhood vaccination schedule differs depending on the area, just as disease exposure does (Figure 6.1).

As of right now, adult vaccination recommendations include a yearly influenza shot, a tetanus-diphtheria booster every 10 years, and a tetanus-diphtheria-acellular pertussis booster at least once during adulthood. The goal of including acellular pertussis once in adulthood is to stop whooping cough from spreading to young children or people who are not able to receive the vaccination.

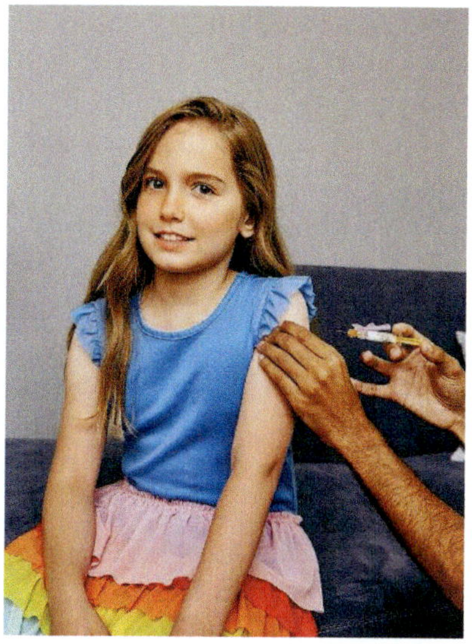

Figure 6.1. *Girl about to be vaccinated in her upper arm.*

Source: By SELF Magazine – Young girl about to receive a vaccine in her upper arm, CC BY 2.0, https://commons.wikimedia.org/w/index.php?curid=81631650.

It is advised that adults born after 1956 who were not vaccinated against measles, mumps, rubella, or varicella as children get these shots as adults. Vaccinations against hepatitis A, hepatitis B, and the human papillomavirus are also advised for adults. Adults at high risk, such as those residing in close quarters (college students living in dorms, military personnel living in barracks), are advised to get the meningococcal vaccine. Adults who are considered high-risk, such as those who already have pulmonary conditions like chronic obstructive pulmonary disease (COPD), should also get vaccinated against pneumococcal disease.

Patients who are immunocompromised or unable to produce antibodies should receive passive immunization. It's also relevant in cases where the illness could manifest before active immunity has a chance to produce antibodies, like in rabies patients. In this case, the patient might contract rabies before the effective production of antibodies by active immunization. Regardless of a history of SARS-CoV-2 infection, vaccination against COVID-19 is recommended for those older than six months. This includes suggestions for those with long-lasting COVID-19 symptoms.

6.1.5. Contraindications

Immunization contraindications are uncommon. An allergy to a vaccine or a component of the vaccine is the main reason not to get it. When receiving a live attenuated vaccine, patients with a history of immune system impairment, such as AIDS or another immune deficiency, should exercise caution. Given that live attenuated vaccines have the potential to infect the fetus, pregnant women should not receive them unless there is an immediate risk (such as a polio epidemic). Generally speaking, live vaccinations shouldn't be given to severely immunocompromised individuals.

When giving a vaccine to a child who has an acute, moderate-to-severe illness—with or without a fever—care should be taken. It might be challenging to identify whether a fever that occurs after vaccination in this population is the direct result of the vaccination or a result of ongoing illness. This could make treating the illness more difficult. Rotavirus vaccinations are contraindicated in cases of severe combined immunodeficiency (SCID) and prior history of intussusception, according to the CDC. The Advisory Committee on Immunization Practices (ACIP) states that patients who have experienced encephalopathy within seven days of receiving a pertussis-containing vaccine shouldn't receive any more doses of that vaccine.

6.1.6. Equipment

Using sterile needles and syringes, vaccinations are given. The vaccination, the precise method of administration, and the preference of the clinician all influence the size and kind of syringe and needle. It is also necessary to wear personal protective equipment, such as medical gloves. Before administering the vaccine, the skin is prepared with alcohol or another topical disinfectant. After administration, the site can be covered with a simple band-aid, gauze, and tape.

6.1.7. Personnel

Healthcare professionals who administer vaccinations include medical assistants, licensed practical nurses and licensed vocational nurses, registered nurses, nurse practitioners, physicians, physicians' assistants, pharmacists, and pharmacy technicians.

6.1.8. Preparation

Depending on the manufacturer, vaccinations are available in different preparations. Combinations of vaccinations are common; examples include the measles, mumps, rubella or tetanus, diphtheria, and vaccine against acellular pertussis. There are two types of vaccine preparations: single-dose and multi-dose. While some vaccines are supplied in vials that need to be drawn into a syringe before administration, others are prefilled syringes. Acyclovir, famciclovir, or valacyclovir use of particular antiviral medications should be discontinued 24 hours before varicella vaccination. Antiviral medication should also be avoided for 14 days following varicella vaccination.

6.1.9. Technique or Treatment

Immunizations are usually given intramuscularly, meaning that the preparation is injected straight into the belly of a muscle. Certain vaccinations are administered transdermally or subcutaneously.

6.1.10. Complications

A minor percentage of vaccines have the potential to cause B-symptoms, such as fever, exhaustion, and myalgias, after injection. These symptoms, which typically last a day or two, are brought on by the immune system mounting a defense against the antigen that the vaccine introduces. The injection site may swell, turn red, and experience localized muscle soreness. Although extremely rare, more serious complications are possible. A vaccination or one of its constituents may cause anaphylaxis.

Guillain-Barre Syndrome is an extremely uncommon but potentially fatal condition that affects the peripheral nervous system and is brought on by vaccinations. It is unknown how vaccinations result in Guillain-Barre syndrome. Ascending paresthesias and paralysis are among the symptoms; respiratory muscle paralysis is a possibility.

6.1.11. Clinical Significance

Maintaining public health requires vaccination. It has been demonstrated that disease prevention increases life expectancy and improves quality of life. Significant outbreaks of diseases once thought to be exterminated or almost exterminated have occurred as anti-vaccination movements gain momentum. Regrettably, patients and primary care physicians frequently overlook preventive measures like vaccinations. Parents frequently don't know when their children should receive their vaccinations because they don't know the proper vaccination schedule. Missed appointments for a variety of reasons is another frequent cause of vaccination misses. Systems for patient recall and reminders have been developed, and they have significantly increased the rates of vaccination compliance.

6.1.12. Enhancing Healthcare Team Outcomes

Immunization administration and compliance monitoring are normally the responsibilities of nurses, pharmacists, and other healthcare professionals. In many cases, patients' parents and other caregivers are not solely to blame for low vaccination compliance. In addition, primary care physicians, nurses, and pharmacists may neglect preventive care because they are preoccupied with appointments related to particular ailments or symptoms or the need to fill prescriptions. Systems for provider recall and reminders have also been developed, and they have also demonstrated an increase in vaccination compliance. To guarantee that everyone in the community is protected by the proper vaccination, the team must cooperate (Demirjian and Levy, 2009; Havelaar et al, 2010; Davis, 2011; Ginsburg et al, 2014; Rappuoli et al, 2017).

6.2. IMMUNIZATION SCHEDULES

For children, vaccination is a crucial and successful health intervention. It has aided in protecting millions of kids from infectious and potentially fatal diseases throughout history. Some diseases that were once thought to be incurable are now either completely eradicated or very easily controlled thanks to vaccinations. However, a lot of new diseases have also been discovered recently. This emphasizes the need to immunize children even more.

Administering vaccines to children at the appropriate age and dosage is essential for their effectiveness. Children are most vulnerable to certain diseases at specific ages, such as polio being more prevalent in children under 5 years old. By vaccinating children within this age group, the risk of harm from the disease is greatly reduced. Failure to vaccinate or delay in vaccination leaves a child unprotected and significantly increases their likelihood of becoming severely ill.

6.2.1. At Birth

6.2.1.1. Bacillus Calmette Guerin (BCG)

- This is a single-dose vaccine.
- Given as an injection to the upper arm.
- The tuberculosis vaccine provides protection from the disease.
- This vaccination may cause the following side effects:
  - discomfort or discharge at the injection site.
  - High temperature
  - Headache
  - swollen glands beneath the armpit on the immunization-affected arm.

6.2.1.2. Oral Polio Vaccine (OPV) – 0 Dose

- At birth, this is the first dose administered. Your child takes the third dose at 10 weeks, the fourth at 14 weeks, and the fifth at six weeks.
- Administered orally
- The poliovirus, a highly contagious illness that attacks the nervous system and can cause complete paralysis, is prevented by this vaccine. The majority of the virus's victims are young children, under five.

- Potential side effects of this vaccine include:
  - There are no common side effects associated with this vaccine.

6.2.1.3. Hepatitis B Birth Dose

- This is a single-dose vaccine.
- Administered via injection
- This vaccine guards against the viral infection known as hepatitis B, which damages the liver and can result in both acute and chronic illness.
- This vaccination may cause the following side effects:
  - Side effects are rare, with the exception of minor redness and soreness where the injection was administered.
  - Since the vaccine is inactivated (dead), it cannot spread the infection.

6.2.2. 6 Weeks

6.2.2.1. Oral Polio Vaccine (OPV) – 1

- At six weeks, this is the second dose of OPV. Your child takes their next dose at 10 weeks, and their last dose at 14 weeks.
- Administered orally
- The poliovirus, a highly contagious illness that attacks the nervous system and can cause complete paralysis, is prevented by this vaccine. The majority of the virus's victims are young children, under five.
- This vaccine doesn't have any typical side effects.

6.2.2.2. Pentavalent – 1

- At six weeks old, this is the first dose administered. Your child takes their next dose at 10 weeks, and their last dose at 14 weeks.
- Administered via injection
- With this vaccine, you can avoid contracting hepatitis B, hepatitis b, pertussis, tetanus, and hib.
- The following are possible adverse effects of this vaccination.
  - Pain, redness, and swelling could appear where the injection was administered.
  - Fever may briefly occur in children following vaccination.
  - Usually starting the day after vaccination, symptoms last one to three days.

6.2.2.3. Rotavirus Vaccine (RVV) – 1

- Of the three doses, this is the first. Your child takes their second dose at 10 weeks, and their final dose at 14 weeks.

- Administered orally
- This vaccine provides defense against rotaviruses, which are the most frequent cause of severe diarrheal illness in young children and newborns.
- Potential side effects of this vaccine include:
  - Side effects are rare and mild
  - May include diarrhea, vomiting and irritation

6.2.2.4. Pneumococcal Conjugate Vaccine (PCV) – 1

- The first of the PCV's two doses. When your child is 14 weeks old, the second dose is administered.
- Administered via injection
- From milder infections like sinusitis and otitis media, this vaccine protects against meningitis, septicemia, and pneumonia.
- This vaccination may cause the following side effects:
  - Redness
  - Swelling
  - Pain or tenderness
  - Fever
  - Loss of appetite
  - Fussiness (irritability)
  - Feeling tired
  - Headache
  - Muscle aches or joint pain
  - Chills

6.2.2.5. Inactivated Polio Vaccine (fIPV) – 1

- The first of the two fIPV doses. Your child receives the second dose at 14 weeks of age.
- Administered via injection
- The poliovirus, a highly contagious viral disease that primarily affects children under the age of five, is protected against by this vaccine.
- Potential side effects of this vaccine include:
  - Soreness
  - Fever

6.2.3. 10 Weeks

6.2.3.1. Pentavalent – 2

- Your child takes their second dose at 10 weeks, and their final dose at 14 weeks.
- Administered via injection
- With this vaccine, you can avoid contracting hepatitis B, hepatitis b, pertussis, tetanus, and hib.
- Potential side effects of this vaccine include:
  - Pain, redness, and swelling could appear where the injection was administered.
  - Fever may briefly occur in children following vaccination.
  - Usually starting the day after vaccination, symptoms last one to three days.

6.2.3.2. Oral Polio Vaccine (OPV) – 2

- When your child is 10 weeks old, this is the third OPV dosage they have taken. When the child is 14 weeks old, the final dosage is administered.
- Administered orally
- The poliovirus, a highly contagious illness that attacks the nervous

system and can cause complete paralysis, is prevented by this vaccine. The majority of the virus's victims are young children, under five.

- There are no typical adverse effects linked to this vaccination.

6.2.3.3. Rotavirus Vaccine (RVV) – 2

- Your child takes their second dose at 10 weeks, and their final dose at 14 weeks.
- Administered via injection
- Administered orally
- This vaccine provides defense against rotaviruses, which are the most frequent cause of severe diarrheal illness in young children and newborns.
- This vaccination may cause the following side effects:
    - There are seldom any negative effects.
    - include nausea, diarrhea, and irritability.

6.2.4. 14 Weeks

6.2.4.1. Pentavalent – 3

- At 14 weeks old, this is the final Pentavalent vaccination dose to be administered.
- Administered via injection
- With this vaccine, you can avoid contracting hepatitis B, hepatitis b, pertussis, tetanus, and hib.
- Potential side effects of this vaccine include:
    - Symptoms such as swelling, redness, and pain may be experienced at the injection site.
    - Fever may briefly occur in children following vaccination.
    - Usually starting the day after vaccination, symptoms last one to three days.

6.2.4.2. Oral Polio Vaccine (OPV) – 3

- When your child is 14 weeks old, this is the final OPV dose that should be given.
- Administered orally
- The poliovirus, a highly contagious illness that attacks the nervous system and can cause complete paralysis, is prevented by this vaccine. The majority of the virus's victims are young children, under five.
- There are no common side effects associated with this vaccine.

6.2.4.3. Rotavirus Vaccine (RVV) – 3

- When your child is 14 weeks old, this is the last dose of RVV that is administered.
- Administered via injection
- Administered orally
- This vaccine provides defense against rotaviruses, which are the most frequent cause of severe diarrheal illness in young children and newborns.
- Potential side effects of this vaccine include:
    - Side effects are rare and mild
    - May include diarrhea, vomiting and irritation

6.2.4.4. Pneumococcal Conjugate Vaccine (PCV) – 2

- the second of two PCV doses administered at 14 weeks of age.
- Administered via injection
- This vaccine provides defense against infections as minor as sinusitis and otitis media, as well as against meningitis, septicemia, and pneumonia.
- Potential side effects of this vaccine include:
  - Redness
  - Swelling
  - Pain or tenderness
  - Fever
  - Loss of appetite
  - Fussiness (irritability)
  - Feeling tired
  - Headache
  - Muscle aches or joint pain
  - Chills

6.2.4.5. Inactivated Polio Vaccine (fIPV) – 2

- The final fIPV dose is given to your child at 14 weeks.
- Administered via injection
- The poliovirus, a highly contagious viral disease that primarily affects children under the age of five, is protected against by this vaccine.
- Potential side effects of this vaccine include:
  - Soreness
  - Fever

6.2.5. 9–12 Months

6.2.5.1. Measles & Rubella (MR) – 1

- The first of the MR vaccine's two doses. The second dosage is given to infants who are 16 to 24 months old.
- Administered via injection
- This vaccine protects against rubella and measles. Measles is frequently a serious illness that is made worse by bronchopneumonia or middle ear infections. Rubella is most common in childhood and causes a mild exanthemous illness with few constitutional symptoms.
- Potential side effects of this vaccine include:
  - Redness, swelling and sore feeling for 2 to 3 days
  - Babies or young children may have a slight fever for two or three days following the injection, or they may feel a little under the weather for 7 to 11 days.

6.2.5.2. Japanese Encephalitis (JE-1)

- The first of the JE-1 vaccine's two doses. Your child receives the second dose between the ages of 16 and 24 months.
- Administered via injection
- The primary cause of viral encephalitis in Asia, Japanese encephalitis, is prevented by this vaccine. The majority of infections are mild or show no symptoms at all, aside from headache and fever. But occasionally, it can lead to a serious clinical illness.

- Potential side effects of this vaccine include:
  - Fever though rarely (more often in children).
  - Headache or muscle aches mainly in adults.
  - Pain, tenderness, redness, or swelling around the vaccine shot.

6.2.5.3. Pneumococcal Conjugate Vaccine – Booster

- This is a single-dose vaccine.
- Administered via injection
- The vaccine provides defense against meningitis, bacteremia, sinus infections, ear infections, and pneumonia.
- Potential side effects of this vaccine include:
  - Redness/swelling
  - Loss of appetite
  - Irritability
  - Fever
  - Increased crying

6.2.6. 16–24 Months

6.2.6.1. Measles & Rubella (MR) – 2

- The second of your child's two doses of the MR vaccine, administered between 16 and 24 months of age.
- Administered via injection
- The vaccination provides defense against rubella and measles. Childhood measles is a nearly universal clinical experience that can be quite severe and often be exacerbated by middle ear infections or bronchopneumonia. German measles, also known as rubella, primarily affects children and causes a mild exanthemous illness with few constitutional symptoms.
- Potential side effects of this vaccine include:
  - The injection site appears red, swollen, and sore for two to three days.
  - Babies or young children may have a slight fever for two or three days following the injection, or they may feel a little under the weather for 7 to 11 days.

6.2.6.2. Japanese Encephalitis (JE-2)

- The last JE vaccination to be given to children aged 16 to 24 months.
- Administered via injection
- The primary cause of viral encephalitis in Asia, Japanese encephalitis, is prevented by this vaccine. The majority of infections are mild or show no symptoms at all, aside from headache and fever. But occasionally, it can lead to a serious clinical illness.
- Potential side effects of this vaccine include:
  - Fever, albeit infrequently (children more frequently).
  - mostly in adults, headaches or aches in the muscles.
  - Redness, swelling, soreness, or pain in the vicinity of the vaccination site.

6.2.6.3. Diphtheria Pertussis & Tetanus (DPT) – Booster 1

- The first of the DPT vaccine's two doses. Your child, who is between the ages of 5 and 6, receives the second dose.
- Administered via injection
- The vaccination provides a defense against tetanus, pertussis, and diphtheria.
- Potential side effects of this vaccine include:
  - Soreness or swelling around the area of the vaccine shot.
  - Fever
  - Irritation
  - Exhaustion
  - Loss of appetite
  - Vomiting

6.2.6.4. Oral Polio Vaccine – Booster

- This is a single-dose vaccine.
- Administered orally
- The poliovirus, a highly contagious illness that attacks the nervous system and can cause complete paralysis, is prevented by this vaccine. The majority of the virus's victims are young children, under five.
- There are no common side effects associated with this vaccine.

6.2.7. 5–6 Years

6.2.7.1. Diphtheria Pertussis & Tetanus (DPT) – Booster 2

- Your child should receive the second dose of the DPT vaccine when they are between five and six years old.
- Administered via injection
- The vaccination provides defense against tetanus, pertussis, and diphtheria.
- Potential side effects of this vaccine include:
  - Soreness or swelling around the area of the vaccine shot.
  - Fever
  - Irritation
  - Exhaustion
  - Loss of appetite
  - Vomiting

6.2.8. 10 Years

6.2.8.1. Tetanus & Adult Diphtheria (Td)

- This is a single-dose vaccine.
- Administered via injection
- The vaccination offers defense against tetanus, which is spread by the spores of the Clostridium tetani bacteria and can result from cuts or wounds. Breathing problems, heart failure, paralysis, or even death are possible outcomes of diphtheria. The majority of cases happen 14 days after infection.
- Potential side effects of this vaccine include:
  - Pain
  - Redness or swelling around the area of the vaccine shot
  - Mild fever
  - Headache
  - Exhaustion
  - Nausea, vomiting, diarrhea, or stomachache

6.2.9. 16 Years

6.2.9.1. Tetanus and Adult Diphtheria (Td)

- This is a single-dose vaccine.
- Administered via injection
- The vaccination offers defense against tetanus, which is spread by the spores of the Clostridium tetani bacteria and can result from cuts or wounds. Breathing problems, heart failure, paralysis, or even death are possible outcomes of diphtheria. The majority of cases happen 14 days after infection.
- Potential side effects of this vaccine include:
  - Pain
  - Redness or swelling around the area of the vaccine shot
  - Mild fever
  - Headache
  - Exhaustion
  - Nausea, vomiting, diarrhea, or stomachache

Please contact your community's health center or your local physician with any urgent medical concerns (Demirjian and Levy, 2009; Havelaar et al, 2010; Davis, 2011; Ginsburg et al, 2014; Rappuoli et al, 2017).

6.3. THE COLD CHAIN FOR VACCINES

A cold chain is a supply chain that maintains a consistent temperature and contains all the tools and processes needed to produce vaccines. The cold chain starts at the manufacturing plant's cold storage unit, continues through the vaccine's transportation and delivery, includes appropriate storage at the provider facility, and concludes with the patient receiving the shot. It is the joint responsibility of vaccine producers, distributors, public health personnel, and healthcare providers to guarantee the preservation of the vaccine cold chain throughout the entire vaccine production and administration process.

6.3.1. Vaccine Storage and Handling Standard Operating Procedures (SOPs)

Standard operating procedures (SOPs) for handling and storing materials should be created and maintained by facilities in a clear, comprehensive, and current manner. All employees should review the SOPs, and the vaccine coordinator should update them once a year.

Plans and data for these three key areas should be included in SOPs.

- General information – Provide job descriptions, frequently used forms, staff training requirements, and contact details for vaccine manufacturers, equipment service providers, and key facility personnel.
- Routine storage and handling – Provide details on managing the vaccine inventory in every way, from ordering to keeping an eye on storage conditions.
- Emergency vaccine storage, handling, and transport – describe what should be done in the event of an emergency that could jeopardize vaccine storage conditions, such as equipment failures, power outages, natural disasters, or other emergencies.

For advice on routine and emergency SOPs, VFC providers or those who possess vaccines purchased with public funds should get in touch with their immunization program.

6.3.1.1. Staff Training

The facility's standard operating procedures (SOPs) should be followed by all employees who handle vaccines or receive deliveries. Staff members should be aware of where SOPs are located and should keep them close to vaccine storage units.

Training in handling and storage needs to be completed:

- as a component of orientation for new hires.
- every year to serve as a refresher for all employees participating in vaccination campaigns.
- when a fresh batch of vaccines is added to stock.
- when recommendations for vaccinations are revised.

6.3.1.2. Vaccine Coordinator

All vaccines should be handled and stored properly, and in the event that the primary coordinator is not available, a backup coordinator should be designated to take over. These people ought to receive thorough training in both standard operating procedures and emergency protocols. Coordinator duties can be carried out by the coordinator themselves or assigned to suitable personnel. In addition to making sure the delegate has training that certifies their proficiency for the particular tasks given, the coordinator needs to make sure the tasks are finished.

Among the coordinator's duties are:

- Ordering vaccines
- Ensuring that vaccine deliveries are received and stored properly.
- Recording data from the vaccine inventory.
- Keeping an eye on and managing the stock of vaccines in storage units, including changing out outdated shots.
- Installing temperature monitors (TMDs) and keeping track of daily readings.
- Reacting to equipment malfunctions and temperature excursions (temperatures outside of range).
- Supervising the transport of vaccines (when necessary).
- Overseeing emergency preparations
- Establishing and maintaining SOPs for handling and storage.

6.3.2. Vaccine Storage and Temperature Monitoring Equipment

A facility must have adequate equipment for monitoring and storage that is properly configured, maintained, and repaired as needed. By using this equipment, patients are shielded from unintentionally obtaining tainted vaccines, and facilities are shielded from the costs associated with revaccinating patients, replacing costly vaccines, and losing the trust of their patients.

6.3.2.1. Refrigerators and Freezers

The following freezer and refrigerator models are suggested by the CDC:

- Preferably, pharmaceutical-grade or purpose-built units that can freeze or refrigerate biologics, including vaccines, are used. These units can be large units or small, under-the-counter models.
- In certain practice settings, a stand-alone, household-grade unit might be a suitable substitute if a purpose-built or pharmaceutical-grade unit is unavailable. A household-grade combination refrigerator/freezer unit should only have its refrigerator section used. It is not advisable to store vaccines in the freezer section of this kind of unit, and there might be sections of the refrigerated section that should not be utilized either. These units have temperature swings and cold spots, and the air coming from the freezer may expose vaccines that have been refrigerated to below-freezing temperatures. For storage, facilities that keep frozen vaccines on hand need a separate freezer unit.

Every unit should be able to accommodate, without being crowded, the largest inventory that is anticipated during the busiest time of the year (such as flu season). Never keep any vaccines in a combined unit designed like a dorm or bar. A single external door and an evaporator plate/

cooling coil, which is typically housed in an icemaker/freezer compartment, are common features of these units. Even in cases where vaccines are used for short-term storage, there is a considerable risk that they could freeze.

6.3.2.2. Temperature Monitoring Devices (TMDs)

Each and every vaccine storage facility needs a trustworthy TMD. A "digital data logger" (DDL), which is recommended by the CDC and mandated by VFC, is a device that records continuously at intervals of no less than 30 minutes. A buffered temperature probe is used by many DDLs. Standard thermometer readings typically reflect air temperature, whereas temperatures obtained using a buffered probe closely match vaccine temperature. DDLs give information about the duration of a temperature excursion—a unit operating outside of the advised temperature range. To guarantee device accuracy, each DDL needs to have a current, valid Certificate of Calibration Testing (sometimes referred to as a "Report of Calibration").

DDLs ought to possess the following qualities:

- Detachable probe (such as one buffered with glycol, glass beads, sand, or Teflon®) that most accurately represents vaccine temperatures.
- Set a temperature alarm when it goes outside of range.
- Low-battery indicator
- Current, minimum, and maximum temperature display
- Recommended uncertainty of +/-0.5°C (+/-1°F)
- The user can program the logging interval, also known as the reading rate, to take and record temperature readings at least once every 30 minutes.

Ensuring vaccine safety requires the ability to download temperature data from a DDL to a computer using specialized software or to be retrieved from a website for user review. The user may also be able to adjust how frequently temperature readings are taken using the software or website.

Every facility ought to have a suggested TMD for:

- Each vaccine storage unit
- Each emergency transport unit
- Backup if the primary device breaks down or is not available for calibration testing (with a different schedule for testing).

Every one to two years or as recommended by the manufacturer, calibration testing should be carried out. The CDC advises that a DDL's valid and current Certificate of Calibration Testing should contain the following:

- Model/device name or number
- Serial number
- Date of calibration (report or issue date)

- Verification that the test was successful for the instrument (or instrument in tolerance).
- Recommended uncertainty of +/–0.5°C (+/–1°F) or less

6.3.2.3. Storage Unit Setup

Storage units need to be positioned with space between them, the ceiling, and any walls in a room with good ventilation. Nothing ought to be able to obstruct the motor compartment cover. The unit needs to be level, sturdy, and have its bottom elevated above the ground. The unit door ought to slide smoothly open and shut and sit flush with the unit's body. According to studies, the majority of units function best in environments with typical indoor room temperatures, which are typically defined as being between 20°C and 25°C (68°F and 77°F). See the owner's manual that comes with the product from the manufacturer for more details on positioning and spacing.

6.3.2.4. Stabilizing Temperatures

A freshly installed or repaired refrigerator may require two to seven days to reach a stable temperature, while a freezer may require two to three days. The lowest and maximum temperatures for each workday for two to seven days should be checked and recorded before using a unit for storing vaccines. Temperatures should be checked and recorded at least twice a workday if they can't be done digitally. The unit is stable and ready for use after two days in a row with temperatures within the advised range.

6.3.2.5. Power Supply

To safeguard the power supply of the storage unit:

- There should only be one storage unit plugged in per outlet.
- To stop the unit from being unplugged, use an outlet cover or a safety-lock plug.
- Put up "DO NOT UNPLUG" signs on storage units and outlets to warn employees, maintenance personnel, electricians, and other workers not to disconnect equipment.
- People should be warned not to turn off the power to storage units by labeling fuses and circuit breakers.
- When using power outlets that can trip or turn off, proceed with caution. Additionally, stay away from multioutlet power strips, built-in circuit switches (which may have reset buttons), and outlets that are turned on by a wall switch.

6.3.2.6. Equipment Maintenance

To guarantee correct operation, maintain necessary temperatures, and increase the equipment's useful life, storage units and temperature monitoring devices require routine maintenance.

- Regularly inspect storage unit door seals for indications of deterioration.
- To ensure a smooth opening and closing of the door and a proper fit against the unit's body, check and adjust the door hinges. The thermostat may react to warmer room temperatures if the door is left open, and the unit will have to work harder

to keep the interior at the proper temperature. Certain areas of the device may experience extremely low temperatures. It could be beneficial to use a self-closing door and an open-door alarm.

- As directed by the manufacturer, clean the motor and unit coils.
- Maintain a clean interior to prevent the growth of bacteria and fungi. To reduce the possibility of the temperature going out of range, cleaning needs to be done quickly.
- When the amount of frost exceeds one centimeter or the recommended limit specified by the manufacturer, manually defrost freezers. As directed by the manufacturer. Vaccines should be temporarily kept in a freezer-temperature-appropriate unit while they defrost.
- The accuracy of temperature monitoring equipment is impacted by "drift" over time. The device should be replaced if calibration testing shows that it is no longer accurate within +/−0.5°C (+/−1°F). Making corrections to ensure accuracy is not advised.
- Temperature adjustments for storage units might be necessary over time. Only a vaccine coordinator should be able to adjust the temperature; this shouldn't happen in the middle of the workday when a lot of doors are being opened. The coordinator needs to make sure there aren't any more problems (e.g., broken TMD, unplugged unit, left door open, etc., before modifying the temperature in any way.
- Use the backup TMD to verify the temperature before making any adjustments if you think there might be a problem with the TMD.

When using a backup generator, it should be serviced once a year and tested every three months, following the manufacturer's instructions.

6.3.3. Organizing and Storing Vaccine in Storage Unit

Refer to the manufacturer's package inserts for the most recent advice on handling and storing particular vaccines and diluents.

6.3.3.1. Storing Vaccine

To confirm vaccines are stored correctly and to minimize the risk of administration errors (Figure 6.2):

- Until they are ready to be administered, keep vaccines in their original packaging in separate containers with closed lids to protect them from light and to add more thermal stability. Keep manufacturer-filled syringes and loose vials sealed in their original packaging. This makes it harder to keep track of expiration dates and manage inventory, raises the possibility of administration errors, and exposes vaccines to light. It is advised that vaccines be stored outside of their packaging for some specially made units. If so, store the vaccine according to the manufacturer's recommendations.
- Prioritize those vaccines and diluents with later expiration dates by placing those with earlier expiration dates first.

- Label and package vaccines and diluents similarly, or arrange adult and pediatric formulations on different shelves.
- Diluent should always be kept in the same refrigerator as the matching vaccine. Do not put diluent in the freezer.
- Place diluents and vaccines two to three inches away from the door, floor, ceiling, and walls of the unit.
- To encourage air circulation, line up vaccines and diluents in rows with space between them.
- Vaccines and diluents should not be kept in any area of a household-grade unit that might not be able to maintain consistent temperatures or adequate airflow, such as right under cooling vents, in deli, fruit, or vegetable drawers, or on refrigerator door shelves.
- Put water bottles in a household-grade unit's door racks, floor, and top shelf. Stable temperature maintenance can be achieved by placing water bottles inside the unit. It is not advised to use water bottles with some pharmaceutical-grade equipment; instead, adhere to the manufacturer's instructions.
- Keep everything outside of vaccines, diluents, and water bottles out of storage units. If biological products and other medications need to be kept in the same unit as vaccines, they need to be properly labeled and kept in different bins or containers. Things that might be contaminated (e.g., blood, pee, and feces) should be stored and contained appropriately beneath vaccinations to prevent contamination from leaks or drips.
- Arrange the TMD at the center of the unit, encircling it with the vaccines. Temperature should be recorded by a DDL no less than once every 30 minutes.

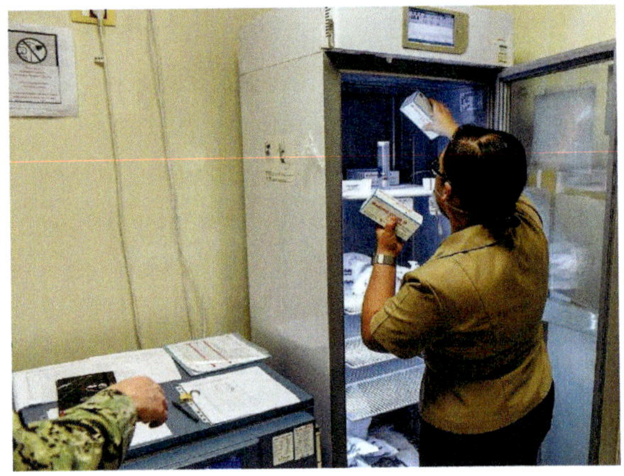

Figure 6.2. *Stand alone refrigerator is being used to store vaccines.*

Source: By Navy Medicine – https://www.flickr.com/photos/navymedicine/50828755263/, Public Domain, https://commons.wikimedia.org/w/index.php?curid=98814900.

6.3.4. Temperature Ranges

The recommended temperature range for refrigerators is 2°C to 8°C (36°F to 46°F). The recommended temperature range for freezers is –50°C to –15°C (–58°F to +5°F). Temperature excursions can be avoided by setting refrigerator or freezer thermostats to the factory-set or midpoint temperature. Thermostats come in a variety of markings and typically display degrees of coldness as opposed to temperatures. The only method to determine the temperature in the vaccine storage area is to use a TMD to measure and record the temperature.

6.3.4.1. Monitoring Vaccine Temperatures

At the beginning of each workday, the minimum and maximum temperatures in the storage unit should be checked and recorded to guarantee the safety of the vaccines. It is recommended to check and record the current temperature at least twice a day (at the beginning and end of the workday) if the TMD being used does not display the minimum and maximum temperatures.

Each storage unit door (or one close by) should have a temperature monitoring log sheet with the following details on it.

- Minimum/maximum temperature (or current temperature if using a device that does not record minimum/maximum temperatures)
- Date
- Time
- The individual's name who took and recorded the temperature.
- Any steps done if a temperature excursion happened.

Leave a blank space in the log if a reading is overlooked. These entries need to be separated from those where the TMD was unable to provide a reading. Make sure the unit doors are securely closed at the end of the day and throughout the day. Check storage unit temperature readings once a week for any variations in temperature patterns that might call for taking appropriate action, such as modifying the unit's temperature or fixing or replacing any damaged storage or temperature monitoring equipment. (Unless state statutes or rules require a longer period) Temperature data should be retained for three years.

6.3.4.2. Temperature Excursions (Out-of-Range Temperatures)

A temperature excursion is defined as any measurement that deviates from the ranges advised in the package inserts provided by the vaccine manufacturers and calls for quick action.

- Report the issue to a supervisor or the primary or backup vaccine coordinator right away.
- Vaccines that have been exposed should be labeled "DO NOT USE" and kept separate from other vaccines in the storage unit (do not discard these vaccines).
- The supervisor or coordinator for vaccines should start recording the event's specifics.
- Follow the SOPs for temperature excursions at your facility, making sure to check the location of temperature monitoring devices and adjust the unit temperature as necessary.
- For advice, follow your SOPs and get in touch with your vaccination program and/or the vaccine manufacturer(s).
- thorough recording of the incident, including the steps taken and the outcomes.

Vaccines should never be kept in a broken-down unit for a long time. If a unit is thought to have failed, emergency SOPs should be put into place.

6.3.5. Vaccine Inventory Management

Ensuring that vaccines are appropriately unpacked, stored, and tracked for each dose received, administered, compromised, expired, or transferred is crucial.

6.3.5.1. Deliveries

- **Scheduling and Receiving Deliveries:** When vaccines arrive, they should be reported right away to the vaccine coordinator or designee. Vaccines should be stored as soon as they are unpacked. Delivery of vaccines should only be planned for days and times when personnel will be available. Never leave a vaccination delivery container unsupervised.
- **Unpacking Deliveries:** Diluents and vaccines should be promptly unpacked and stored at the recommended temperatures. It is not advisable to keep them in an unopened shipment box.
  - Look for any indications of damage on the shipping container and its contents.
  - Verify the contents with the packing list. The packing list for frozen vaccines may indicate the longest period of time the vaccines can be in transit based on the date of shipment.
  - Verify that the right kind and amount of diluents were included with the lyophilized vaccines.
  - Verify the expiration dates of vaccines and diluents to make sure that nothing is nearing or has already expired.

The vaccine manufacturer should be contacted right away if there are any differences between the contents and the packing list or if there are any other concerns regarding the contents (such as temperature excursion). Vaccines should be marked "DO NOT USE" and kept apart from other vaccines in the proper vaccine storage unit until vaccine viability is determined if a temperature excursion is suspected. Regarding any VFC or other vaccines acquired with public funds, get in touch with the state or local immunization program.

6.3.5.2. Inventory Accounting

To make sure there are enough vaccines and diluents on hand, conduct an inventory assessment of the vaccine stock at least once a month and before placing orders. Factors such as current vaccine supplies, storage capacity, and projected demand are taken into consideration when placing an order. It may be necessary for VFC providers to use the immunization information system (IIS) to track inventory since many state and local IISs have vaccine inventory accounting features.

6.3.5.3. Stock Rotation and Removal

Rotating vaccine supplies and routinely checking for expired doses are important. Vaccines and diluents that have expired should be taken out right away to prevent accidental administration.

6.3.5.4. Understanding Expiration Dates

One of the most important aspects of handling and storing vaccines properly is knowing when a vaccine or diluent expires. Staff members must learn how to read expiration dates in order to prevent patients from receiving incorrect doses of vaccines, as administering expired vaccines continues to be one of the most common vaccine storage and handling errors.

The product may be used up until and including the last day of the month if the expiration date is just one month or one year. The product can only be used until the end of the day if a day is included along with the month and year. Regardless of the expiration date, goods that have been tainted or compromised should not be used. In certain cases, vaccines must be used before the expiration date listed on the label, such as when a manufacturer indicates a beyond-use date (BUD). The date the vial is first punctured and the storage details found in the package insert are used to compute the BUD. The vaccine should be used by the manufacturer's specified expiration date if it has no BUD.

The BUD, along with the initials of the person performing the calculation, should be written on the label in place of the expiration date. Some instances are as follows:

- After being combined with a diluent, reconstituted vaccines have a limited shelf life. For instance, the reconstituted vaccine needs to be used within 30 minutes, according to the package insert, and if it's not used by then, it needs to be thrown away. The package insert should be carefully examined because this time frame might only apply while the reconstituted vaccine is still in the vial and not after it is drawn into a syringe.
- Once a needle has been inserted, multidose vials (MDVs) may have a limited amount of time before they can be used. For instance, the package insert might specify that the vaccination needs to be thrown out 28 days after it is administered. The BUD is June 29, 2020 if the vial is entered on June 1, 2020.
- Inappropriate storage conditions can cause vaccines to expire before their manufacturer-specified dates. The vaccine's manufacturer may decide that it is still safe to use even though the label's expiration date is earlier.

Certain MDVs have a maximum number of doses that can be stopped in addition to a BUD. Even if there is still vaccine in the vial after the maximum number of doses has been removed, it should be thrown away.

6.3.5.5. Vaccine and Equipment Disposal

Even though they have to be thrown away, occasionally unopened vials, expired vials, compromised vaccines, and unused doses of vaccine and diluent can be returned for credit. Information specific to a particular vaccine can be obtained from the manufacturer or from the state or local immunization program. Syringes and vials that are open or broken, syringes that have been activated by the manufacturer, and vaccines that have been predrawn by the provider are not returnable and must be disposed of following state regulations.

All syringe/needle devices must be stored in biohazard containers that are labeled or color-coded, closable, puncture-resistant, and leakproof on the sides and bottom as soon as they are used. This procedure aids in avoiding reuse and unintentional needlesticks. Before being disposed of, used needles shouldn't be cut, recapped, or removed from syringes. Vials of vaccines that are compromised, empty, or have expired are typically not regarded as hazardous or pharmaceutical waste and do not need to be disposed of in a biomedical waste container. Nonetheless, one should adhere to the state's disposal regulations. State environmental agencies determine the requirements for disposing of medical waste.

6.3.5.6. Predrawing Vaccines

Only at the moment of administration should vaccinations be administered. Rather than being stored, general-purpose syringes are meant to be administered right away. Without a preservative, predrawn vaccine syringes may become contaminated and harbor microorganisms. Furthermore, over time, the interaction between vaccine components and the polymers in a plastic syringe may result in a reduction of the vaccine's potency. Vaccine waste can also arise from predrawing vaccinations.

Vaccine manufacturers do not recommend predrawing vaccines, not even for off-site clinics. For large immunization clinics, the CDC suggests using manufacturer-filled syringes (MFSs) as an alternative.

If vaccines must be predrawn:

- Assist in preventing medication errors by setting up a distinct administration station for every type of vaccine.
- Only after reaching the clinic location or mass immunization event should vaccines be prepared.
- No more than one MDV or 10 doses should be drawn up at once by each person giving vaccinations.
- Monitor the flow of patients to prevent preparing unnecessary doses.
- When the vaccine is ready to be administered, only then should it be predrawn into a syringe.
- If a predrawn vaccine is not used within 30 minutes of being reconstituted, store it according to the manufacturer's instructions, taking note of the storage duration.

After the workday, any vaccine that is still in predrawn syringes should be thrown away. It is never appropriate to put a predrawn, reconstituted vaccine back into a vial for storage.

6.3.6. Vaccine Transport

The vaccine should be delivered straight to the location where it will be used to safeguard the supply of vaccines. However, for an occasion such as an on-site immunization clinic, vaccines may occasionally need to be transported to an off-site or satellite facility. In addition, transportation might be necessary in the event of prolonged blackouts, flooding, or other natural calamities that could endanger the vaccine supply. In these cases, specific steps need to be taken to safeguard the vaccine supply. Transporting vaccines to satellite or off-site locations differs from both shipping and emergency transportation. When shipping vaccinations between locations, a professional carrier and a lengthy transit duration are typically involved. Transport is the transportation of vaccines over short distances and times between providers. The best mode of transportation may change depending on the circumstances. When transferring vaccines, trained personnel should use an organization's standard operating procedures (SOPs), which should explicitly outline the transport protocols for every scenario.

6.3.6.1. Preparing Vaccines for Transport

The supplies required for transporting the largest annual inventory of vaccines should be on hand at the facility. It is acceptable to use soft-sided containers designed especially for the transportation of vaccines (which may be a component of an approved container and packout system). Soft-sided food or beverage coolers that are sold commercially should not be used since the majority of them have inadequate insulation and are susceptible to changes in ambient or outdoor temperature. In addition to using the proper coolants and transport materials based on the particular transport system(s) being used, each transport container should have a TMD. The vaccines may, as a last resort, be transported in the same shipping containers that they were originally shipped in for emergencies. Vials that have been partially used cannot be transferred between providers or states.

6.3.6.2. Transport of Refrigerated Vaccines to Off-Site or Satellite Facilities

Best practices for transport include:

- A maximum of eight hours should be allotted for either transport alone or transport plus the clinic workday.
- To guarantee that there are always equal quantities of vaccines and diluents for reconstitution, transport diluents alongside the corresponding vaccines.
- Carry only the necessary quantity of vaccine for the working day.
- The passenger compartment, not the trunk, should hold the transport containers if a noncommercial vehicle must be used.

6.3.6.3. Transport of Vaccines in Emergencies

In addition to the previously mentioned steps, in an emergency:

- Before packing any vaccines, make sure the alternative vaccine storage facility can store vaccines.
- Make a note of any safety precautions taken at the time of the incident, such as water bottles, TMDs that run on batteries, transportation to a different location, etc.
- When the power has returned or you are prepared to pack vaccines in transport containers, only then should you open the door of the vaccine storage unit.

If it is possible to predict an emergency (e.g., weather event), halt vaccination campaigns before the start of an emergency to give enough time for transportation and packing.

6.3.6.4. Storing Vaccines at the Destination

Vaccines should be kept in a suitable storage unit with a TMD as soon as they are at the off-site site. Observe and document storage unit temperatures following the following guidelines:

- If the device shows the lowest and maximum temperatures, this data needs to be verified and noted.
- At the beginning and conclusion of the workday, at least two temperature checks and records should be made if the device does not show the minimum or maximum temperature.

The following instructions should be followed when storing vaccines in a portable vaccine storage unit if an on-site storage unit is not possible.

- As close to the vaccines as possible, place a TMD (ideally with a probe) in a thermal buffer, and check and record the temperatures every hour.

As much as possible, keep the container closed (Demirjian and Levy, 2009; Havelaar et al, 2010; Davis, 2011; Ginsburg et al, 2014; Rappuoli et al, 2017).

6.4. DISEASE SURVEILLANCE

Despite their shortcomings, conventional, passive disease surveillance systems are typically sufficient to meet program requirements in routine disease control programs. On the other hand, routine surveillance efforts fall short of the mark in disease elimination or eradication programs. Every case matters in sophisticated disease eradication and elimination programs. It is impossible to attain and maintain the eradication of diseases that can be prevented by vaccination without proper surveillance.

Programs for the surveillance of communicable diseases have typically depended on passive reporting, in which medical professionals and other providers submit reports. In many jurisdictions, laboratory-based reporting has essentially supplanted traditional provider-based reporting for diseases and conditions for which laboratory confirmation is regularly obtained due to the far more thorough case ascertainment. Still, reporting in conventional passive surveillance systems is insufficient, even when lab-based reports are added. Notwithstanding this drawback, the fact that the primary purpose of these data is to track disease occurrence trends rather than to launch public health initiatives in reaction to individual cases means that they are still valuable.

In programs aimed at eliminating diseases, surveillance plays a distinct role. Aggressive efforts must be made to identify factors that allow cases to continue occurring despite the low incidence of disease to achieve the goal of zero cases. These cases may point to the need for new preventative measures, but surveillance data are necessary to monitor the effectiveness of any such measures. Furthermore, prompt notification is required to limit the spread of disease through public health measures. This was demonstrated during the global campaign to eradicate smallpox. The persistence of smallpox cases despite widespread vaccination led to the creation of a novel smallpox eradication plan; i.e., a large circle of contacts surrounding each case-patient was found and immunized, encircling the remaining patients in a protective shield of immunity. In the end, smallpox was eradicated worldwide as a result of these efforts. Without the ability to quickly identify and address specific cases as well as the recognition of the need for an additional strategy, this goal would not have been possible. In 1963, Andrews and Langmuir wrote, "To achieve and maintain the eradication status of a specific disease within an area, it is necessary to: 1) prevent or nullify the reestablishment of the disease from carriers, relapsing cases, or imported sources of infection, and 2) obstruct transmission until endemicity ceases. In light of this, it is necessary to establish a sufficient surveillance system to recognize and address these risks to the goal of eliminating disease."

6.4.1. Development of Surveillance Indicators

The Pan American Health Organization (PAHO) developed techniques to track the quality of surveillance in 1988 as part of the Western Hemisphere polio eradication effort, given the critical role that surveillance plays in the elimination of disease. Ampleness of case investigation (e.g., percentage of cases with properly timed laboratory specimens obtained) and timeliness of laboratory testing were among the surveillance indicators. Measures of surveillance infrastructure included the number of reporting units reporting on a weekly basis, the interval between case onset and notification, and the timeliness of laboratory testing. While these attributes aren't typically monitored outside of evaluation projects in regular disease control programs, doing so would surely yield valuable data for any surveillance system. These characteristics coincide with those that the CDC suggests assessing surveillance systems based on.

6.4.1.1. Indicators of Reporting Completeness

Due to the particular need for surveillance in disease elimination programs, PAHO also created an indicator that made it possible to keep track of how comprehensive reports were. Measures of the effectiveness of case ascertainment and the quality of case investigation after a case is reported as suspected are essential components of disease elimination programs. If the majority of cases go unreported, then a thorough investigation into those that are is insufficient. More importantly, it gets harder to understand why there aren't any reported cases when disease incidence drops. What does zero mean exactly? Does it indicate that no cases were reported, or that no one searched?

To tackle this issue, PAHO created a successful plan of action during the Latin American polio eradication campaign. Instead of monitoring for paralytic poliomyelitis, surveillance was conducted for a syndrome affecting children under the age of 15 that encompasses paralytic polio and other conditions, such as Guillain-Barré Syndrome (GBS). In other words, the surveillance system was set up to find cases that were clinically consistent with polio (suspected cases), and then monitor those cases while laboratory testing was conducted to confirm or deny a diagnosis of polio caused by wild poliovirus. In cases where sufficient laboratory testing was not obtained to confirm or exclude the diagnosis of polio, the case was deemed compatible and the case investigation and surveillance process was deemed unsuccessful. Tracking the incidence of acute flaccid paralysis (AFP) in children under the age of 15 years old can help determine how accurately cases of suspected polio are identified. In the absence of polio, GBS and other conditions causing AFP in children occur at a fairly constant rate over time. One could be fairly certain that the absence of reported polio cases actually meant the absence of polio in countries or regions reporting rates of AFP of 1 per 100,000 children under the age of 15 and without confirmed or compatible polio cases. On the other hand, the lack of cases could be due to insufficient surveillance rather than the absence of polio if AFP rates among children in this age group were less than 1 per 100,000. One important aspect of PAHO's attempt to assess the effectiveness of polio surveillance was tracking the frequency of AFP reporting in Latin America. Investigators could locate, support, and record areas with insufficient surveillance by closely monitoring this at the regional and national levels.

Regretfully, there aren't many more instances of vaccine-preventable illnesses that have indicators that are comparable to the AFP rate. For instance, there is no external benchmark that compares to the rate of AFP in polio surveillance to assess the comprehensiveness of measles surveillance. Although keeping an eye on every instance of AFP is extremely sensitive, it is not targeted. The PAHO approach's classification of cases with incomplete evaluations as "compatible" is another crucial component. "The goal of a disease elimination program is to identify all true cases through the use of an extremely sensitive case definition; however, it's also critical to identify non-cases through sufficient case investigation and laboratory testing. Both of these components were included in the PAHO strategy, which improved the surveillance system's sensitivity and specificity.

6.4.2. Surveillance Indicators in the United States

Indicators of vaccine-preventable diseases are used in the US to make sure the fundamental elements of case investigation and surveillance are carried out as intended, as well as to pinpoint areas in which each needs to be improved. The

Council of State and Territorial Epidemiologists (CSTE) approved surveillance indicators for a subset of vaccine-preventable diseases in 1994, following recommendations made by the Centers for Disease Control. The indicators have been improving ever since to increase their utility. Currently, CDC regularly keeps an eye on the following indicators.

Indicators for measles surveillance:

- The percentage of confirmed cases that were fully reported to the NNDSS, including the date of reporting to the health department, the hospitalization, laboratory testing, immunization history, transmission setting, epidemiologic linkage, date of birth, and onset date.
- the time span between the start of the symptoms and the public health announcement date.
- the percentage of cases that have been verified through laboratory testing.
- the percentage of cases with an external source.
- the percentage of cases for which the CDC received at least one clinical specimen for viral isolation.
- The quantity of measles-like illness (MLI) reports that were discarded (as of January 2006).

Mumps surveillance indicators:

- The percentage of confirmed cases reported to NNDSS includes complete information such as clinical case definition, hospitalization, laboratory testing, vaccination history, date reported to the health department, transmission setting, outbreak related, epidemiologic linkage, date of birth, and onset date.
- The time span between the start of the symptoms and the public health announcement date.
- The percentage of cases that have been verified through laboratory testing.
- The percentage of cases with an external source.

Indicators for rubella surveillance:

- The percentage of confirmed cases that were fully reported to NNDSS, including all relevant details such as the date of report to the health department, hospitalization, vaccination history, laboratory testing, clinical case definition, transmission setting, epidemiologic linkage, date of birth, and onset date.
- The time span between the start of the symptoms and the public health announcement date.
- The percentage of cases that have been verified through laboratory testing.
- The percentage of cases with an external source.
- The percentage of confirmed cases among reproductive age women who are aware of their pregnancy status.

Indicators for the surveillance of invasive diseases caused by *Haemophilus influenzae* type B:

- The percentage of cases that were fully reported to the NNDSS, including the species, specimen type, vaccination history, and serotype testing (clinical case definition).

- The percentage of cases among children under five who have received all recommended vaccinations.
- The percentage of cases in which an isolate was serotyped among children under the age of five.

Indicators for pertussis surveillance:

- The percentage of instances that were fully reported to the NNDSS, including the clinical case definition, complications, antibiotic course, laboratory results, vaccination history, and epidemiologic information [e.g., epidemiologic connection/outbreak].
- The time span between the start of the symptoms and the public health announcement date.
- The percentage of cases that are laboratory tested and meet the criteria for a clinical case.
- The percentage of case patients who have received all recommended vaccinations.

Indicators for invasive pneumococcal disease surveillance:

- The percentage of cases that were fully reported (clinical case definition, serotype, and vaccination history) to the NNDSS.
- The percentage of serotype-classified cases.
- The percentage of case patients who have received all recommended vaccinations.

Meningococcal disease surveillance indicators:

- The percentage of cases that were fully reported (birthdate, age, and event date) to the NNDSS.
- The percentage of cases that are officially reported as verified.
- The percentage of cases where the outcome is known.
- Percentage of cases that have been verified through serogroup testing.
- The percentage of case patients who have received all recommended vaccinations.

Indicators for varicella disease surveillance:

- The percentage of cases that were hospitalized, had multiple lesions and were fully reported to the NNDSS.
- The percentage of cases that are officially reported as verified.
- Percentage of cases that have been verified through laboratory testing.
- The percentage of cases connected to an outbreak.
- The percentage of case patients who have received all recommended vaccinations.

6.4.3. Additional Approaches and Future Directions

Given the low number of cases of most vaccine-preventable diseases currently reported in the United States, these indicators have helped identify significant issues with case investigation and reporting; however, a crucial issue that still needs to be addressed is the sensitivity of the surveillance system, i.e., does the lack of cases from a specific jurisdiction mean that there weren't any cases at all?

Using active surveillance, or contacting and requesting reports from all providers and institutions accountable for reporting regularly, is one strategy to enhance the completeness of reporting. In demonstration projects, active surveillance has been demonstrated to increase the reporting of measles, rubella, salmonellosis, and hepatitis; however, it is typically too costly to carry out on a regular basis.

The following presumptions justify active surveillance:

- There are incidents in the neighborhood.
- Case-patients are people who seek medical care or who otherwise come into contact with organizations that are required by law to report information.
- The provider or institution is aware of the condition.
- Cases remain unreported because it is too difficult to complete reporting forms or make phone calls to the health department.
- Cases will be reported if providers' administrative reporting burden is lessened.

These requirements are rarely met for rare diseases, which include the majority of vaccine-preventable diseases in the U.S. In fact, illnesses that were relatively common or at the very least endemic in the population being watched have been the subject of earlier examples of the value of active surveillance. Active surveillance for measles and rubella is unlikely to be of much interest to providers in the absence of a significant, ongoing outbreak, as there have been few cases of these illnesses in many towns and states in recent years.

To track the surveillance infrastructure—that is, the number of clinics and other facilities that took part in the surveillance system—PAHO established a weekly negative reporting system as part of the Western Hemisphere's polio eradication effort. Every reporting unit was required to submit a negative report for AFP exclusively if no cases were found that week (i.e., "no cases of acute flaccid paralysis") in addition to any cases of the disease that were discovered in the weekly report on notifiable diseases. It was implicitly assumed that since the patient would seek medical attention, any such cases would be acknowledged. To avoid allocating the resources required for active surveillance, this was an attempt to obtain the advantages of active surveillance within a passive surveillance system. However, according to an assessment conducted in one nation, case finding efforts were not always made in conjunction with negative reporting at the local level, and significant training was required to give negative reporting any real significance there.

Methods such as application of external standards, identification of imported cases, monitoring the level of reporting for suspected cases that are ruled out as cases by epidemiologic and laboratory investigation, monitoring diagnostic effort, and monitoring circulation of the organism may be helpful, but none of them can give conclusive evidence that the absence of reported cases indicates the absence of disease in the population.

6.4.3.1. Application of External Standards

As was previously mentioned, keeping an eye on the rate of AFP in children under the age of 15 was found to be an effective way to guarantee adequate surveillance throughout the Western Hemisphere's polio eradication program. Regretfully, neither the measles nor the majority of other diseases that can be prevented by vaccination have an equivalent external standard. On the other hand, invasive disease caused by *Haemophilus influenzae* type b might have an external standard. According to data from an ongoing laboratory-based surveillance system, non-type B invasive disease affects children under the age of five at a rate of roughly 1 in 6 per 100,000. If this rate remains largely constant over time across various regions, it can be used as an external benchmark to assess the caliber of type B invasive disease reports. In the year 1991, cases of *H. influenzae* invasive disease, both those caused by type B and non-type B strains, are included in the Nationally Notifiable Disease System (NNDSS). due to invasive illness brought on by non-type b *H. influenzae* vaccination does not protect against strains in any age group, and since adult cases of type B are still common, the lack of documented cases of invasive *H. influenzae*. Any kind of influenza illness in any age range within a jurisdiction clearly indicates a lack of surveillance.

6.4.3.2. Identification of Imported Cases

The ability of a surveillance system to identify imported cases is one indirect indicator of the caliber of case ascertainment at the national level. If no importations are found and reported at the state level, this could indicate that there is no disease or that there is no effort being made to find cases. For a variety of reasons, cases involving non-permanent residents of the country are likely less likely to be reported and thoroughly investigated than cases involving permanent residents. These reasons include visitors' lack of access to healthcare, their temporary stay in the country, which makes it challenging to conduct a thorough case investigation, and their potential to avoid contact with law enforcement if they are in the country without the proper documentation. In the US, measles cases are frequently reported, looked into, and confirmed; these cases typically have little to no spread. In jurisdictions where there are no reported cases of US acquisition, the presence of imported cases serves as strong proof of a functional surveillance system. This idea is included in the list of indicators for measles surveillance (the percentage of cases with an imported source).

The effectiveness of the surveillance system provides evidence that endemic transmission of the measles has been eradicated in the United States. While measles is no longer common throughout the Western Hemisphere, it is still endemic in many Western European and Asian nations. Rubella endemic transmission has also been eradicated in the US, though cases of importation from other countries are still being reported. Travelers from other countries are likely to bring measles or rubella with them, especially from those where the illness is endemic and there are a lot of foreign visitors. If such cases are not found, it may be the case that surveillance is not sensitive enough at the national level to find unique cases that were acquired in the US.

6.4.3.3. Monitoring Cases that are Ruled Out

Monitoring the number of suspected disease cases that are reported, looked into, and rejected as cases is another method for keeping tabs on the accuracy of case ascertainment. PAHO used this strategy to eradicate polio throughout the Western Hemisphere. Even though polio had become an extremely rare disease, reports of suspected cases persisted throughout the region, and cases were thoroughly investigated, including the collection of laboratory specimens at the right time. In this way, the effectiveness of the system was measured by proving thousands of cases were not polio. Similar to this, cases of acute flaccid paralysis that were not thoroughly examined were categorized as compatible, demonstrating a deficiency in both case investigation and surveillance.

The quality of measles surveillance and case investigation at the state level has been monitored since 1997 through the establishment of surveillance for discarded measles-like illness (MLI). When such data was available, it offered some reassurance that attempts were being made to identify cases of measles and that, once a case was reported, an investigation was sufficient because it simultaneously demonstrated that: (1) many cases were reported; and (2) nearly all were ruled out as measles by appropriate investigation. The surveillance system's assurance of strength supported the conclusion that measles transmission within the United States had been eradicated.

As of January 1, 2006, there was no longer any indigenous measles transmission in the United States, making the use of discarded MLI as a surveillance indicator obsolete. MLI data collection was challenging in some areas and necessitated gathering a lot of information on cases that were eventually rejected, which might be viewed as an inefficient use of scarce resources outside of special evaluation projects. Furthermore, there is a lot of variation in the United States when it comes to who is responsible for which case investigation; in many states, the task falls to the city and county health departments. It was difficult to mandate that every suspected case of measles be reported to the state when cases were diagnosed locally and the illness was nearly always ruled out. As a result, even though state employees might have understood the value of gathering this data as a performance indicator, it's possible that the relevant data wasn't accessible to them. Currently, there is no external standard to determine the number of suspected measles cases that need to be reported and looked into in a population if the measles virus is not introduced and spreads.

6.4.3.4. Monitoring Diagnostic Effort

Measuring diagnostic effort could be an additional strategy for surveillance assessment, given the challenges in gathering data on reported cases that are rejected as cases. The level of suspicion of a vaccine-preventable disease is indicated by the diagnostic effort; if the disease is suspected, appropriate laboratory testing should be performed to confirm or rule out the suspicion. This could be applied, for instance, to the assessment of pertussis surveillance; monitoring the number of specimens submitted over time, even in the absence of a positive result, offers solid proof that the diagnosis is being explored if no cases are discovered. By monitoring the submission of laboratory requests for diagnostic testing (such as IgM antibody tests for measles, mumps, or rubella), a similar strategy could be used for other vaccine-preventable diseases. Nobody is looking if testing is not taking place.

This strategy is possible without creating new data collection systems through the consolidation of laboratory functions and the creation of standards and systems for electronic reporting of laboratory data. The lack of documented cases is more likely to represent the absence of disease since testing indicates that the diagnosis is being explored. The amount of testing that is deemed "enough" in the absence of an external standard is still debatable, but this method does account for suspected cases that are assessed in the private sector but are not labeled as such.

6.4.3.5. Monitoring Circulation of the Organism

Surveillance for the agent, or the bacteria or virus that causes the disease, is one addition to case surveillance. Measles, mumps, rubella, diphtheria, pertussis, invasive pneumococcal and meningococcal diseases, varicella, and polio can all be detected by molecular typing techniques, which have been used to augment case surveillance data. Monitoring the organism can reveal details about its origins, evidence of endemic transmission, and evidence of repeated introduction from various sources.

For instance, evidence of an ongoing public health issue even in the absence of documented cases was shown by the demonstration of endemic transmission of multiple strains of the toxigenic Corynebacterium diphtheriae in a Northern Plains Indian community. The cessation of endemic measles transmission in the US and the growing significance of measles case importation have both been proven by molecular epidemiology. Similar techniques used on rubella virus isolates from individuals with the disease and infants with congenital rubella syndrome in the US have been crucial in proving that endemic rubella transmission has been eradicated in this nation. Eventually, tracking the organism's movement becomes a crucial part of surveillance efforts as diseases move closer to eradication (Demirjian and Levy, 2009; Havelaar et al, 2010; Davis, 2011; Ginsburg et al, 2014; Rappuoli et al, 2017).

6.5. INFECTIOUS DISEASES IN CHILDREN

The main causes of death in children differ according to age. Children under the age of five are particularly susceptible to contracting infectious diseases such as tuberculosis, pneumonia, diarrhea, and HIV. Conflict, injuries, and non-communicable diseases are major threats to older children. Even though common infectious diseases are completely preventable and treatable, a significant number of young children still die from them. In 2019, diarrhea, malaria, and pneumonia accounted for about 30% of all deaths worldwide in children under the age of five. Children in the poorest parts of the world suffer disproportionately, with sub-Saharan Africa having a higher prevalence of infectious diseases.

It is possible to buck these trends. UNICEF works to save and stop disease-related deaths of children all over the world. We assist nations in bolstering their basic healthcare infrastructure, particularly in the community, and battling prevalent infectious illnesses like tuberculosis, HIV, malaria, and pneumonia.

6.5.1. Childhood Tuberculosis

Chronic tuberculosis (TB) is a bacterial infection that primarily affects the lungs, though it can also occasionally affect the kidneys, spine, or brain. The main way that TB spreads is by air. Being asymptomatic of tuberculosis is not the same as having an active case of the disease.

The stages of tuberculosis can be explained in three key ways. They are listed below:

- **Exposure:** When someone has come into contact with or been exposed to someone who is suspected of having tuberculosis, this happens. The individual who was exposed will not have any symptoms of the illness, a normal chest X-ray, and a negative skin test result.
- **Latent TB Infection:** This happens when a person has tuberculosis bacteria in their body but does not exhibit any disease symptoms. The TB organisms are blocked by the immune system of the infected person, and in the majority of cases, the infection is lifelong dormant. This individual would have a normal chest X-ray but a positive skin test result.
- **TB Disease:** The person exhibiting symptoms and indicators of an ongoing infection fits this description. Both the skin test and the chest X-ray would be positive for this individual.

Mycobacterium tuberculosis is the main TB bacteria (M. TB). Numerous M-infected individuals. tuberculosis stays in the latent stage of the disease and never progresses to active TB. However, TB organisms can withstand the body's defenses, multiply, and cause an active disease in people with weakened immune systems, such as those with HIV (human immunodeficiency virus) or diabetes, as well as those receiving treatment with drugs that can weaken the immune system, like corticosteroids and chemotherapy. Compared to older children and adults, very young children are more likely to have TB that spreads through their bloodstream and results in complications like meningitis.

TB affects people of all ages, races, and genders. Those who are more vulnerable include the following:

- Those who cohabit or work with TB-affected individuals.
- Populations underserved by medicine.
- Homeless people
- Individuals from other nations where tuberculosis is common.
- People residing in communal places like nursing homes.
- People who abuse alcohol
- People who use intravenous drugs
- People with impaired immune systems
- The elderly
- Healthcare professionals who interact with populations at high risk.

6.5.1.1. Symptoms of TB

Symptoms of TB can vary depending on the age of the affected child. The most common symptoms of active TB include, but are not limited to:

- In children:
    - Fever
    - Unintended weight loss
    - Poor growth
    - Sweating at night
    - Cough
    - Swollen glands
    - Chills
- In adolescents:
    - A prolonged cough lasting more than three weeks.
    - Productive cough
    - Pain in the chest
    - Blood in their sputum
    - Weakness and fatigue
    - Swollen glands
    - Unintended weight loss
    - Decrease in appetite
    - Fever
    - Chills or night sweats

The signs and symptoms of tuberculosis can mimic those of other illnesses or lung disorders. Always get a diagnosis from your child's physician.

6.5.1.2. Causes

When an infected person coughs, sneezes, speaks, sings, or laughs, the TB bacteria is released into the air; however, an individual must typically be exposed to the germs multiple times before contracting the infection. Personal objects like clothes, bedding, glasses, cutlery, handshakes, toilets, and other things that a person with tuberculosis has touched are unlikely to spread the infection. The best defense against tuberculosis spread is adequate ventilation.

6.5.1.3. Diagnosis

A TB skin test is used to diagnose TB. A tiny amount of testing material is injected into the skin's outermost layer during this examination. Within two or three days, the test could come back positive for tuberculosis infection if a particular size bump appears. Sputum tests and X-rays are two more tests that can be performed to identify if a child has TB disease. Interferon-gamma release assays are another type of blood test that can help diagnose *Mycobacterium tuberculosis*.

Skin tests for TB are advised for those who:

- In high-risk categories.
- Who work or reside near individuals who pose a high risk.
- Who haven't had a skin test for TB.

According to the American Academy of Pediatrics, children should have skin testing done.

- Immediate testing:
    - If it's believed that the child has been exposed within the previous five years.
    - If the child's X-ray appears to be TB-related.
    - If the child exhibits any tuberculosis symptoms.
    - If the child is from a nation where tuberculosis is common.
- Yearly skin testing:
    - For children with HIV.
    - For kids housed in juvenile detention centers.
- Testing every 2 to 3 years:
    - For kids who come into contact with high-risk individuals.
- Consider testing in children from ages 4 to 6 and 11 to 16:
    - If the parent of the child is from a nation where there is a lot of risk.
    - If the young person has visited dangerous places.
    - If the young person resides in a heavily populated area.

6.5.1.4. Treatment

Your child's physician will decide on a specific course of treatment based on:

- Age, general health, and medical background of the individual
- Extent of the disease
- His or her tolerance to particular drugs, treatments, or procedures.
- Anticipations regarding the disease's progression.
- Your opinion or preference

Treatment may include:

- Short-term hospitalization
- Medications
- For children between the ages of 2 and 11 who may have latent tuberculosis. To eradicate the TB organisms from the body, an isoniazid course lasting 6 to 12 months is typically administered.
- For children with active TB. In order for a medication to be effective, doctors may prescribe three or four different drugs at once, such as isoniazid, rifampin, pyrazinamide, or streptomycin, for a duration of up to six months or longer.

Within a few weeks of starting treatment, patients typically start to get better. If the patient follows a doctor's instructions and completes the recommended course of treatment, they should not be contagious after two weeks of treatment with the appropriate medications.

6.5.2. Poliomyelitis

Children under the age of five are primarily affected by poliomyelitis, also known as polio, a highly contagious viral disease. Person-to-person transmission of the virus occurs primarily through the fecal-oral route or, less frequently, through a shared vehicle (e.g., contaminated food or water), grows in the colon, and then has the ability to enter the nervous system and paralyze people.

The Global Polio Eradication Initiative was started in 1988 when the World Health Assembly adopted a resolution calling for the complete eradication of polio worldwide. It was subsequently joined by the Bill and Melinda Gates Foundation, Gavi, the Vaccine Alliance, national governments, Rotary International, and the US Centers for Disease Control and Prevention (CDC).

From an estimated 350,000 cases in over 125 endemic countries in 1988 to 6 reported cases in 2021, wild poliovirus cases have decreased by over 99%. Wild poliovirus type 2 was eliminated in 1999, while wild poliovirus type 3 was eliminated in 2020 out of the three strains of the virus (type 1, type 2, and type 3). As of 2022, Pakistan and Afghanistan are the only two nations where endemic wild poliovirus type 1 still exists.

6.5.2.1. Symptoms

The poliovirus spreads widely. Though it can vary from 4 to 35 days, the incubation period is typically 7 to 10 days. Through the mouth, the virus enters the body and grows in the intestines. After then, the nervous system is invaded. Up to 90% of infected people show no symptoms or very minor ones, and the illness is typically not diagnosed. Others have fever, exhaustion, headache, nausea, neck stiffness, and limb pain as their initial symptoms. These symptoms typically last two to 10 days, and in the majority of cases, recovery is total. The virus, however, results in paralysis in the remaining percentage of cases, usually affecting the legs, and this paralysis is typically permanent. After infection, paralysis can develop as quickly as a few hours later. 5 to 10% of paralyzed people die as a result of their breathing muscles becoming immobile.

The virus is spread quickly, particularly in places with inadequate sanitation and hygiene systems, by the feces of infected individuals, who are typically children.

6.5.2.2. Treatment

Polio cannot be cured; vaccination is the only way to avoid contracting it. When given repeatedly, the polio vaccine can give a child lifelong protection. Since the Global Polio Eradication Initiative was started in 1988, more than 20 million people who would have otherwise been paralyzed are now able to walk. During polio vaccination campaigns, vitamin A has been systematically administered to prevent an estimated 1.5 million childhood deaths.

The goal of polio treatments is to reduce and eliminate symptoms. Antispasmodic medications are used to relax the affected muscles, while heat and physical therapy are used to stimulate the muscles. While permanent polio paralysis cannot be reversed, this can increase mobility. In the battle against polio, vaccination is essential. The virus continues to spread when strategic approaches are not put into practice. Cases of wild poliovirus endemic transmission are still occurring in border regions of Pakistan and Afghanistan. If polio is not eradicated in these last areas, there could be up to 200 000 new cases annually worldwide in the next 10 years. For this reason, it is imperative to guarantee the total eradication of polio, permanently.

6.5.3. Diphtheria

Bacteria that produce toxins are the cause of the infectious disease diphtheria. When an infected person coughs or sneezes, it can spread from one person to another. Even though they may not show any symptoms of the disease, some people can still spread the bacteria to other people. Although severe disease, complications, and death can also occur, others will experience mild disease.

Although it can afflict anyone, children who were not vaccinated were most frequently afflicted. The respiratory system is harmed by the diphtheria toxin, which can also spread throughout the body. Fever, sore throats, and swelling of the neck glands are typical symptoms. The greatest defense against contracting diphtheria or infecting others is vaccination. The vaccination aids in your body's defense against the infection and is safe. Worldwide cases of diphtheria occurred prior to the 1930s, when the vaccine was developed and widely administered. Despite the availability of a safe and effective vaccine, outbreaks have been happening more frequently recently due to under vaccination (Figure 6.3).

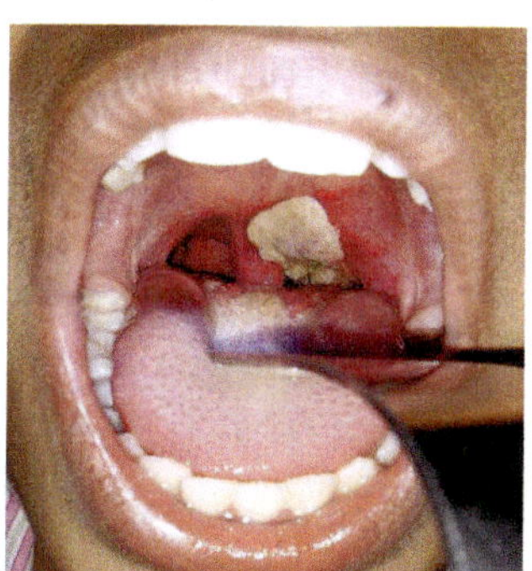

Figure 6.3. *An adherent, dense, gray pseudomembrane covering the tonsils is classically seen in diphtheria.*

Source: By Dileepunnikri – Own work, CC BY-SA 3.0, https://commons.wikimedia.org/w/index.php?curid=27093567.

6.5.3.1. Effects of the COVID-19 Pandemic

Delivery of regular immunization services and surveillance operations were impacted by the COVID-19 pandemic. These setbacks have made a lot of kids more vulnerable to diseases like diphtheria that can be prevented with vaccinations. No WHO region is totally free of diphtheria, and places, where the diphtheria toxoid-containing vaccine is not widely used, allow the bacteria to spread, raising the possibility of outbreaks and putting everyone who is not vaccinated or has not received enough vaccinations at risk. In primary healthcare, immunization and surveillance programs should be reinforced. Additionally, every child should receive three doses of the diphtheria toxoid-containing vaccine during infancy, childhood, and adolescence. To quickly close immunity gaps and identify and confirm cases, countries should also put in place strong surveillance systems.

6.5.3.2. Signs and Symptoms

Diphtheria symptoms typically appear two to five days after bacterial exposure. Fever, swollen neck glands, weakness, and sore throat are typical signs of the infection. It becomes difficult to breathe and swallow when dead tissue in the respiratory tract covers tissues in the tonsils, throat, and nose within two to three days of infection. The majority of severe cases and fatalities resulting from diphtheria are caused by the toxin and its consequences. Nerve and cardiac inflammation are examples of complications. About 30% of cases of diphtheria can be fatal for those who are not vaccinated and receive insufficient treatment; children under the age of five are particularly vulnerable.

6.5.3.3. Who Is at Risk?

Any individual who lacks immunity—whether through vaccination or not—can contract the infection. Recurrences of diphtheria have been observed whenever vaccination rates drop.

Regular immunization is disrupted in nations experiencing or recovering from natural disasters or conflicts due to damaged health infrastructure and services. In residential camps, there is an increased risk of infection due to overcrowding.

6.5.3.4. Treatment

Early intervention with appropriate treatment reduces the risk of complications and death significantly. This is the reason that, in the event that diphtheria is suspected, rapid confirmation testing and treatment should be initiated. Antibiotics and diphtheria antitoxin are typically used to treat cases of diphtheria. Blood circulation toxin is neutralized by a diphtheria-specific antitoxin. Antibiotics hasten the removal of the bacteria, stop them from reproducing and producing toxins, and stop them from spreading to other people. Unfortunately, a number of contemporary diphtheria strains have shown resistance to a number of widely used antibiotics. Following the resolution of the acute stage of the disease, anyone who has experienced diphtheria should also get vaccinated.

Antibiotics should be administered prophylactically to people who have come into contact with cases of diphtheria in order to prevent illness. All of their contacts' immunization records should also be examined. They ought to be offered vaccinations as well if they haven't received them all.

6.5.3.5. Prevention

Vaccines against diphtheria are available and are frequently administered in conjunction with tetanus, pertussis, and other illnesses. In order to offer long-term protection, the World Health Organization advises administering six doses of the diphtheria vaccine, beginning at age 6 weeks and continuing through adolescence. The best approach to prevent diphtheria is to vaccinate the entire community with a high coverage rate as part of routine immunization services integrated into primary health care. For long-term protection, all children should receive a full primary series of vaccinations against diphtheria along with three booster doses. The vaccine works and is safe.

Most frequently, the diphtheria vaccine is administered in conjunction with immunizations against tetanus, pertussis, hepatitis B, *Hemophilus influenzae*, and inactivated polio. Combining vaccinations adds the benefit of protection against additional childhood illnesses that can cause tetanus, pertussis, meningitis, and polio, but also slightly raises the cost and permits sharing of delivery and administration expenses. 84% of children in 2022 received all three doses of the primary series of the diphtheria vaccination. Nonetheless, there are significant differences in coverage levels between and within nations. Inadequate immunization in subsequent child cohorts may result in diphtheria cases and outbreaks.

6.5.4. Pertussis

A dangerous bacterial infection of the lining of the breathing passages, especially the area around the windpipe, is called pertussis. *Bordetella pertussis* is the bacteria that causes pertussis, commonly known as whooping cough, and it is highly contagious. Whooping cough can affect anyone, although it typically affects infants and young children. It poses a particular risk to infants. Babies may find it difficult to breathe, eat, or drink due to severe coughing fits.

6.5.4.1. Symptoms

After exposure, pertussis symptoms can appear 3 to 12 days later and linger up to two weeks. Nasal congestion, runny nose, sneezing, mild fever, and watery eyes are some of the early symptoms. Pertussis causes a two-week course of illness that starts with a dry, hacking cough that develops into prolonged spasms of coughing. The tongue may stick out, the eyes may enlarge, and the face may turn discolored during these spasms. Vomiting and the production of mucus are possible. Whooping noises are frequently heard after coughing fits. Adults and infants under three months old might not make this distinctive sound when they inhale.

6.5.4.2. Diagnosis

The diagnosis is made based on the patient's medical history and physical examination. It can then be verified by looking for the bacteria in smears or cultures of secretions from the upper throat and nose.

6.5.4.3. Treatment

Antibiotic therapy is the mainstay of treatment; in order to stop the infection from spreading, it may also be prescribed to other family members of the afflicted individual. After starting antibiotic therapy, the infected person should be kept isolated for five days, and contact with infants should be strictly avoided. When a baby has pertussis, they are admitted to the hospital; this is also the case for babies who have the illness between three and six months of age.

6.5.5. Tetanus

Spores of the bacterium *Clostridium tetani* are the source of the acute infectious disease tetanus. Spores can be found all over the environment, but they are most common in soil, ash, animal and human intestines and feces, skin, and rusty objects like barbed wire, nails, and needles. Since the spores are resistant to heat and most antiseptics, they can last for many years.

Tetanus can strike anyone, but it is especially common and dangerous in young infants and expectant mothers who have not received enough tetanus-toxoid-containing vaccinations. Maternal tetanus occurs during pregnancy or within 6 weeks of the end of the pregnancy, while neonatal tetanus occurs within the first 28 days of life. The illness is still a major public health concern throughout much of the world, but it is particularly prevalent in low-income nations or areas where vaccination rates are low and unhygienic birth practices are widespread. When contaminated material is used to cover the umbilical stump or nonsterile instruments are used to cut the umbilical cord, neonatal tetanus results. Deliveries made on contaminated surfaces or by persons with dirty hands pose additional risks.

Approximately 25.000 newborns perished from neonatal tetanus in 2018, which is a 97% decrease from the approximate 787,000 newborn deaths from the disease in the first month of life in 1988. However, waning immunity and limited opportunities for males to receive booster doses in many countries increase the risk of tetanus in adolescent and adult male circumcised populations.

6.5.5.1. Symptoms and Diagnosis

Tetanus incubation lasts anywhere from three to 21 days following infection. Most cases happen in a span of 14 days.

Symptoms can include:

- jaw twitches or difficulty opening the mouth.
- cramps in the back, abdomen, and limbs that occur frequently.
- sudden noise-induced painful muscle spasms.
- trouble swallowing
- seizures
- headache
- fever and sweating
- variations in heart rate or blood pressure.

Muscle spasms, which are frequently accompanied by the infant's incapacity to suckle or breastfeed, and prolonged crying are signs of neonatal tetanus. Laboratory confirmation is not necessary for the diagnosis of tetanus; instead, it is made based on clinical features. According to the World Health Organization, a confirmed case of neonatal tetanus is defined as an illness that strikes an infant who, during the first two days of life, is able to suckle and cry normally, but loses this ability between days three and 28 and exhibits rigidity or spasms.

According to the WHO, a person must exhibit at least one of the following symptoms in order to be diagnosed with non-neonatal tetanus: painful muscle contractions or a prolonged facial spasm that looks like a smile. Tetanus can strike patients even if they are unable to remember a specific wound or injury, despite the fact that this definition depends on a history of injury or wound.

6.5.5.2. Treatment

A medical emergency involving tetanus necessitates:

- care in the hospital
- prompt administration of the medication known as human tetanus immune globulin (TIG).
- aggressive wound care
- drugs to control muscle spasms
- antibiotics
- tetanus vaccination.

Individuals who recover from tetanus require vaccination because they lack natural immunity and are susceptible to infection again.

6.5.5.3. Prevention

Immunization with tetanus-toxoid-containing vaccines (TTCV), which are given during prenatal care contacts and are part of routine immunization programs worldwide, can prevent tetanus. The WHO advises that a person receive 6 doses of TTCV (3 primary plus 3 booster doses) to be protected for the rest of their life. As early as 6 weeks of age is recommended for the start of the 3-dose primary series, with a minimum of 4 weeks separating each subsequent dose. It is best to administer the three booster doses in the second year of life (12–23 months), at ages 4–5, and at ages 9–15. The ideal interval between booster doses is four years or more.

Tetanus vaccinations come in a variety of forms, all of which are mixed with vaccinations against other illnesses.

- vaccines against tetanus and diphtheria (DT).
- DTaP vaccines: diphtheria, tetanus, and pertussis (whooping cough).
- vaccines against tetanus and diphtheria (Td).
- vaccinations against tetanus, diphtheria, and pertussis (Tdap).

Women of reproductive age can avoid neonatal tetanus by receiving the TTCV vaccination, either before or after becoming pregnant. Strong medical procedures, such as clean delivery, cord care during childbirth, and appropriate wound care for dental and surgical procedures, can also prevent tetanus. Tetanus incidence rates are extremely low in nations where national immunization programs have sustained high immunization coverage for several decades.

6.5.6. H. Influenzae B Infection

Haemophilus influenzae (*H. influenzae*) is a group of bacteria that can cause various infections in infants and young children, including ear, eye, sinus, and pneumonia infections. The more severe type, known as *H. influenzae* type b (Hib), which used to cause significant disease in the U.S., is now rare thanks to the Hib vaccine. Before widespread vaccination, up to 130 out of 100,000 children were affected by serious Hib infections, but now that number has decreased to less than 1 out of 100,000. Hib infections, such as meningitis and epiglottitis, were life-threatening, but are now uncommon due to the vaccine. However, there is still a small risk of Hib infection in children who have not completed their vaccine series or in older children who did not receive the vaccine as infants. Traveling to countries where the Hib vaccine is not widely used can also pose a risk. Most *H. influenzae* infections today are caused by non-type b strains of the bacteria.

6.5.6.1. Types of Haemophilus influenzae Infections

One particular type of bacteria that can cause a wide range of infections is called *Haemophilus influenzae*. These infections can be minor, like infections in the ears, or serious, like infections in the bloodstream. Physicians think about some "Invasive" *H. influenzae* infections. When bacteria infiltrate areas of the body that are typically germ-free, invasive disease results. As an illustration, *H. influenzae* can enter the bloodstream and cause bacteremia, or they can infect the fluid surrounding the brain and spine and cause meningitis. Most invasive diseases are dangerous, necessitating hospital care, and occasionally they can be fatal.

The prevalent forms of invasive illnesses brought on by *H. influenzae* are:

- Pneumonia (lung infection)
- Bloodstream infection
- The swelling of the lining of the brain and spinal cord is known as meningitis.
- Epiglotittis (swelling in the throat)
- Cellulitis (skin infection)
- Infectious arthritis, or joint inflammation.

In addition, *H. influenzae* frequently causes bronchitis in adults and ear infections in children.

6.5.6.2. Causes of Hib Infection

Most healthy individuals have hives in their throats and noses, but they don't get sick from them. *Haemophilus influenzae* bacteria come in different varieties, and infection with the type b (Hib) bacterium can cause a variety of symptoms in susceptible individuals, some of which are life-threatening.

The primary means of transmission for the Hib disease is direct contact with infected droplets from coughing or sneezing, as well as secretions from an infected person's nose and throat. Usually, two to four days pass between coming into contact with the bacteria and the illness starting. For as long as the bacteria is present in the throat or nose, the Hib carrier remains contagious. To eradicate the infection, 24 to 48 hours of the right antibiotic treatment are usually needed. Your child should not be allowed to attend daycare or school if they have a Hib infection until after they have finished taking the recommended course of antibiotics and your doctor has determined that they are no longer contagious. Living with an individual who has Hib infection can sometimes necessitate the use of prophylactic antibiotics. In such a scenario, medical professionals will receive guidance from the Department of Health.

6.5.6.3. Diagnosis of Hib Infection

It is crucial to specifically test for the presence of Hib because other bacteria can cause infections that are similar to those caused by Hib. One's diagnosis could be:

- physical examination

- blood test
- test of the cerebrospinal fluid, which is obtained through lumbar punctures and involves the use of needles.
- tests of other specimens.

When symptoms of a life-threatening condition appear suddenly in a previously healthy child, it is usually an emergency diagnosis.

6.5.6.4. Treatment for Hib infection

The course of treatment may vary depending on the illness.

- admission to hospital
- an antibiotic course that is appropriate.

In order to help a child with epiglottitis breathe, a breathing tube may be placed and they may receive care in an intensive care unit.

6.5.6.5. Immunization Against Hib

Immunization is advised for all newborns, young children, and individuals with specific medical risk conditions as it offers the best defense against Hib infection. The National Immunization Program Schedule offers protection against Hib. The Hib vaccination is free in Victoria for the following reasons.

- The first three main doses of the Hib vaccine are administered to all babies at two (starting at six weeks), four, and six months of age. This is done as part of a six-in-one vaccine that also includes the polio, hepatitis B, pertussis (whooping cough), diphtheria, and tetanus shots.
- Every child receives their fourth booster dose of the Hib vaccine at 18 months of age.
- A single catch-up dose is necessary for children who have not received any previous doses and are between the ages of 18 and 59 months.
- Catch-up doses of the combined vaccine (diphtheria, tetanus, pertussis, whooping cough), hepatitis B, polio, and Hib vaccine) are available for children up to and including nine years of age.

For those without a spleen or with a malfunctioning spleen who have not received a prior Hib vaccination, a single dose of the vaccine is advised. It is advised that recipients of stem cell transplants be vaccinated against Hib, with a recommended course of three doses.

6.5.6.5.1. Before Hib Immunization

Make sure you inform your doctor or nurse before receiving an immunization if you (or your child):

- are sick on the day of the vaccination (higher than 38°C).
- possess experienced a severe reaction to a vaccination in the past.
- possess a severe allergy to all things.
- are pregnant.

6.5.6.5.2. Pregnancy and Hib Immunization

The Hib vaccine is not advised for women who are nursing or pregnant, but you should still consult your doctor if you are expecting a child and do not have a spleen.

6.5.6.6. Side Effects of Hib Vaccine

Although all medications can have unwanted side effects, immunizations containing vaccines against diphtheria, tetanus, Hib, and other infectious diseases (including the six-in-one, four-in-one, three-in-one, and two-in-one vaccines) are generally effective and safe. Side effects from these combined vaccines are rare and typically mild, but may include:

- localized injection site swelling, redness, and pain.
- sporadically a lump (nodule) at the injection site that may persist for several weeks without requiring treatment.
- low grade (fever) temperature.
- Children can be drowsy, exhausted, agitated, tearful, and generally unhappy.

Muscle aches may also be felt if a combined immunization also includes the polio vaccine (the six-in-one and the four-in-one vaccine).

6.5.6.6.1. Managing Fever after Immunization

Typically, vaccination-related side effects are minor and transient, happening within the first 48 hours of the shot. Typically, special care is not needed. Several treatment options are available to mitigate the side effects of the vaccine, such as:

- Give them more water to drink.
- Infants and kids should not be overdressed if they are hot.
- While it is not advised to take paracetamol on a regular basis following vaccination, it can be administered if there is a fever. When administering paracetamol to children in particular, make sure you consult your pharmacist or check the label for the appropriate dosage.

6.5.6.6.2. Managing Injection Site Discomfort

For one to two days following an injection, many vaccines can cause pain, redness, itching, swelling, or burning at the injection site. It may be necessary to take paracetamol to relieve the discomfort. A hard, tiny lump called a nodule may occasionally remain at the injection site for a few weeks or months. There is no need for treatment and this shouldn't be concerning.

6.5.6.6.3. Concerns about Immunization Side Effects

See your doctor or immunization nurse as soon as possible, or proceed straight to a hospital, if an adverse event that follows immunization is sudden, severe, or persistent, or if you have concerns about your child's or your own health following immunization. It's also crucial to consult a doctor if you or your child are feeling sick, as this could be the result of another illness rather than the vaccination.

The Victorian Surveillance of Adverse Events Following Vaccination in the Community (SAEFVIC) Line is the place to report adverse events that follow immunization. The central reporting service for any major adverse events that occur after vaccinations in Victoria is called SAEFVIC. You can talk about reporting adverse events in other states or territories with your immunization provider.

6.5.6.6.4. Rare Immunization Side Effects

Any vaccination carries a very small risk of causing a life-threatening allergic reaction (anaphylaxis). Because of this, it is recommended that you remain at the clinic or doctor's office for at least 15 minutes after receiving your vaccination in case more care is needed. For more information or if you are concerned, get in touch with your doctor if any other reactions are severe and ongoing (Demirjian and Levy, 2009; Havelaar et al, 2010; Davis, 2011; Ginsburg et al, 2014; Rappuoli et al, 2017).

6.5.7. Measles

A virus causes a childhood infection known as measles. Measles was once fairly common, but vaccinations almost always prevent it. Measles, also known as rubeola, is contagious, dangerous, and sometimes fatal in young children. Even though measles death rates have been declining globally as more kids get the vaccine, the illness still claims the lives of over 200,000 people annually, the majority of whom are children. The measles hasn't been common in the US for roughly 20 years due to high vaccination rates overall. Recent cases of measles in the U.S. started outside the nation and affected individuals who were either unvaccinated or unaware of their vaccination status.

6.5.7.1. Symptoms

Signs and symptoms of measles usually manifest 10 to 14 days following viral exposure. The following are typical measles signs and symptoms.

- Fever
- Dry cough
- Runny nose
- Sore throat
- Inflamed eyes (conjunctivitis)
- Koplik's spots are tiny white spots on the inner lining of the cheek that have bluish-white centers on a red background. They are located inside the mouth.
- A skin rash consisting of big, flat patches that frequently merge together.

The infection progresses for two to three weeks.

- Infection and incubation. The first 10 to 14 days following infection are when the measles virus multiplies within the body. During this period, there are no measles signs or symptoms.
- Nonspecific signs and symptoms. A mild to moderate fever, along with other symptoms like a runny nose, sore throat, swollen eyes, and conjunctivitis, are the usual first signs of measles. This rather minor ailment could linger for two to three days.
- Acute illness and rash. Little red spots, some of which are slightly elevated, make up the rash. The skin appears splotchy red due to spots and bumps in tightly clustered formations. First, the face gets red.

The rash appears on the arms, chest, and back over the course of the following few days, before moving on to the thighs, lower legs, and feet. Simultaneously, the temperature increases significantly, frequently reaching 104 to 105.8 F (40 to 41 C).

- Recovery. One may experience a seven-day rash from measles. The face rash disappears first, followed by the thighs and feet. The cough and skin darkening or peeling where the rash was may persist for approximately 10 days after other symptoms of the illness go away.

For approximately eight days, beginning four days before the rash's appearance and concluding four days after it does, a person who has the measles can transmit the virus to others.

6.5.7.2. Causes

The measles is a highly transmissible disease. It can thus be transmitted to other people very easily. A virus that is present in an infected child or adult's nose and throat is what causes measles. Infectious droplets spray into the air when a person with the measles coughs, sneezes, or talks, where they can be inhaled by other people. The contagious droplets have an hour or so to hang in the atmosphere. It is also possible for the contagious droplets to land on a surface, where they can survive and propagate for a few hours. Touching an infected surface and then rubbing your eyes or putting your fingers in your mouth or nose can spread the measles virus. Between four days before and four days following the rash's appearance, measles is extremely contagious. When exposed to someone who has the measles virus, about 90% of people who have not had the disease or received the vaccination will contract it.

6.5.7.3. Diagnosis

The characteristic rash of measles and Koplik's spot, a small, bluish-white spot on a bright red background on the inside lining of the cheek, are usually enough to confirm the diagnosis. Your doctor might inquire about any measles vaccinations you or your child have received, any international travel outside of the U.S. recently, as well as if you've come into contact with anyone who's feverish or rashy. But many healthcare professionals have never encountered measles. Numerous other illnesses can be mistaken for the rash. If required, a blood test can determine if the rash is indeed the measles. Measles virus confirmation can also be achieved by a test that typically requires a urine sample or throat swab.

6.5.7.4. Treatment

Once contracted, there is no particular treatment for measles. Treatment entails treating or avoiding complications in addition to offering comfort measures like rest to relieve symptoms. After being exposed to the virus, there are steps that can be taken to safeguard those who are not immune to the measles.

- **Post-Exposure Vaccination:** Within 72 hours of being exposed to the measles virus, anyone who is not immune to the disease, including infants, may receive the measles vaccine as a preventative measure. In most cases, the symptoms of measles are milder and disappear faster if the illness persists.
- **Immune Serum Globulin:** Immunoglobulin, a protein injection, is a possible treatment for individuals exposed to the virus who are pregnant, nursing babies, or have compromised immune systems. These antibodies can either prevent measles or lessen its symptoms when administered within six days of virus exposure.

6.5.7.4.1. Medications

Among the possible courses of treatment for measles are:

- **Fever Reducers:** Over-the-counter drugs like acetaminophen (Tylenol, etc.), ibuprofen (Advil, Motrin IB, Children's Motrin, etc.), or naproxen sodium (Aleve) can help reduce fevers associated with measles if they are causing discomfort for you or your child. Carefully read the labels, or get advice from your pharmacist or healthcare provider regarding the right dosage.

When giving aspirin to kids or teenagers, proceed with caution. Even though aspirin is safe to use in kids over three, it should never be given to kids or teenagers who are recovering from the flu or chickenpox. This is because aspirin has been connected to Reye's syndrome in these kids, a rare but potentially fatal illness.

- **Antibiotics:** Your doctor may prescribe an antibiotic if you or your child contracts a bacterial infection during the measles, such as pneumonia or an ear infection.
- **Vitamin A:** Youngsters who are deficient in vitamin A are more likely to contract the measles severely. Vitamin A administration may mitigate the severity of a child's measles infection. For children older than a year, a large dose of 200,000 international units (IU) is typically administered. Younger children may receive smaller doses.

6.5.7.5. Prevention

In the U.S. to avoid contracting measles, the Centers for Disease Control and Prevention (CDC) advises both adults and children to get the vaccine.

6.5.7.5.1. Measles Vaccine in Children

Usually, a combination measles-mumps-rubella (MMR) vaccine is administered in place of the measles vaccine. The measles, mumps, rubella, varicella, or MMRV vaccine may also be included in this vaccination. It is advised by medical professionals that children get the measles, mumps, and rubella (MMR) vaccination between the ages of 12 and 15 months and again between the ages of 4 and 6 before starting school. The two doses of the MMR vaccination have a 97% lifetime protection rate against measles. The symptoms of measles are usually not too severe in the few individuals who contract it after receiving vaccinations.

Keep in mind:

- If you'll be traveling internationally outside the U. S. See your child's doctor about receiving the measles vaccination earlier if your child is between 6 and 11 months old.
- Your child may require two vaccinations spaced four weeks apart if they did not receive the two doses of the vaccine at the prescribed times.

For roughly six months following delivery, infants born to mothers who have had the vaccination or who are immune due to past measles infections are typically shielded from the disease. The vaccination can be administered as early as six months of age if a child needs to be protected against the measles before the age of 12 months, for instance, to travel abroad. Even so, children who receive their vaccinations before the recommended age still need to receive them later.

In addition to requiring fewer shots, giving a child the MMR vaccine as part of a recommended vaccination series can stop them from developing immunity to measles, mumps, and rubella later on. The combined vaccination is equally safe and effective as the individual shots. Fever and a sore arm from the injection site are possible side effects, though they are usually not severe.

6.5.7.5.2. Measles Vaccine in Adults

If you are an adult without evidence of immunity, you may require the measles vaccination and:

- possesses a higher risk of contracting the measles due to factors like working in a hospital, going to college, or visiting countries outside of the U.S.

- was born, at most, in 1957. You cannot contract the measles again if you have already had the illness because your body has strengthened its defenses against the virus. The majority of those born or residing in the U.S. are resistant to the measles because they have already had it before 1957.

Evidence of immunity, or defense against contracting the measles, consists of:

- Measles vaccination records that are properly documented in writing.
- tests in the lab that demonstrate immunity.
- test results indicating a history of measles infection.

See your doctor if you're unsure if you require the measles vaccination.

6.5.7.5.3. Preventing Measles During an Outbreak or Known Infection

To safeguard friends and family who lack immunity, take the following actions if someone in your home has the measles:

- **Isolate:** People who have the measles should stay at home and avoid going back to social situations during the four days leading up to the rash appearing because this is a highly contagious period.

Siblings, for example, who have not received the vaccination, should also avoid contact with the infected individual.

- **Vaccinate:** As soon as possible, make sure that anyone who is susceptible to contracting the measles but has not received all recommended vaccinations gets the vaccine. This covers all infants older than six months as well as anyone born after 1957 who does not possess proof of immunity.

6.5.7.5.4. Preventing New Infections

It is crucial to receive the measles vaccination for the following reasons.

- **Maintaining and Fostering General Immunity:** Since the introduction of the measles vaccine, measles has virtually been eliminated in the U.S., even though not everyone has been vaccinated. This effect is called herd immunity.

But because vaccination rates are probably declining, herd immunity may be waning a little bit at this point. The incidence of measles in the U.S. recently increased significantly.

- **Preventing a Measles Outbreak:** Measles starts to resurface shortly after vaccination rates start to drop, which is why stable vaccination rates are crucial.

Here's an illustration. A now-discredited study that erroneously connected autism to the measles, mumps, rubella (MMR) vaccine was published in 1998. The study's original country, the United Kingdom, saw a record low vaccination rate in 2003–2004, with roughly 80% of children receiving vaccinations. In England and Wales, there were almost 1,400 cases of measles with lab confirmation in 2008.

6.5.7.5.5. No Proven Link between the MMR Vaccine and Autism

Following the MMR study in 1998, there were some vaccination declines observed in the UK and other countries, leading some individuals to speculate that a connection might exist. Since then, there have been many concerns expressed regarding a potential connection between autism and the MMR vaccine. The MMR vaccine and autism, however, are not linked by science, according to a number of comprehensive reports from the American Academy of Pediatrics, the National Academy of Medicine, and the Centers for Disease Control and Prevention (CDC). These organizations observe that toddlers with autism are frequently diagnosed between the ages of 18 and 30 months, which coincides with when children receive their first dose of the MMR vaccine. However, this timing coincidence shouldn't be interpreted as a cause-and-effect relationship (Demirjian and Levy, 2009; Havelaar et al, 2010; Davis, 2011; Ginsburg et al, 2014; Rappuoli et al, 2017).

6.5.8. Mumps

Before the introduction of the MMR vaccine, children were frequently afflicted with the contagious viral infection known as mumps.

6.5.8.1. Symptoms of Mumps

The painful swellings in the side of the face beneath the ears, known as the parotid glands, are the most noticeable sign of mumps, giving a victim of the disease a recognizable hamster face. Headaches, joint pain, and fever are some additional signs of the mumps that may appear a few days prior to parotid gland swelling.

6.5.8.2. How Mumps Is Spread

Similar to how colds and the flu are spread, mumps is also contracted by inhaling or contacting infected saliva droplets that land on surfaces and enter the mouth or nose. A person is most contagious in the days just prior to the onset of symptoms and in the days that follow. It's critical to stop the infection from spreading during this time, especially to unvaccinated teens and young adults.

If you already have the mumps, you can stop it from spreading by:

- Frequently use soap to wash your hands.
- sneezing into a tissue and discarding it.
- When your symptoms initially appear, stay away from work and school for at least five days.

6.5.8.3. Preventing Mumps

Make sure your child receives the combined MMR vaccine for rubella, measles, and mumps to protect them against the mumps. The standard childhood immunization schedule of the NHS includes the MMR vaccination. A booster dose should be given to your child twice, once around the age of 12 to 13 months and again at 3 years and 4 months. The vaccination offers about 88% protection against the mumps after both doses are administered. To schedule a vaccination, anyone who was not administered both doses of the MMR vaccine as a child should speak with their doctor.

6.5.8.4. Treatment for Mumps

The mumps infection should go away in one or two weeks, but there is currently no treatment for it.

To reduce symptoms, treatment consists of:

- consuming plenty of fluids and resting in bed.
- utilizing pain relievers like ibuprofen and paracetamol; children under the age of 16 shouldn't be given aspirin.
- using a warm or cold compress to ease the pain in the enlarged glands.

6.5.8.5. Complications

The majority of the time, mumps passes without seriously harming a person's health. Severe consequences are not common. However, if the mumps virus penetrates the outer layer of the brain, it can result in viral meningitis. Testicular or ovarian swelling is another complication (assuming the patient has completed puberty).

6.5.9. Rubella

The viral disease rubella results in a skin rash and a low fever. Although it is not brought on by the same virus that causes measles (rubeola), it is also known as German measles. Contact with fluid from the nose and throat can transmit rubella. A vaccine can stop it from happening. Rubella typically causes only a mild case of rash and a few respiratory symptoms in babies and children. However, it may pose a serious infection risk to a developing fetus. Birth defects or miscarriage may result from it.

6.5.9.1. Causes of Rubella in A Child

A virus is the cause of rubella. The virus is transmitted by secretions from an infected person's throat and nose. It can also transfer from a pregnant woman to her fetus. Up until the age of one, a newborn diagnosed with rubella is thought to be contagious. Infections with rubella are most prevalent in late winter and early spring.

6.5.9.2. Symptoms of Rubella in a Child

After being exposed to the virus, a child may not exhibit any symptoms of rubella for 14–21 days. Each child may experience symptoms slightly differently. The most typical signs begin with:

- A period of not feeling well
- Low fever
- Runny nose
- Diarrhea

These signs could linger for one to five days.

Next, a rash shows up. The pimple:

- begins as a pink rash with patches of tiny, raised lesions on the face.
- As the face rash goes away, it extends to the arms, legs, and torso.
- Fades in 3 to 5 days

Additionally, your child might have enlarged neck lymph nodes. An older child's joints might be painful and inflamed. When the rash is first developing, a child is most contagious. However, a child may spread the rash seven days before it appears and seven days after it does. This means that a child may infect others with the virus before you even realize they are ill. Rubella symptoms can resemble those of other illnesses. Ensure that your child visits their physician to receive a diagnosis.

6.5.9.3. Evaluation

Due to the possibility of mild and non-specific symptoms, the clinical diagnosis of rubella can be challenging. Consequently, in order to confirm rubella, doctors must rely on serological testing. Using an enzyme immunoassay, the most popular diagnostic procedure for recent postnatal infection is the identification of IgM antibodies specific to rubella. IgM antibodies specific to rubella are typically detectable four days after the rash appears. Furthermore, a four-fold or higher increase in rubella-specific IgG titers between acute and convalescent sera is indicative of both infection and reinfection. Rubella-specific low avidity IgG can also be used to confirm recent primary rubella infections.

If a pregnant woman has been exposed to someone with suspected rubella, it is important to test her blood for rubella-specific IgG antibodies promptly. A positive result means she is likely immune, while a negative result requires further testing for rubella-specific IgG and IgM antibodies three weeks later to rule out an asymptomatic primary rubella infection. Congenital rubella infection can be diagnosed during pregnancy by finding specific IgM in fetal blood or detecting rubella RNA in amniotic fluid, fetal blood, or chorionic villus biopsy with

RT-PCR. In newborns, congenital rubella is diagnosed by finding rubella-specific IgM within the first 6 months of life or by observing an increase or persistence of rubella-specific IgG after 6 to 12 months. Laboratory evidence of CRS can also be provided by detecting the viral genome in nasopharyngeal swabs, urine, and oral fluid using RT-PCR.

6.5.9.4. Treatment / Management

When treating non-gravid individuals for postnatally acquired rubella, non-steroidal anti-inflammatory drugs are typically used to treat fever, arthralgia, and/or arthritis. The gestation age at the onset of infection determines the course of treatment for pregnant women. Pregnancy termination should be considered in accordance with local ethical and legal regulations, as the fetus is at high risk of infection and subsequent malformation if the infection develops before 18 weeks of gestation. With ultrasound monitoring and specialized neonatal care, the pregnancy may be continued if the infection develops after 18 weeks of gestation. Children with congenital rubella syndrome should receive organ-specific and symptomatic treatment. A multidisciplinary approach is typically used, and evaluations in the areas of pediatrics, ophthalmology, cardiology, audiology, and neurodevelopment are necessary. To keep an eye out for any delayed manifestations, long-term monitoring is required.

6.5.9.5. Differential Diagnosis

It is necessary to differentiate rubella from other infections that present with similar maculopapular rashes, such as measles, infectious mononucleosis, cytomegalovirus, enteroviruses, scarlet fever, mycoplasma infection, arboviruses (Zika virus, West Nile fever, Ross River fever, and Chikungunya virus), and human herpesvirus 6 and 7. In the differential diagnosis of rubella, non-infectious causes such as drug eruption, contact dermatitis, and Kawasaki disease should also be taken into account.

6.5.9.6. Prognosis

Rubella postnatal infection is usually mild, self-limited, and has a very good prognosis. Children with congenital rubella syndrome, on the other hand, have a less favorable prognosis that varies based on the severity and number of organs affected. Infants with thrombocytopenia, pulmonary hypertension, hepatosplenomegaly, and interstitial pneumonia have a significant mortality risk. Congenital rubella syndrome sufferers may also experience long-term consequences such as heart failure, blindness, developmental delays, and shortened lifespans.

6.5.9.7. Complications

The most frequent consequence of a rubella infection is the development of polyarthritis and polyarthralgia, which affects up to 70% of adolescent and adult females. It affects the wrists, fingers, knees, and ankles and is typically symmetrical. Thrombocytopenia, hemolytic anemia, myocarditis, pericarditis, hepatitis, orchitis, retinopathy, uveitis, Guillain-Barré syndrome, and post-infection encephalitis are other, albeit uncommon, symptoms. Premature labor, congenital rubella syndrome, intrauterine fetal death, miscarriage, and intrauterine growth retardation are all possible outcomes of rubella infection during pregnancy. If the infection is caught during the first 12 weeks of pregnancy, there is a greater chance of complications.

6.5.10. Varicella

Chickenpox, also known as varicella, is a contagious disease caused by the varicella-zoster virus (VZV), a DNA virus belonging to the herpesvirus group. After the initial infection, the virus remains in the body, specifically in the sensory nerve ganglia, in a dormant state. The primary infection results in chickenpox, while reactivation of the dormant virus leads to shingles, a condition also known as herpes zoster.

6.5.10.1. Clinical Features

6.5.10.1.1. Incubation Period and Prodrome

Varicella typically takes 14 to 16 days, with a range of 10 to 21 days, to incubate after exposure to a varicella or herpes zoster rash. Particularly in adults, a mild prodrome of fever and malaise may manifest one to two days prior to the onset of rash. The rash is frequently the initial indication of illness in children.

6.5.10.1.2. Varicella in Unvaccinated Persons

The rash is itchy and widespread. Before crusting, the lesions move quickly from macular to papular to vesicular. Usually, lesions occur simultaneously in every developmental stage. Usually, the rash starts on the face, back, and chest before spreading to every part of the body. Typically, the back and chest are where the lesions are most prevalent. A typical case lasts four to seven days. Varicella is typically mild in healthy children, causing an itchy rash, malaise, and a temperature as high as 102°F for two to three days. Pregnant women, immunocompromised individuals, adults, adolescents, and infants are more susceptible to more severe disease and complications. Lifelong immunity is typically conferred upon recovery from a primary varicella infection. It is rare for varicella to recur in otherwise well individuals. Immunocompromised individuals may be more susceptible to a second varicella infection. Re-exposure to natural (wild-type) varicella may result in re-infection that increases antibody titers without resulting in disease or observable viremia, similar to other viral infections.

6.5.10.1.3. Varicella in Vaccinated Persons (Breakthrough Varicella)

When a vaccinated person contracts the wild-type varicella-zoster virus (VZV) more than 42 days after receiving their varicella vaccination, this condition is known as breakthrough varicella. Typically, breakthrough varicella is not severe. Less than 50 skin lesions and afebrile or mildly fevered conditions are typical in patients. When compared to those who are not vaccinated, they typically experience a shorter illness. Rather than vesicular, the rash is more likely to be primarily maculopapular. However, 25–30% of individuals receiving a single dose vaccination and developing breakthrough varicella will exhibit clinical characteristics akin to those of varicella patients who have not received a vaccination. It can be challenging to diagnose breakthrough varicella based solely on clinical presentation because the illness's symptoms are frequently mild. Confirming varicella and managing patients and their contacts appropriately depend more and more on laboratory testing. Compared to individuals who have only received one dose of the vaccine, recipients of two doses experience a lower incidence of breakthrough varicella; in fact, there is some evidence that the disease may be even milder in two-dose recipients.

6.5.10.2. Transmission

The varicella virus spreads easily. Direct contact, inhaling aerosols from vesicular fluid of acute varicella or zoster skin lesions, and possibly through infected respiratory secretions that may also be aerosolized are the three ways that the virus can transfer from one person to another. A varicella patient is contagious for one to two days prior to the rash appearing and until all lesions have crusted. Vaccinated individuals may experience non-crusting lesions. Until no new lesions have developed for a full day, these individuals are regarded as contagious.

The time interval between virus exposure and varicella development is 10 to 21 days. Research on the spread of varicella among family members indicates that approximately 90% of vulnerable close contacts will contract the illness after coming into contact with an infected individual. One household study discovered that the risk of VZV transmission from herpes zoster was roughly 20% of the risk for transmission from varicella, despite the fact that there is insufficient data to evaluate the risk of VZV transmission from zoster. Individuals who have breakthrough varicella are also communicable. People with mild breakthrough varicella (less than 50 lesions) who received a single dose of the varicella vaccine were found to be one-third more contagious than those who had not received the vaccine, according to a study on the spread of varicella in households. On the other hand, individuals with 50 lesions or more from breakthrough varicella were no less contagious than those who had not received the vaccination. Compared to measles, varicella is less contagious, but it is more contagious than rubella and the mumps.

6.5.10.3. Complications

The most typical varicella-related side effects are:

- **In Children:** soft tissue and skin bacterial infections.
- **In Adults:** Pneumonia

Viral pneumonia, encephalitis, cerebellar ataxia, and hemorrhagic conditions are among the virus's severe side effects. Bacterial infections also cause the following serious side effects:

- Septicemia
- Toxic shock syndrome
- Necrotizing fasciitis
- Osteomyelitis
- Bacterial pneumonia
- Septic arthritis

6.5.10.4. People at High Risk for Severe Varicella

Those listed below are susceptible to severe varicella.

- individuals with compromised immune systems who do not exhibit varicella immunity, such as:
  - those who have lymphoma or leukemia.
  - those taking immune-suppressive drugs, such as chemotherapeutic agents or systemic steroids at high dosages.
  - those suffering from immune system disorders or cellular immune deficiencies.
- infants whose moms contract varicella between five days before delivery and two days thereafter.
- Premature infants exposed to zoster or varicella, in particular:
  - hospitalized premature babies whose mothers do not exhibit any signs of immunity and who were born at less than 28 weeks gestation.
  - hospitalized premature babies, regardless of their mothers' varicella immunity status, who are born before 28 weeks of pregnancy or who weigh more than 1,000 grams at birth.
- pregnant ladies who don't show any signs of varicella immunity.

6.5.10.4.1. Immunocompromised People

When immunocompromised individuals contract varicella, they run the risk of internal organ infection, or visceral dissemination, which can result in pneumonia, encephalitis, hepatitis, and disseminated intravascular coagulopathy. They may experience more lesions in their atypical varicella rash and a longer illness than immunocompetent varicella patients. It is possible for new lesions to develop on the palms and soles, to be hemorrhagic, and to persist in developing for longer than seven days.

6.5.10.4.2. People with HIV or AIDS

Children infected with HIV often have an unusual rash, with new lesions appearing every few weeks or months. The lesions may begin as normal maculopapular vesicular lesions but may progress to necrotic, crusted, hyperkeratotic, non-healing ulcers. Children with low CD4 counts who are HIV-positive are more likely to experience this. According to certain research, children with HIV have a lower incidence of VZV dissemination to the visceral organs than do other immunocompromised individuals infected with the virus. Additionally, children receiving antiretroviral therapy or adults with higher CD4 counts at the time of varicella infection may experience a lower rate of complications. Children and adolescents with HIV infection may develop retinitis. The majority of adults, including those with HIV, have already experienced varicella and have tested positive for VZV. Consequently, varicella is comparatively rare in adults with HIV infection.

6.5.10.4.3. Pregnant Women

When pregnant women contract varicella, they run the risk of developing serious complications, most commonly pneumonia, and in rare instances, varicella may even be fatal. While other research has not corroborated this finding, some studies have indicated that varicella contracted during the third trimester increases the incidence and severity of VZV pneumonia. There is a tiny chance that a baby born to a pregnant woman who contracts varicella in the first or early second trimester will have congenital varicella syndrome (0.4 to 2.0%). The infant might be born underweight, with abnormalities in the brain, eyes, and limbs, as well as skin scarring.

The newborn is susceptible to neonatal varicella if the mother has varicella rash between five days prior to delivery and two days following delivery. Neonatal varicella death rates used to be estimated to be around 30%, but with the introduction of VZV immune globulin and intensive supportive care, the mortality rate has dropped to roughly 7%.

6.5.10.5. Managing People at High Risk for Severe Varicella

Varicella-Zoster Immune Globulin: Varicella-zoster immune globulin can stop varicella from developing or lessen the severity of the disease in people exposed to varicella or herpes zoster who are unable to receive the varicella vaccine. It is advised to give varicella-zoster immune globulin to those who cannot get the vaccine and who: 1) do not show any signs of immunity to varicella; 2) are at high risk of contracting an infection from exposure; and 3) are not immune to varicella.

VariZIGTM is the varicella-zoster immune globulin product that has been licensed for use in the US. VariZIG can be administered within 10 days of exposure to VZV and should be administered as soon as possible.

- **Acyclovir Treatment:** The AAP suggests that individuals at higher risk for moderate to severe varicella should be considered for treatment with oral acyclovir or valacyclovir. These groups at increased risk include:
  - healthy adults over the age of 12.

- people suffering from long-term lung or skin conditions.
- Individuals undergoing extended salicylate treatment.
- those getting corticosteroid courses that are brief, sporadic, or aerosolized.

Oral acyclovir or valacyclovir may be chosen by certain medical professionals to treat secondary cases that occur in a household. Oral acyclovir or valacyclovir therapy should be administered within the first 24 hours following the onset of the varicella rash for optimal benefit.

The American Academy of Pediatrics advises against administering oral acyclovir or valacyclovir therapy to otherwise healthy children who have typical varicella without any side effects. Drug category B includes acyclovir according to the U.S. Food and Drug Administration's Drug Risk Classification in pregnancy. For pregnant women who have varicella, some experts advise taking valacyclovir or acyclovir orally, especially in the second and third trimesters. If a pregnant patient has serious varicella-related viral complications like pneumonia, intravenous acyclovir is advised.

Treatment with intravenous acyclovir is advised for severe illness (e.g., encephalitis, pneumonia, thrombocytopenia, and severe hepatitis) as well as varicella in patients with compromised immune systems (including those receiving high-dose corticosteroid therapy for longer than 14 days).

Adults with VZV infections can be treated with famciclovir; however, children's safety and effectiveness have not been determined. Foscarnet should be used to treat VZV infections caused by acyclovir-resistant strains of the virus, which typically affect immunocompromised individuals. However, it is advised to consult an infectious disease specialist before starting treatment.

6.5.10.6. Assessing Immunity to Varicella

For all children, adolescents, and adults without proof of varicella immunity, two doses of the vaccine are advised. For optimal protection against the illness, individuals who have already received one dose of the varicella vaccine ought to receive their second dose.

Any of the following could be a sign of varicella immunity.

- Documentation of age-appropriate varicella vaccination.
  - Children in preschool (ages 12 months to 3 years): one dosage.
  - Individuals of school-age, adolescents, and adults are recommended to receive two doses.
- proof of immunity from the lab or proof of illness from the lab*.
- Births in the United States prior to 1980 should not be regarded as proof of immunity for healthcare personnel, pregnant women, and individuals with compromised immune systems.
- diagnosis or confirmation by a medical professional of a history of varicella or herpes zoster.

*While commercial assays are useful for evaluating immunity induced by disease, they are not sensitive enough to identify immunity induced by vaccinations (i.e., they could produce erroneous negative outcomes).

To confirm a varicella history, medical professionals should ask about:

- An epidemiological connection to a laboratory-confirmed varicella case, or another typical varicella case.
- Proof of laboratory validation, if tests were carried out while the illness was acute.

Individuals without laboratory confirmation of varicella nor an epidemiologic connection should not be recognized as having a legitimate medical history. If these individuals have only received one dose of the vaccine, a second dose is advised. There is no need for vaccination if a medical professional confirms the diagnosis using the aforementioned standards. It is not advised to routinely test for varicella immunity following two vaccination doses. Commercial assays currently on the market are not sensitive enough to always detect antibodies following vaccination. The outcomes of later serologic testing take precedence over the documented receipt of two doses of the varicella vaccine.

6.5.10.7. Preventing Varicella in Healthcare Settings

6.5.10.7.1. Nosocomial Transmission of VZV

It is commonly known that nosocomial transmission of VZV can pose a serious risk to a patient's life in some circumstances. Nosocomial transmission cases are rare in the US since the varicella vaccine was introduced. In hospitals, long-term care facilities, and other healthcare settings, patients, healthcare providers, and visitors who have varicella or herpes zoster can infect susceptible patients and healthcare providers with VZV. Transmissions in healthcare environments have been linked to a lack of prompt implementation of control measures and a delay in the diagnosis or reporting of varicella and herpes zoster. Certain patients without evidence of immunity are at increased risk for severe varicella and its complications, even though all susceptible patients in healthcare settings are at risk:

- premature babies born to mothers who are vulnerable.
- infants, regardless of mother immune status, born at less than 28 weeks gestation or weighing less than 1,000 grams.
- Individuals with compromised immune systems, such as those receiving immunosuppressive treatment, suffering from cancer, or lacking sufficient immune function.
- Pregnant women

6.5.10.8. Management of Patients with Varicella

Until lesions are dry and crusted, healthcare providers should take all standard precautions in addition to airborne (negative air-flow rooms) and contact precautions. Patients with varicella should be isolated in closed rooms with no contact with people who do not exhibit proof of immunity if negative air-flow rooms are not available. Personnel with proof of immunity should tend to patients who have varicella.

6.5.11. Enteric Fever

Acute, potentially fatal, feverish infection known as enteric fever is brought on by *Salmonella typhi* (typhoid fever) or *S. paratyphi* (paratyphoid fever). Food and water tainted by the excrement and urine of an acutely ill or recovering individual, or by a long-term asymptomatic carrier, are the means of transmission.

6.5.11.1. Clinical Clues

Enteric fever can present with a variety of clinical manifestations, ranging from a mild case (low-grade fever, malaise, occasionally a slight dry cough) to a severe case (severe abdominal pain, serious complications). The infecting dose determines the length of the incubation time. While incubation can range from three days to three months, the typical range is one to three weeks.

Enteric fever manifests clinically as:

- Sustained fever to 40°C
- Malaise
- Abdominal pain
- Constipation or diarrhea
- Severe headache
- Change in mental status
- Especially on the trunk, erythematous, slightly elevated lesions that blanching are called evanescent rose spots.
- Hepatomegaly
- Splenomegaly
- Dactylitis

6.5.11.2. Severity of Infection

In 10% to 15% of cases, complications from enteric fever usually arise in the second or third week of sickness. Within the hospitalized typhoid fever patient population, 3% may experience potentially fatal intestinal bleeding and perforations. Less common side effects include endocarditis and meningitis. Hemolysis during typhoid fever is possible in patients with thalassemia or glucose-6-phosphate dehydrogenase deficiency (G6PD).

The severity and course of an enteric infection can be influenced by several factors.

- length of the illness prior to receiving treatment
- selection of an antimicrobial therapy.
- Age
- Previous exposure
- Typhoid vaccination history
- Virulence of the bacterial strain
- Quantity of inoculum ingested
- Features of the patient, including the type of human leukocyte antigen (HLA), immunosuppression (e.g., AIDS).
- Drugs that reduce stomach acid (e.g., antacids, H2 blockers, etc.).

6.5.11.3. Diagnosis

All febrile children who have traveled to or returned from endemic areas in the previous three months should have a diagnosis considered. Early in the illness, multiple blood cultures are best collected in order to make an accurate diagnosis of enteric fever. Just 50% of blood cultures result in a positive result. It is recommended to send at least one stool sample for bacterial culture and sensitivity testing, with a 30–50% yield. Urine culture yields the least. Children who have experienced a history of Schistosoma hematobium or tuberculosis infection of the urinary tract, which may predispose them to chronic urinary carriage following typhoid fever, may benefit from urine culture. A bone marrow aspirate for culture may be required on occasion; the yield is 90%. There could be leukopenia.

The Widal test is a serologic assay used to detect IgM and IgG antibodies to the O and H antigens of Salmonella. This test is considered unreliable and is not recommended in Canada. Unfortunately, newer serologic assays are not easily accessible. Since there is no definitive serologic test for enteric fever and cultures may yield negative results, the diagnosis often has to be based on clinical evaluations.

6.5.11.4. Management

6.5.11.4.1. Infection Control

Contact precautions must be taken by hospitalized patients diagnosed with enteric fever until three consecutive stool specimen cultures yield negative results. The collection of specimens needs to happen at least 48 hours after antimicrobial therapy is stopped.

6.5.11.4.2. Antimicrobial Therapy

Typhoid fever's clinical course is shortened, and the mortality rate is decreased, with specific antibiotic therapy. Although strains obtained in developing nations are typically susceptible to ceftriaxone, they are frequently resistant to numerous antibiotics. In the 1980s, multidrug resistance (to ampicillin, co-trimoxazole, and chloramphenicol) appeared. In the 1990s, ciprofloxacin susceptibility decreased, and more recently, there have been isolated instances of extended-spectrum cephalosporinase-producing strains. Though it is beginning to spread to other regions of Asia and Africa, resistance is most problematic in South Asia and the Middle East.

If bacteria are susceptible, ampicillin, cotrimoxazole, azithromycin, or ciprofloxacin can be used in place of empirical parenteral ceftriaxone antibiotic therapy; however, this will also depend on the infection site, the host, and the clinical response. Ciprofloxacin has benefits for susceptible S. typhi, there is a decreased incidence of stool carriage, fewer relapses, and a quicker recovery from the fever. It is not authorized for children under the age of 18 to use fluoroquinolones. However, Salmonella species that are resistant to multiple drugs could be a possible use case for ciprofloxacin. Azithromycin might be the most effective oral antibiotic in simple situations where *Salmonella typhi* or *Salmonella paratyphi* is resistant to ciprofloxacin, provided that the organism is susceptible.

Although shorter courses of antibiotics (7 to 10 days) have been successful in treating uncomplicated enteric fever, 10 to 14 days of treatment is recommended for enteric fever. Osteomyelitis should be treated for 4 to 6 weeks, and meningitis for at least four.

6.5.11.4.3. Additional Supportive Measures

For the treatment of patients with enteric fever, further supportive measures could be:

- Oral or intravenous hydration
- Acetaminophen
- Intensive care
- Appropriate nutrition
- Blood transfusion

In the past, patients with severe enteric fever—which is characterized by delirium, obtundation, stupor, coma, or shock—have been recommended corticosteroids. But a recent review indicates that in order to verify their usefulness, larger trials may be necessary.

6.5.11.4.4. Relapse

Even with appropriate therapy, the relapse rate is between 5 and 10%. Relapses are usually milder than the original illness and happen two to three weeks after the fever has subsided. Similar to the first illness, cultures are repeated prior to starting antibiotics. Usually, the pattern of antibiotic susceptibility remains consistent from the initial episode. Differential diagnosis should be further considered based on clinical signs and symptoms.

6.5.11.4.5. Notifying Public Health and Exclusion

Cases of *Salmonella typhi* and *Salmonella paratyphi* infection must be reported to public health authorities, who will then decide how best to manage the cases and contacts in accordance with local regulations. Until three consecutive stool cultures are negative, obtained at least 48 hours after the end of antibiotic treatment, children and staff at child care centers are excluded (Demirjian and Levy, 2009; Havelaar et al, 2010; Davis, 2011; Ginsburg et al, 2014; Rappuoli et al, 2017).

6.5.12. Malaria

A common infection in hot, tropical regions is malaria. Rarely, mild climates can also experience it. Some people may develop mild symptoms from malaria, while others may develop potentially fatal symptoms. Malaria is treatable with the right care.

6.5.12.1. Causes

The parasites that mosquitoes carry are what cause malaria. When an insect bites a person who is already ill, they take up the parasite. The mosquitoes then bite other people, spreading malaria to them. Rarely, malaria can spread from person to person through shared needles, blood transfusions, organ donation, or congenital malaria, which affects mothers and their children. Malaria affects millions of people annually throughout the world. Sub-Saharan Africa is where most cases occur. Malaria causes more than 500,000 deaths worldwide each year. In the United States, malaria is uncommon, and the majority of cases occur in immigrants, travelers, and military personnel. All ages can be affected by malaria, but young children and expectant mothers are more susceptible to serious illness.

6.5.12.2. Signs & Symptoms

In addition to lethargy and irritability, early signs of malaria can also include poor appetite and difficulty sleeping. Chills typically accompany these symptoms, which are followed by a fever and rapid breathing. The fever may either increase very quickly to 105°F (40°C) or higher, or it may rise gradually over the course of one to two days. There is then a severe sweating episode as the fever subsides and the person's body temperature swiftly returns to normal.

Symptoms such as chills, fever, and sweating may recur every two to three days, contingent on the type of malaria parasite causing the infection. Additional symptoms include an enlarged spleen, headache, nausea, and aches and pains throughout the body, particularly in the back and abdomen. Malaria can cause seizures or even cause a person to lose consciousness. In certain instances, the kidneys may also be impacted.

6.5.12.3. Diagnosis

Based on a patient's symptoms, examination results, and place of residence or travel, doctors may suspect malaria. Using a microscope, doctors may extract a sample of blood to look for malaria parasites, which are found inside infected red blood cells. If a patient has a fever with no apparent cause, doctors in nations where the disease is common may treat them for malaria without ordering laboratory work.

6.5.12.4. Treatment

Antimalarial medications can be injected intravenously, orally, or administered through an IV line to treat malaria. A patient may receive treatment at home over a few days or in the hospital with IV medication where they can be monitored more carefully, depending on the parasite causing the malaria and the severity of the illness. In addition, medical professionals keep an eye out for symptoms of dehydration, seizures, anemia, and other issues that could impact the spleen, kidneys, or brain. A patient might require blood transfusions, oxygen support, and fluids. Malaria usually heals in two weeks if caught early and treated. However, those who reside in regions where malaria is prevalent may contract the disease again and never fully recover from one bout of illness to the next. In children who are malnourished, the disease can be lethal if left untreated.

6.5.12.5. Prevention

By employing mosquito-control initiatives targeted at eliminating malaria-carrying mosquitoes, health authorities attempt to prevent malaria. When visiting a region where malaria is a major concern, you can:

- Install window screens.
- Use insect repellent.
- Cover beds with mosquito netting. Bed nets treated with insecticides have significantly reduced the number of African children who die from malaria.
- Put on long sleeves and long pants to cover your skin.
- When mosquitoes are most active, which is usually at dawn and dusk, stay inside.

Before traveling to any tropical or subtropical region where there is a high risk of malaria, consult your doctor. To stop the illness, your doctor can prescribe antimalarial medications to your family. These are taken prior to, during, and following a trip. Around the world, numerous vaccines against malaria are being developed and tested. However, the malaria parasite has a convoluted life cycle, making vaccine development challenging.

6.5.13. Dengue Illness

A virus spread by mosquitoes is the cause of the tropical illness known as dengue fever. Fever, headaches, rashes, and generalized body pain can all be caused by the virus. The majority of dengue fever cases are mild and resolve on their own within a week or so.

Despite sporadic outbreaks in Texas, Florida, and Hawaii, dengue fever is not common in the continental United States. However, dengue fever is widespread in American Samoa, Puerto Rico, and the U.S. Virgin Islands. It is also widespread in many tropical nations in Asia, Africa, and Central and South America. Be cautious of dengue fever if you are planning a trip abroad, particularly to a tropical nation. The risk of infection can be reduced by applying insect repellent, covering sleeping areas with netting, and staying indoors between the hours of dusk and dawn when mosquitoes are most active.

6.5.13.1. Causes of Dengue Fever

Four related viruses that cause dengue fever are transmitted by Aedes mosquitoes, which are widespread in tropical and subtropical regions across the world. Aedes mosquitoes can spread the dengue virus to humans they bite, and the mosquito itself may contract the virus. Someone else may contract the dengue virus and become ill with dengue fever if they are bitten by this mosquito. There is no direct way for the virus to infect someone. Rarely, dengue fever can develop into dengue hemorrhagic fever (DHF), a more severe form of the illness. DHF requires immediate medical attention because it may be fatal.

6.5.13.2. Signs & Symptoms of Dengue Fever

When a child has dengue fever for the first time or in younger age, symptoms are usually mild. Moderate to severe symptoms may be present in older children, adults, and people who have previously had an infection.

The following are typical dengue fever signs and symptoms.

- high fever, possibly as high as 105°F (40°C)
- discomfort in the bones, muscles, joints, and/or behind the eyes.
- severe headache
- rash covering most of the body.
- slight bleeding in the gums or nose.
- bruising easily

The term "breakbone fever" was once used to describe dengue fever, which may help you understand the extreme pain it can occasionally cause in the muscles and bones. Although it doesn't truly break bones, the fever can occasionally give the impression that it does. After being bitten by an infected mosquito, symptoms can appear anywhere between four and two weeks later and usually last for two to seven days. Following the reduction of the fever, additional symptoms may worsen and result in more severe bleeding; gastrointestinal issues such as nausea, vomiting, or intense abdominal pain; and respiratory issues such as breathing difficulties. If DHF is left untreated, severe bleeding, dehydration, and a sharp drop in blood pressure (shock) may occur. These symptoms are potentially fatal, so you should get medical attention right away. A person who has contracted that specific strain of the virus develops immunity to it (though they remain susceptible to infection from any of the other three types).

6.5.13.3. Diagnosis

Make an immediate doctor's appointment if you suspect your child has dengue fever. If your kid has had dengue fever recently and is experiencing a fever or excruciating headache, you should also get them checked out by a physician. The doctor will examine your child and assess the symptoms in order to diagnose the condition. Your child's medical history, recent travels, and a blood sample for testing will all be questioned by the doctor.

6.5.13.4. Treatment

There is no particular treatment for dengue fever. Mild cases are treated with plenty of rest and fluids to avoid dehydration. Acetaminophen-containing pain relievers can lessen dengue fever-related headaches and discomfort. Aspirin and ibuprofen-containing pain relievers should be avoided as they increase the risk of bleeding. The majority of dengue fever cases clear up in a week or two and don't result in any long-term issues. Seek immediate medical attention if someone exhibits severe disease symptoms or if symptoms worsen in the first few days after the fever subsides. This could be a sign of a medical emergency called DHF.

In hospitals, intravenous (IV) fluids and electrolytes (salts) to replenish those lost through vomiting or diarrhea are administered to treat severe dengue fever cases. This is typically sufficient to treat the disease effectively when started early. In more complex cases, a blood transfusion might be necessary for the medical team.

Efforts should be made to prevent mosquito bites on anyone infected with dengue fever in all cases. This will lessen the chance of the sickness infecting more people.

6.5.13.5. Prevention

A dengue vaccine is recommended for kids and teens 9–16 years old who have already had dengue fever and who live in the U.S. territories where it is common. It is not advised for visitors to these regions. However, the vaccine is insufficient on its own. Keeping yourself safe from mosquito bites is still crucial. Make certain to:

- Install screens on windows and doors, and fix any damaged or broken screens right away. Keep windows and doors without screens closed.
- When your children go outside, make sure they have on long sleeve shirts, long pants, shoes, and socks. At night, cover their beds with mosquito netting.
- Apply insect repellent to children as instructed. Select the one containing lemon eucalyptus oil.
- Restrict the amount of time that children spend outside during the day, especially during mosquito season, which runs from dawn to dusk.
- Keep areas free of mosquito breeding grounds. Remove any standing water from items like containers and abandoned tires, and replace the water in birdbaths, dog bowls, and flower vases at least once a week, as they lay their eggs in the water.

Travelers from abroad can reduce their risk of contracting dengue fever by following these precautions and avoiding areas where the disease is currently spreading.

6.5.14. Pediatric HIV Infection and Disease

The immune system is weakened by the human immunodeficiency virus (HIV), which reduces the body's capacity to fight infections and cancers. If treatment is not received, HIV multiplies further within the body, resulting in acquired immunodeficiency syndrome (AIDS), an advanced stage of HIV infection. At this point, the body is extremely susceptible to malignancies and infections that are normally combated by a functioning immune system, which can result in chronic illness and even death. However, antiretroviral medications are typically costly, and in low- and middle-income nations, access to diagnostic procedures and therapies is limited. HIV-positive infants and young children are especially susceptible; the majority do not live to be five years old without treatment. Current treatments make it easy to prevent HIV transmission from a pregnant mother to her unborn child, but despite global advancements in mother-to-child transmission prevention, a high rate of pediatric infections persists in certain developing nations.

- Causes
    - 90% of infants living with HIV received the virus from their HIV-positive mothers either through breastfeeding or during pregnancy.
    - Not all pregnant HIV-positive women have access to effective treatment, which can stop HIV transmission from a mother to her child.
- **Symptoms:** HIV affects babies in the same ways that it affects adults, but the illness advances more quickly in babies. Among the symptoms are:
    - sluggish development and weight increase.
    - severe wasting
    - diarrhea and infections of the upper respiratory tract that lead to more serious health issues and even death.
    - infections such as tuberculosis
- **Diagnosis:** Rapid HIV antibody testing has reduced the cost and improved the feasibility of HIV field diagnosis in underprivileged areas.

- **Treatment:** HIV infection does not have a treatment. However, early diagnosis of infants is crucial. Administering antiretroviral therapy (ART) to children with HIV at an early stage of the infection can help them live longer, healthier lives. When taken daily, these medications can significantly lower the blood level of HIV and raise CD4 cell counts, which will slow the disease's progression.
- **Prevention:** Antiretroviral therapy (ART) should be started as soon as possible for HIV-positive pregnant women in order to prevent mother-to-child transmission (PMTCT). By lowering the amount of virus in the mother's blood, antiretroviral therapy (ART) lowers the likelihood that the mother will infect her child. A child should receive ART both before and after delivery; this will strengthen the infant's immune system.

6.5.15. Rabies

Some warm-blooded animals can contract rabies, a virus belonging to the Rhabdoviridae family. The nervous system is attacked. If treatment is not received, the disease is 100% fatal in animals once symptoms appear. The primary carriers of rabies in North America are skunks, raccoons, foxes, coyotes, and bats. These untamed creatures can infect livestock, dogs, and domestic cats in some areas. In the US, rabies is more common in cats than in dogs. Each state keeps records on animals that could be rabies carriers. If a child has been bitten by a particular animal and you are unsure about it, it is best to look up information specific to the area.

6.5.15.1. How Does Rabies Occur?

Via cuts, scratches, or mucous membranes (such as the lining of the mouth and eyes), the rabies virus enters the body and makes its way to the central nervous system. After entering the brain, the infection spreads to other organs by entering the nerves and multiplying there. The primary organ involved in the transmission of rabies from one animal to another is the salivary gland. Through the saliva of the infected animal, the rabies virus is spread when an infected animal bites another animal. Because rabid animals lick their claws, scratches caused by their claws can be dangerous as well. When an animal carrying the rabies virus licks an area that is openly scratched or sore on a human, the human may become infected.

6.5.15.2. Symptoms of Rabies

While the average incubation period in humans is roughly two months, it can vary from five days to over a year from the time of exposure to the onset of illness. The most typical signs and symptoms of rabies are listed below. However, each child may have a unique set of symptoms. Symptoms could consist of:

- Rabies: Stage 1
  - First phase of hazy symptoms, which lasted for two to 10 days.
  - Vague symptoms may include:
  - Fever
  - Headache
  - Malaise
  - Decreased appetite
  - Vomiting
- It is possible for there to be tingling, pain, or itching at the wound site.
- Rabies: Stage 2:

Due to their incapacity to swallow saliva, children frequently experience difficulty swallowing (also known as foaming at the mouth); in fact, the mere sight of a glass of water may frighten them.

Certain children experience agitation and disorientation, while others experience paralysis.

There could be an immediate death or a coma that leads to death from other complications.

Rabies symptoms can mimic those of other illnesses or medical issues. Always get a diagnosis from your child's physician.

6.5.15.3. Diagnosis

The direct fluorescent antibody test (dFA) is a commonly used diagnostic tool for rabies in animals. Typically, test results are known in a matter of hours. If the animal is not rabid, knowing these results could prevent a child from needing medical attention. Since no single test can definitively rule out rabies in humans, several tests are required to either confirm or rule out the disease. Samples of serum, saliva, spinal fluid, and skin biopsies obtained from the nape of the neck are used for testing.

6.5.15.4. Treatment for Rabies

A customized rabies treatment plan will be determined by your child's physician. Unfortunately, once symptoms of the disease appear, there is no recognized, reliable treatment for rabies. However, when administered soon after an exposure, certain vaccines (HDCV, PCEC) are effective and provide immunity against rabies. In cases where rabies exposure is suspected, treatment consists of a single immunoglobulin dose and multiple rabies vaccine injections spaced out over a two-week duration. It can also be used to protect people like veterinarians and animal handlers before an exposure happens.

6.5.15.5. Prevention

One way to lower the risk of animal bites is to practice safety when around animals, even your own pets. The following are some broad recommendations to prevent rabies and animal bites:

- When in public, keep pets on a leash or in a fenced yard.
- Choose your family's pets wisely.
- A young child and a pet should never be left alone.
- Maintain up-to-date vaccination records and rabies vaccinations for your pets.
- Keep an eye on your pets to make sure they don't encounter any wild animals. To get rid of any stray animals, give your local animal control agency a call.

Preventing animal bites may also be achieved by teaching your kids about animal safety. Here are some things to keep in mind:

- Avoid attempting to divide combatant animals.
- Steer clear of any odd or sick animals.
- When an animal is eating, leave them alone.
- Never approach or engage in play with any kind of wild animal.

Remember to give your healthcare provider the following information if you or someone you know has been bitten or scratched by an animal:

- The incident's location (backyard, forest, etc.)
- What kind of animal is involved (wild or domesticated).
- Kind of exposure (licking an open wound, cutting, or scratching).

- The body part that is affected (hand, leg, face, etc.).
- Number of exposures
- Whether or not the animal (if known) has received a rabies vaccination.
- Whether the animal is ill or not, and if it is, what symptoms did it exhibit?
- Whether the animal can be quarantined or used for testing.

Animal control officers should be notified if your child has been bitten by a wild or sickly-looking animal; do not try to catch it yourself (Demirjian and Levy, 2009; Havelaar et al, 2010; Davis, 2011; Ginsburg et al, 2014; Rappuoli et al, 2017).

A Closer Look

Economics of Immunizations

- **Positive Externality:** Immunizations force upon society what is referred to as a positive consumer externality. Through herd immunity, an individual not only shields themselves from specific antigens but also enhances the protection of everyone else in the community. We observe an undervaluing of the marginal benefit of each vaccination because the market transactions for immunizations do not account for this additional protection. People who base their decisions on their personal marginal benefit rather than the social marginal benefit are to blame for this market failure. Due to society's undervaluing of vaccinations, we end up with a quantity that is less than what is socially optimal through regular market transactions.

For instance, if person A values their own immunity to a particular antigen at $100 but the vaccination costs $150, person A will choose not to get the shot. On the other hand, if person B values person A's immunity at $70 due to the additional benefit of herd immunity, then the total social marginal benefit of their immunization is $170. Immunization underconsumption results from Individual A's private marginal benefit being less than her social marginal benefit.

- **Socially Optimal Outcome:** Underconsumption of any good is always the result of private marginal benefits being lower than social marginal benefits. The value that society assigns to each distinct vaccination determines how much of a difference there is. Immunization rates frequently fall short of the socially optimal level required to completely eradicate the antigen. Rather, they arrive at a social quantity that permits the ideal number of ill people. The majority of diseases that are routinely immunized in the US still only occasionally cause significant outbreaks and have a minor prevalence. Measles is an excellent illustration of a disease whose social optimum allows for outbreaks in the US that frequently result in a small number of fatalities.

There are other instances of diseases, like smallpox, that were so serious that the virus's eradication brought an end to the social ideal. In these situations, the social marginal benefit is so great that the cost of reaching an immunization level that prevents the disease from spreading and surviving is accepted by society. Complete eradication is not always the aim of immunization, despite the severity of some diseases, due to the cost of vaccination compared to the social marginal benefit. We know that the socially optimal outcome is not the complete eradication of all diseases for which there is an immunization, even though it can be difficult to pinpoint exactly where this point is.

- **Internalizing the Externality**: Payments equal to the marginal benefit must be made in order to internalize the positive externality imposed by vaccinations. These payments are typically made by the government in the form of subsidies in nations like the United States. In the United States, immunization programs were administered by municipal and state governments prior to 1962. Due to the uneven distribution of subsidies, certain areas of the US reached the socially optimal level of immunization while other areas were left without them and stuck at the level of private marginal benefit. The United States has been gradually shifting toward the larger-scale socially optimal result since 1962 and the passage of the Vaccination Assistance Act. It is challenging to determine when the social optimum has been reached, even with government support. Cultural movements are causing private marginal benefit curves to shift in addition to the difficulties in estimating the true social marginal benefit of vaccinations. Certain private citizens now see the marginal benefit of vaccination differently as a result of vaccine scandals. Individual A will not be willing to pay for or receive vaccinations if they feel that there is a significant health risk—possibly greater than the antigen itself—associated with immunization. It becomes more challenging for governments to reach a social optimum through subsidies as there are fewer willing participants and a wider marginal benefit.

Nonprofit groups can also influence a society toward the socially ideal result without the help of the government by giving free vaccinations to underdeveloped areas. Developing societies will not be able to reach a quantity set by private marginal benefits if they are unable to initially afford the vaccinations. Organizations can help privately under-immunized communities move toward the social optimum by administering immunization programs.

Summary

- Immunity is the ability of the human body to tolerate the presence of material indigenous to the body and to eliminate foreign substances. This discriminatory ability to eliminate foreign substances is performed by a complex system of interacting cells called the immune system.
- Vaccines affect the immune system, primarily through B-lymphocytes and T-lymphocytes.
- Passive immunity is protection by antibody or antitoxin produced by one animal or human and transferred to another. Passive immunity provides immediate protection against infection, but that protection is temporary. The antibodies will degrade during a period of weeks to months, and the recipient will no longer be protected.
- Active immunity is protection produced by a person's own immune system. The immune system is stimulated by an antigen to produce antibody-mediated and cell-mediated immunity. Unlike passive immunity, which is temporary, active immunity usually lasts for many years, often for a lifetime.
- Childhood vaccinations are indicated for the prevention of a multitude of viral and bacterial infections and their sequelae. Specific vaccination recommendations for children vary by region, as exposure to diseases varies by region.
- Immunization is an important and effective health intervention for children. Over the course of history, it has helped keep millions of children protected against infectious and life-threatening diseases.
- A cold chain is a temperature-controlled supply chain that includes all vaccine-related equipment and procedures. The cold chain begins with the cold storage unit at the manufacturing plant, extends to the transport and delivery of the vaccine and proper storage at the provider facility, and ends with administration of the vaccine to the patient.
- It is important to make sure vaccines are unpacked and stored correctly and to account for every dose received and used, whether administered, wasted, compromised, expired, or transferred.
- To protect the vaccine supply, vaccine should be delivered directly to the facility where it will be used. However, sometimes, vaccine needs to be transported to an off-site or satellite facility for an event like an on-site vaccination clinic.
- Major causes of death among children vary by age. Children under 5 are especially vulnerable to infectious diseases like malaria, pneumonia, diarrhea, HIV and tuberculosis. For older children, non-communicable diseases, injuries and conflict pose significant threats.

References

1. Adegoke, A. A., Mvuyo, T., & Okoh, A. I. (2012). Ubiquitous *Acinetobacter* species as beneficial commensals but gradually being emboldened with antibiotic resistance genes. *Journal of Basic Microbiology, 52*(6), 620–627. https://doi.org/10.1002/jobm.201200132.

2. Ahmad, T. A., Tawfik, D. M., Sheweita, S. A., Haroun, M., & El-Sayed, L. H. (2016). Development of immunization trials against *Acinetobacter baumannii. Trials in Vaccinology, 5*, 53–60. https://doi.org/10.1016/j.trivac.2016.02.002.
3. Avorn, J. (2015). The $2.6 billion pill–Methodologic and policy considerations. *New England Journal of Medicine, 372*(20), 1877–1879. https://doi.org/10.1056/NEJMp1503006.
4. Bruxvoort, K., Sy, L. S., Luo, Y., & Tseng, H. F. (2018). Real-world evidence for regulatory decisions: Concomitant administration of Zoster vaccine live and Pneumococcal polysaccharide vaccine. *American Journal of Epidemiology*. https://doi.org/10.1093/aje/kwy076.
5. Chiang, M., et al. (2015). Identification of novel vaccine candidates against *Acinetobacter baumannii* using reverse vaccinology. *Human Vaccines & Immunotherapeutic, 11*(5), 1151–1158. https://doi.org/10.1080/21645515.2015.1017410.
6. Custovic, A., et al. (2014). Epidemiological monitoring of nosocomial infections caused by *Acinetobacter baumannii. Medical Archives, 68*(5), 402–406. https://doi.org/10.5455/medarh.2014.68.402-406.
7. Davis, M. M., et al. (2011). Failure-to-success ratios, transition probabilities, and phase lengths for prophylactic vaccines versus other pharmaceuticals in the development pipeline. *Vaccine, 29*(52), 9414–9416. https://doi.org/10.1016/j.vaccine.2011.10.052.
8. Demirjian, A., & Levy, O. (2009). Safety and efficacy of neonatal vaccination. *European Journal of Immunology, 39*(1), 36–46. https://doi.org/10.1002/eji.200838585.
9. Enne, V. I., Personne, Y., Grgic, L., Gant, V., & Zumla, A. (2014). Aetiology of hospital-acquired pneumonia and trends in antimicrobial resistance. *Current Opinion in Pulmonary Medicine, 20*(3), 252–258. https://doi.org/10.1097/MCP.0000000000000055.
10. Gadsby, N. J., et al. (2016). Comprehensive molecular testing for respiratory pathogens in community-acquired pneumonia. *Clinical Infectious Diseases, 62*(7), 817–823. https://doi.org/10.1093/cid/ciw065.
11. Ginsburg, A. S., Meulen, A. S. T., & Klugman, K. P. (2014). Prevention of neonatal pneumonia and sepsis via maternal immunization. *The Lancet Global Health, 2*(11), e679–e680. https://doi.org/10.1016/S2214-109X(14)70318-6.
12. Harris, G., KuoLee, R., Xu, H. H., & Chen, W. (2017). Mouse models of *Acinetobacter baumannii* infection. *Current Protocols in Microbiology, 46*(1), 6G.3.1–6G.3.23. https://doi.org/10.1002/cpmc.40.
13. Havelaar, A. H., et al. (2015). World Health Organization global estimates and regional comparisons of the burden of foodborne disease in 2010. *PLOS Medicine, 12*(12), e1001923. https://doi.org/10.1371/journal.pmed.1001923.
14. Hay, S. I., et al. (2018). Measuring and mapping the global burden of antimicrobial resistance. *BMC Medicine, 16*(1), 78. https://doi.org/10.1186/s12916-018-1083-9.
15. Helal, S., El Anany, M., Ghaith, D., & Rabeea, S. (2015). The role of MDR-*Acinetobacter baumannii* in orthopedic surgical site infections. *Surgical Infections (Larchmt), 16*(5), 518–522. https://doi.org/10.1089/sur.2015.037.
16. Jansen, K. U., Knirsch, C., & Anderson, A. S. (2018). The role of vaccines in preventing bacterial antimicrobial resistance. *Nature Medicine, 24*(1), 10–19. https://doi.org/10.1038/nm.4456.

17. Kennedy, D. A., & Read, A. F. (2017). Why does drug resistance readily evolve but vaccine resistance does not? *Proceedings of the Royal Society B: Biological Sciences, 284*(1860), 20162562. https://doi.org/10.1098/rspb.2016.2562.

18. Kingwell, K. (2018). Vaccines take a shot at antimicrobial resistance. *Nature Reviews Drug Discovery, 17*(4), 229. https://doi.org/10.1038/nrd.2018.11.

19. Kotloff, K. L., et al. (2013). Burden and aetiology of diarrhoeal disease in infants and young children in developing countries (the Global Enteric Multicenter Study, GEMS): A prospective, case-control study. *The Lancet, 382*(9888), 209–222. https://doi.org/10.1016/S0140-6736(13)60844-2.

20. LaVergne, S., et al. (2018). Phage therapy for a multidrug-resistant *Acinetobacter baumannii* craniectomy site infection. *Open Forum Infectious Diseases, 5*(1), ofx275. https://doi.org/10.1093/ofid/ofx275.

21. Laxminarayan, R., Duse, A., Wattal, C., Zaidi, A. K., Wertheim, H. F., & Sumpradit, N. (2016). Access to effective antimicrobials: A worldwide challenge. *The Lancet, 387*(10014), 168–175. https://doi.org/10.1016/S0140-6736(15)00474-2.

22. Lipsitch, M., & Siber, G. R. (2016). How can vaccines contribute to solving the antimicrobial resistance problem? *mBio, 7*(3), e00760–16. https://doi.org/10.1128/mBio.00760-16.

23. Marais, E., de Jong, G., Ferraz, V., Maloba, B., & Dusé, A. G. (2004). Interhospital transfer of pan-resistant *Acinetobacter* strains in Johannesburg, South Africa. *American Journal of Infection Control, 32*(5), 278–281. https://doi.org/10.1016/j.ajic.2003.12.001.

24. Miller, M., Checkley, W., Kirkpatrick, B. D., McCormick, B. J., Lima, A. A., & Bourke, C. D. (2014). The MAL-ED study: A multinational and multidisciplinary approach to understand the relationship between enteric pathogens, malnutrition, gut physiology, physical growth, cognitive development, and immune responses in infants and children up to 2 years of age. *Clinical Infectious Diseases*. https://doi.org/10.1093/cid/ciu653.

25. Morris, M. C., & Surendran, N. (2016). Neonatal vaccination: Challenges and intervention strategies. *Neonatology, 109*(3), 161–169. https://doi.org/10.1159/000441195.

26. Nielsen, T. B., Smedsgaard, J., & Petersen, R. F. (2017). Monoclonal antibody protects against *Acinetobacter baumannii* infection by enhancing bacterial clearance and evading sepsis. *Journal of Infectious Diseases, 216*(4), 489–501. https://doi.org/10.1093/infdis/jix275.

27. O'Neill, J. (2016). Tackling drug-resistant infections globally: Final report and recommendations. *Review on Antimicrobial Resistance*. https://doi.org/10.1016/j.jpha.2015.11.005.

28. Oikonomou, O., Daikos, G. L., & Spanakis, N. (2015). Rapid dissemination of colistin and carbapenem resistant *Acinetobacter baumannii* in Central Greece: Mechanisms of resistance, molecular identification, and epidemiological data. *BMC Infectious Diseases, 15*, 559. https://doi.org/10.1186/s12879-015-1400-4.

29. Peleg, A. Y., Seifert, H., & Paterson, D. L. (2008). *Acinetobacter baumannii*: Emergence of a successful pathogen. *Clinical Microbiology Reviews, 21*(3), 538–582. https://doi.org/10.1128/CMR.00058-07.

30. Perez, F., & Bonomo, R. A. (2014). Vaccines for *Acinetobacter baumannii*: Thinking "out of the box". *Vaccine, 32*(20), 2537–2539. https://doi.org/10.1016/j.vaccine.2014.01.047.

31. Plotkin, S., Robinson, J. M., Cunningham, G., Iqbal, R., & Larsen, S. (2017). The complexity and cost of vaccine manufacturing–An overview. *Vaccine, 35*(33), 4064–4071. https://doi.org/10.1016/j.vaccine.2017.06.002.

32. Qiu, H., Choi, Y., & Wang, Z. (2016). Host resistance to intranasal *Acinetobacter baumannii* reinfection in mice. *Pathogens and Disease, 74*(1), ftw048. https://doi.org/10.1093/femspd/ftw048.

33. Rappuoli, R., Bloom, D. E., & Black, S. (2017). Deploy vaccines to fight superbugs. *Nature, 552*(7683), 165–167. https://doi.org/10.1038/552165a.

34. Reindel, R., & Fiore, C. R. (2017). Phage therapy: Considerations and challenges for development. *Clinical Infectious Diseases, 64*(12), 1589–1590. https://doi.org/10.1093/cid/cix187.

35. Saleem, A. F., Ahmed, I., Mir, F., Ali, S. R., & Zaidi, A. K. (2009). Pan-resistant *Acinetobacter* infection in neonates in Karachi, Pakistan. *Journal of Infection in Developing Countries, 4*(1), 30–37. https://doi.org/10.3855/jidc.317.

36. Serota, D. P., Sexton, M. E., Kraft, C. S., & Palacio, F. (2018). Severe community-acquired pneumonia due to *Acinetobacter baumannii* in North America: Case report and review of the literature. *Open Forum Infectious Diseases, 5*(2), ofy044. https://doi.org/10.1093/ofid/ofy044.

37. Sherman, R. E., Anderson, S. A., Dal Pan, G. J., Gray, G. C., & Gross, T. (2016). Real-world evidence–What is it and what can it tell us? *New England Journal of Medicine, 375*(23), 2293–2297. https://doi.org/10.1056/NEJMp1608502.

38. Simonsen, K. A., Anderson-Berry, A. L., Delair, S. F., & Davies, H. D. (2014). Early-onset neonatal sepsis. *Clinical Microbiology Reviews, 27*(1), 21–47. https://doi.org/10.1128/CMR.00031-13.

39. Thompson, A., Yu, S., Green, S., & Schick, R. (2013). Safety of 13-valent pneumococcal conjugate vaccine in infants and children: Meta-analysis of 13 clinical trials in 9 countries. *Vaccine*. https://doi.org/10.1016/j.vaccine.2013.08.025.

40. Tsai, W. C., Yang, Y. L., & Lee, C. C. (2012). Clinical characteristics, pathogens implicated and therapeutic outcomes of mixed infection in adult bacterial meningitis. *Kaohsiung Journal of Medical Sciences, 28*(10), 531–537. https://doi.org/10.1016/j.kjms.2011.12.008.

41. Warfel, J. M., Papin, J. F., Wolf, R. F., Zimmerman, L. I., & Merkel, T. J. (2014). Maternal and neonatal vaccination protects newborn baboons from pertussis infection. *Journal of Infectious Diseases, 210*(4), 604–610. https://doi.org/10.1093/infdis/jiu167.

42. Yakupogullari, Y., Dilek, A., & Sahin, M. (2016). Is airborne transmission of *Acinetobacter baumannii* possible: A prospective molecular epidemiologic study in a tertiary care hospital. *American Journal of Infection Control, 44*(12), 1595–1599. https://doi.org/10.1016/j.ajic.2016.05.004.

Chapter 7

COMMON DISORDERS IN CHILDREN

Contents

INTRODUCTION

A child is the center of any household. Every parent finds immense happiness in witnessing their child flourish and grow healthily. A child's physical health promotes healthy growth and development. Nonetheless, it is equally critical to recognize that children's emotional health is just as vital as their physical health. Children are both the future and the young minds of today, so ensuring their health now will help them meet the long-term needs of tomorrow. A good balance between the two gives kids the resilience to face life's obstacles at different stages and even serves as a solid foundation for growing up to be healthy adults.

Various factors, such as surroundings, parent-child relationships, genetic inheritance, peer pressure, and stress, can impact a child's emotional and behavioral well-being. In today's world, mental illnesses affect children and young adults worldwide quite frequently. Typically, one out of every 10 children experiences some sort of emotional or behavioral abnormality. Early detection and intervention are crucial because, once a pattern forms, it becomes ingrained in the child's behavior and can be challenging to address.

Orientation and Directional Terms

Term	Definition	Illustration
Bronchiolitis	Bronchiolitis is a common viral lower respiratory tract infection that affects babies and young children under two years old. Most cases of bronchiolitis aren't serious, but sometimes a more serious infection such as pneumonia may be present.	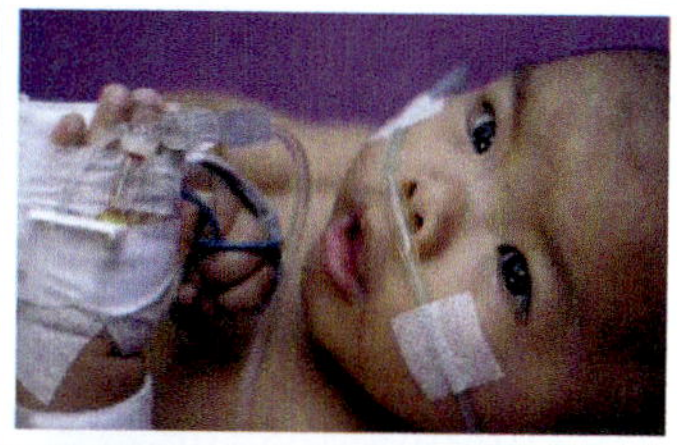
Chickenpox	Chickenpox is a mild and common childhood illness that most children catch at some point. Chickenpox is caused by a virus. It's spread quickly and easily from someone who is infected.	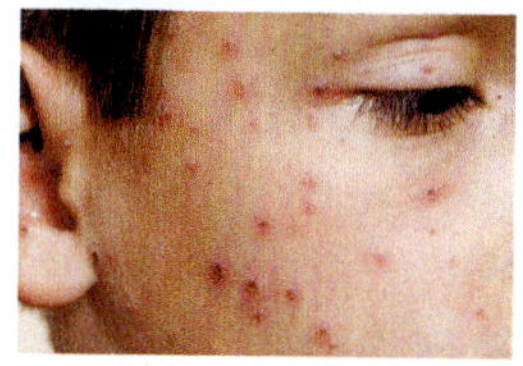
Common cold	A cold is a mild viral infection of the nose, throat, sinuses and upper airways. It's a common infection and usually clears up on its own within a week or two. If you are fit and healthy, it's unlikely to be serious. Painkillers can help reduce the symptoms of colds.	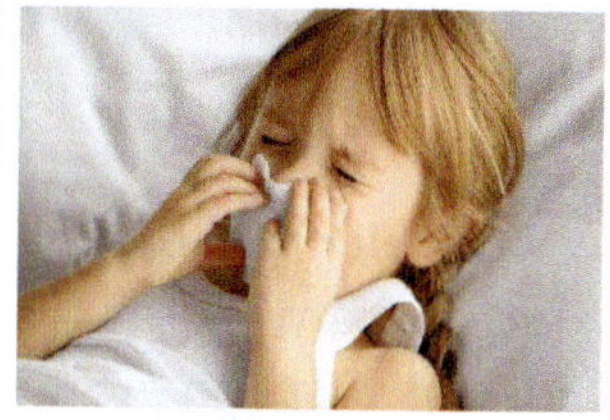
Earache	Earache is a common problem, particularly in children. It can be worrying, but it's usually caused by a minor infection and will often get better in a few days without treatment. Find out common causes of earache.	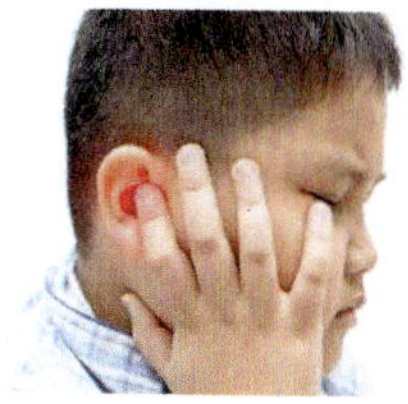
Kawasaki disease	Kawasaki disease is a rare condition that mainly affects children under the age of five. It's also known as mucocutaneous lymph node syndrome.	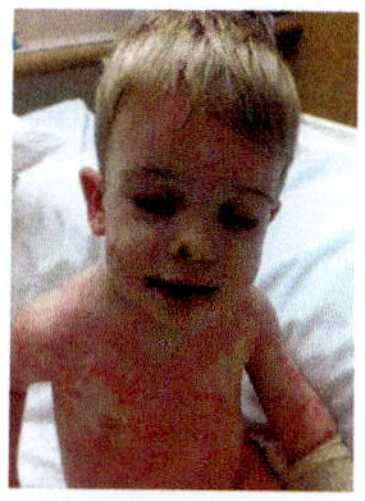
Measles	Measles is a highly infectious viral illness. It can be unpleasant and sometimes leads to serious complications. It's now uncommon because of the effectiveness of the measles, mumps and rubella (MMR) vaccination program. Anyone can get measles if they haven't been vaccinated or they haven't had it before.	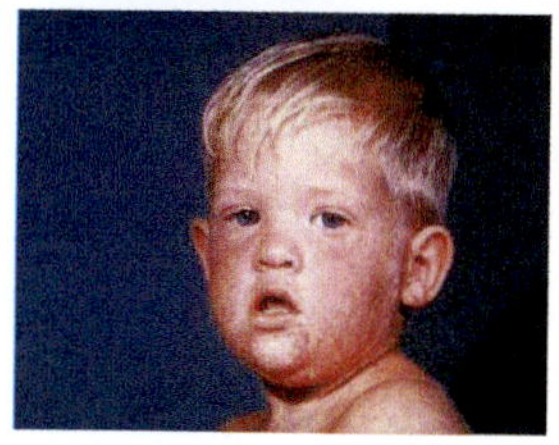

7.1. RESPIRATORY PROBLEMS

Children's health problems are the same as adults. Although their illnesses may be similar, there may be some differences in how severe they are. As a result, knowing what to look out for in particular as a caregiver is crucial because children of different ages will have different problems.

Early childhood is the age group in which children most commonly experience health problems. For this reason, during their time in that age group, it is essential to give them more careful attention. Their respiratory system is frequently the source of an issue. The diagnosis and treatment of the illness may benefit if the caregiver can spot the warning indicators. This can be crucial in avoiding further issues that could affect the kids' general health, like their development and growth at the right age, as well as the right psychological and behavioral characteristics.

7.1.1. Warning Signs for Your Little Ones

The following signs suggest that your children may be experiencing more serious health problems than you had anticipated.

- Excessive coughing that interferes with daily activities or annoys those around them.
- Coughing fits lasting more than 1- 2 weeks.
- Breathing difficulties, wheezing, or coughing during physical activity or during a change in the weather.
- Snoring and/or haltingly irregular breathing.
- Mucus buildup, frequent or persistent stuffiness of the nose, or noisy breathing.
- Discomfort in the nose, chest, or ears.
- Bleeding from the nose or coughing up blood often.

7.1.2. Respiratory Diseases in Children

If your child exhibits any of the symptoms listed above, they could have one of the following serious repository diseases.

- **Acute or Chronic Bronchitis:** Coughing can be brought on by inflammation and can occur day or night, whether it is a dry cough or one that produces phlegm. Similar to a common cold, acute bronchitis can cause prolonged and more frequent coughing. Either bacteria or viruses are frequently the cause of illness, but during the rainy season, common viruses like rhinovirus and RSV typically cause bronchitis in children. This might be so bad that it causes lung inflammation, which results in fever, listlessness, rapid breathing, dyspnea, and dyspnea. You should take your child to the doctor if you observe any of these symptoms; in particular, if the child has a persistent dry cough, as this can also indicate asthma.
- **Rhinitis from Allergy/Allergic to Weather:** Today, due to the warmer climate around the world, the weather has become more unpredictable. With more people living in cities, it is common for children to experience allergy symptoms such as excessive mucus, itchy nose, frequent sneezing, or stuffy nose. Some children may also have itchy eyes, recurring nose

bleeds, discomfort or ringing in the ears, or repeated ear infections. These issues may run in the family as well. All of these problems can disrupt children's daily routines, impacting their ability to learn and sleep. If your child is experiencing these symptoms, it is important to bring them to a doctor for proper treatment. In the meantime, it is advised to keep them away from air pollution sources like automobile exhaust, PM2.5 dust, and smoke from various sources (cigarettes, incense, chemicals, etc.). If they must be in areas with air pollution, they should wear a mask and rinse their nose frequently.

- **Inflammation of the Nasal Cavity and Sinusitis:** These illnesses can develop gradually or suddenly, and they can be caused by allergies or infections. Both bacteria and viruses can cause an infection. Should it be caused by a fungus, the child will cough up thick mucus that runs down their throat. He or she may experience intermittent or prolonged fever, facial pain, and bad breath lasting more than one to two weeks. Any of these signs could indicate sinusitis or nasal cavity inflammation.
- **Upper Airway Obstruction:** When they are sleeping, snoring, labored breathing, restlessness, lying on their stomach, or maintaining a straight head are significant indicators. In a severe situation, the child might not be able to breathe at all and would have to sit up to go to sleep. In severe situations, the child is unable to get enough sleep, feels agitated and sleepy during the day, has trouble concentrating, and has diminished learning potential. Obesity, disfigurement of the face, enlarged tonsils and adenoid glands, chronic sinusitis, persistent nasal cavity infections, and other conditions are the common causes of upper airway obstruction. Any of these ailments may affect a child's growth, development, capacity for learning, and emotional stability if they become chronic.
- **Bronchial Hyperresponsiveness or Asthma:** If your child has a history of allergies (skin, nasal cavity, or food), respiratory system contacts, or shortness of breath, coughing, or wheezing sounding when breathing, especially during exercise or in the early evening, or if your child has a cold and coughs a lot but feels better after taking a bronchodilator, you should take them to see a specialist for allergies and respiratory systems.
- **Foreign Items Inside the Airway:** Youngsters have a tendency to be mischievous and stick foreign objects, like beads or other materials, up their noses, where they may stay for a long time before getting sick. The object may cause a pulmonary infection if it gets lodged in the airway. This infection may recur there. It is best to instruct your kids on appropriate behavior and manners when they are eating.

7.1.3. Preventing Respiratory Diseases in Children

To help prevent respiratory infections in yourself and your children, it is important to follow some simple tips. These include covering your cough or sneeze with your elbow or a tissue, washing your hands frequently with soap and water, and avoiding touching your eyes, nose, and mouth. It's also important to limit contact with sick individuals and ensure that you and your child are up-to-date on vaccinations recommended by healthcare professionals. As a caregiver, it is your duty to prioritize the health and well-being of your children in order to promote their happiness and proper development. If you notice any signs of illness in your children, it is crucial to seek medical advice promptly for appropriate care (Abdulla, 2011; Berni Canani et al, 2016; Colby, 2017; Murray et al, 2019).

7.2. GASTROINTESTINAL PROBLEMS

While occasional indigestion or stomachaches in children are common, you should see a doctor if this occurs frequently or on a regular basis. These days, digestive disorders are inevitable for kids because of the unhealthy diet most of them eat and the abundance of junk and processed food they consume. It is crucial that kids receive the proper amount of nutrients and vitamins from each and every food group. Children can have a variety of digestive disorders, and although they all have different causes, the symptoms—vomiting, nausea, vomiting, dehydration, and diarrhea—are often the same.

7.2.1. Common Pediatric Gastrointestinal Disorders

The most common GI disorders in children are as follows:

7.2.1.1. Gastroenteritis

Gastroenteritis, a common gastrointestinal disorder in children, is caused by viral or bacterial infections. Symptoms of pediatric gastroenteritis include:

- Nausea
- Vomiting
- Diarrhea
- Abdominal pain
- Pyrexia

Children who lose fluids through frequent vomiting and diarrhea may also become dehydrated. The common ways that the bacteria or virus that causes gastroenteritis spread are through contaminated food, water, or contact with an infected individual. Due to their close contact with other children, children who attend daycare centers or schools are more likely to become ill.

7.2.1.2. Inflammatory Bowel Disease

Chronic inflammatory bowel disease, or IBD, is linked to persistent inflammation of the entire gastrointestinal tract or specific sections of it. Children may experience a range of clinical symptoms as a result of the illness. The two primary forms of IBD are ulcerative colitis and Crohn's disease. IBD's clinical signs and symptoms include the following.

- Abdominal pain
- Diarrhea
- Rectal bleeding
- Weight loss
- Fatigue

Inflammation of the eyes, skin rashes, and joint pain can also affect some kids. Although the precise etiology of IBD is still unknown, medical professionals believe a combination of immunological, environmental, and genetic factors are likely at work. Youngsters who have an IBD family history are more likely to get the illness. Living in an urban environment, eating a diet heavy in fat and sugar, and being exposed to certain viruses or bacteria can all raise an individual's risk of developing IBD.

7.2.1.3. Irritable Bowel Syndrome

Common clinical manifestations of IBS in children include the following:

- Abdominal pain and distention
- Constipation
- Diarrhea
- Nausea
- Fatigue
- a feeling of unfinished bowel motions.

Although the precise cause of pediatric IBS is unknown, researchers think stress, diet, and heredity may play a role. Children are more likely to develop the syndrome if they have a family history of IBS or other digestive disorders.

7.2.1.4. Celiac Disease

An immune response to the protein gluten is the hallmark of the autoimmune disease celiac disease. A child suffering from this illness may experience damage and malabsorption of nutrients as a result of their immune system attacking the lining of their small intestine when they eat gluten, which is present in wheat, barley, and rye.

- The following are typical secondary symptoms and clinical manifestations of celiac disease in children.
- Diarrhea
- Abdominal pain
- Bloating
- Weight loss
- Fatigue
- Delayed growth and development

The exact cause of celiac disease is unknown, although a mix of environmental and hereditary factors may be involved. Children who have celiac disease may also have a family history of the condition or other autoimmune diseases.

7.2.1.5. Gastroesophageal Reflux Disease

The condition known as gastroesophageal reflux disease (GERD) is brought on by the reflux of stomach acid and contents back into the esophagus, which causes discomfort and swelling. Children with GERD often report experiencing the following symptoms.

- Heartburn — an intense burning feeling in the throat or chest.
- Regurgitation — a sour taste in the mouth.
- Dysphagia — having trouble swallowing liquids or food.

GERD may also be caused by a hiatal hernia, a weak lower esophageal sphincter, and certain medications, though the precise cause of the condition is still unknown.

7.2.1.6. Crohn's Disease

IBDs such as Crohn's disease can affect any part of the digestive system. Healthcare professionals generally believe that a combination of genetic, environmental, and immunological factors is at play, even though the precise etiology is still unknown. Children of any age can develop Crohn's disease, and the severity and location of the inflammatory response in the digestive tract can affect the clinical manifestations. Children that have Crohn's disease frequently go through:

- Persistent diarrhea
- Abdominal pain
- Weight loss
- Rectal bleeding
- Fever
- Fatigue
- Reduced appetite

Complications from Crohn's disease can occasionally include malnourishment, stunted growth, and fistulas or abscesses in the digestive tract.

7.2.2. Causes of GI Disorders in Children

Numerous bacterial, viral, and parasitic pathogens have been connected to gastrointestinal disorders in children:

- **Bacterial Pathogens:** *Enterobacter coli* (*E. coli*) is a common pathogen that can be transmitted by contaminated food or water and cause pyrexia, diarrhea, and cramping in the abdomen. Salmonella can spread through contaminated food or water and produce symptoms that are similar to these. A third pathogen that can lead to gastrointestinal problems in children is campylobacter, which is frequently transmitted through tainted poultry products.
- **Viral Pathogens:** A frequent cause of pediatric GI disorders is rotavirus. Rotavirus infections are contracted by coming into contact with contaminated surfaces or objects, and they can result in diarrhea, emesis, and pyrexia. Norovirus can also result in gastrointestinal disorders and is spread by tainted food or water, as well as by direct contact with sick people.
- **Parasitic Pathogens:** Children's gastrointestinal disorders can also be caused by parasitic pathogens such as Giardia. Giardia is transmitted by tainted food, water, or contact with an infected individual. Nausea, cramping in the abdomen, and diarrhea can all be caused by infections. Cryptosporidium has comparable symptoms and spreads via comparable routes.

7.2.3. Challenges of Diagnosing GI Diseases in Children with Traditional Testing

There are various difficulties in diagnosing GI disorders in children when using traditional stool testing methods. Due to the difficulty in collecting sufficient stool samples from children—a child's fear or discomfort may compromise the sample, leading to inaccurate test results—one of the main challenges is sample collection. Furthermore, some rare pediatric gastrointestinal disorders may be difficult to detect using conventional testing methods due to their lack of sensitivity. These obstacles might call for specialized testing, such as PCR testing. Additionally, certain long-term medical conditions might call for more thorough diagnostic techniques like endoscopy or colonoscopy. While conventional stool testing has its uses in the diagnosis of pediatric gastrointestinal disorders, it's critical to understand its limitations and, when appropriate, explore alternative testing options.

7.2.4. The Importance of Diagnosing Pediatric GI Disorders

Finding the root cause of a gastrointestinal disorder is critical for healthcare providers to develop an effective treatment plan that can greatly enhance a child's quality of life. Misidentifying a GI disorder can result in a wrong diagnosis and worsen the child's condition. Some GI disorders can lead to severe complications if not treated or managed correctly. For example, inflammatory bowel disease (IBD) can cause serious inflammation and damage to the digestive system, resulting in malnutrition, stunted growth, and potentially life-threatening issues. Additionally, certain GI illnesses may have genetic origins necessitating specialized treatment. Children with conditions like cystic fibrosis may require enzyme replacement therapy, nutritional supplements, and other specialized care to address their GI issues (Abdulla, 2011; Berni Canani et al, 2016; Colby, 2017; Murray et al, 2019).

7.3. NEUROLOGICAL PROBLEMS

One of the most vital and sensitive organs in the human body is the brain. Neurological disorders are problems resulting from a malfunction of the nervous system or the brain itself. Depending on the part of the brain that is affected, these conditions can cause physical or psychological symptoms. The human brain grows from conception to adolescence, starting while the child is still inside the mother. The majority of brain cells are formed prior to birth, but nerve connections do not form until later. There is a large range in the causes, complications, symptoms, and outcomes of neurological disorders. Every neurological ailment affects the nervous system, which includes the spine and brain. Everything in the human body, including movement, vision, and hearing, is managed by the nervous system. The affected area of the brain determines the symptoms and prognosis.

All age groups are susceptible to these conditions, though some neurological disorders are limited to presenting in the early stages of development. They may show up as birth defects, or in other situations, the symptoms are not identified until a child is much older. When a child fails to meet a developmental milestone or exhibits symptoms of a brain injury or infection, most of these neurological symptoms and indicators are detected. Headaches and other brain-related complaints are frequently ignored and only momentarily occur. On the other hand, symptoms such as persistent vertigo or weakness that manifest abruptly and without apparent reason may be signs of neurological disorders.

7.3.1. Various Neurological Disorders

Numerous neurological conditions impact the pediatric population. The most prevalent neurological conditions that affect children include headaches, epilepsy, cerebral palsy, autism, and the aftereffects of brain injuries. Every child has a different combination of symptoms related to each disorder. The neurological conditions that affect children most frequently are:

- **Autism:** The neurodevelopmental disorder known as autism is becoming more and more recognized on a global scale. Impaired social interaction, verbal (spoken) and non-verbal (unspoken) communication impairment, restricted, repetitive pattern of behavior with excessive adherence to routines, and restricted interests are the three main manifestations of the disease. Compared to other kids their age, autistic children have a distinct perspective on the world around them. Although there isn't a single cause for autism, a child may develop the disorder as a result of several behavioral, genetic, and environmental factors. A child with autism may struggle with speech, have emotional problems, and have trouble with social and communication skills. Depending on their age and developmental stage, children require varying interventional techniques. The condition does not have a single treatment that works for everyone. Since every patient with the illness is different, various treatment approaches, such as pharmacological and behavioral therapies, or a mix of the two, are needed.

- **Attention Deficit Hyperactivity Disorder (ADHD):** ADHD is one of the most prevalent neurological conditions that affect kids and can even persist into adolescence. Given the symptoms they encounter, such as forgetfulness and daydreaming, children in schools are frequently labeled as mischievous and left undiagnosed. A child with ADHD has trouble paying attention and has trouble controlling their impulses. These kids struggle to complete assignments and are frequently sidetracked. Brain injury, poor nutrition, drug abuse, and hereditary factors can all contribute to this condition. Since there are precise diagnostic standards and not every hyperactive child fits the mold for ADHD, an expert evaluation is necessary before a diagnosis can be made. Therapy and medication can be used to manage the symptoms of a disease.
- **Dyspraxia:** Although not much is known about it, this condition affects children quite frequently. One condition that makes it difficult to coordinate physical movements is dyspraxia. It can be challenging for kids with this illness to keep their balance and posture. Since it is thought that each person's nerve cells controlling muscle movement develop differently, there is no known cause for the condition. If the disease is identified early and treated with a particular intervention, such as process-oriented occupational therapy, affected children can recover.
- **Epilepsy:** People of all ages can suffer from epilepsy, which is a common disorder. The multiple seizures that are a characteristic of this chronic condition. A brief disruption in brain cell activity results in a seizure. Genetics, neurological injuries sustained before birth, developmental disorders, and infectious diseases are among the possible causes of epilepsy. Seizures can range widely in intensity from person to person. Medication for seizures and lifestyle changes are available as treatments.

- **Headaches:** The majority of headaches aren't signs of neurological conditions, but occasionally they could be brought on by a dangerous underlying problem. A headache may be brought on by modifications to the brain or body that cause the brain to receive pain signals. Children's headaches should be closely watched, especially if they are accompanied by other symptoms like vomiting, clumsiness, decreased alertness, etc.
- **Dyslexia:** A common learning disability in children is dyslexia, which makes it difficult for them to write, spell, read, and understand written material. The precise cause of the ailment remains unidentified. Children with the condition are helped by specialized teaching methods from a variety of professionals during treatment. When dyslexic children receive an early diagnosis, they can read at above-average levels.
- **Cerebral Palsy:** This disorder, which affects a child's motor skills, is brought on by brain damage that develops in the early stages of infancy or before birth. One of the most prevalent neurodevelopmental disorders in children, it can be further classified into different types based on neurological symptoms. Children with this condition struggle with standing, walking, eating, talking, controlling their bladder and bowels, and even with coordination. The illness doesn't get worse with age and is not progressive. Although the exact cause of the illness is unknown, it is thought to be pregnancy-related brain damage or improper fetal development. Although there is no known cure for this illness, therapies and treatment can help make it better.

Every neurological disorder presents itself in a unique way in children. While some illnesses are curable, others can only be controlled. It is imperative to identify all conditions at an early stage to prevent any additional complications. When a child exhibits strange symptoms, parents need to be aware of them and make sure they always take their concerns seriously. When in doubt, it is always advisable to seek medical advice. Your specialist wants to collaborate with you to address your child's needs, so be honest and communicate your concerns to them at all times.

7.3.2. Causes and Risk Factors of Neonatal Neurological Disorders

Sometimes the child has an abnormality in his or her chromosomes, or the condition is inherited from one or both parents. Prematurity, infections, genetic disorders, labor and delivery complications, and maternal health and toxin exposure are additional factors that can occasionally play a role. Inappropriate growth within the brain or spinal cord can also result in neurological conditions; this improper growth can impact the brain's veins, the brain itself, or the spinal cord. Brain disorders are especially common in premature babies. Metabolic disorders that can lead to neurological issues, like phenylketonuria, are frequently identified from birth.

Numerous problems during birth may contribute to the development of a neurological condition. These consist of:

- An oxygen shortage during or soon after birth.
- Certain genital tract infections in mothers that are transferred to the fetus during delivery.
- A head injury that results in internal bleeding in the brain.

These disorders can be brought on by the following during the early postpartum period, but only after the child is born.

- Illnesses such as immunological disorders.
- Infections caused by bacteria or viruses, such as encephalitis or meningitis.
- Head injury

7.3.3. Complications

A neurological disorder can cause mild to severe complications. While some kids will experience disabilities that last a lifetime, others might just take longer to reach developmental milestones. If left untreated, certain illnesses, most notably pseudotumor cerebri, can cause blindness. The best strategy to reduce the consequences or side effects of these brain disorders is to receive an early diagnosis and receive efficient treatment (Abdulla, 2011; Berni Canani et al, 2016; Colby, 2017; Murray et al, 2019).

7.4. MUSCULOSKELETAL AND RHEUMATIC DISORDERS

A variety of musculoskeletal, arthritic, and connective tissue conditions that can manifest in childhood are referred to as pediatric rheumatic diseases. These conditions can impact a child's gastrointestinal system, muscles, joints, skin, and eyes. Each of these inflammatory and autoimmune disorders has distinct symptoms in addition to the common ones, which include pain, heat, and swelling. Any age and any ethnic background of children can be impacted by rheumatic diseases.

7.4.1. Common Pediatric Rheumatic Disease

Pediatric rheumatic disease is classified into four main categories:

i. **Juvenile Idiopathic Arthritis (JIA):** The most prevalent type of juvenile arthritis. It comprises the subsequent subcategories:

- oligoarthritis (up to four joints are affected)
- polyarthritis (five or more joints are affected)
- systemic (joint inflammation, rashes, fever, fatigue, aches)
- enthesitis-related (joint arthritis and tendon swelling)
- juvenile psoriatic (joint arthritis and scaly skin rash).

ii. **Juvenile Dermatomyositis:** An inflammatory autoimmune disease that results in knuckle and eyelid skin rashes as well as muscle weakness.

iii. **Systemic Lupus Erythematosus:** An immune system disorder that typically affects the blood, kidneys, joints, skin, and other body parts. The illness is hard to diagnose and can be confused with juvenile idiopathic arthritis or multiple sclerosis.

iv. **Juvenile Scleroderma:** Describes a set of illnesses that result in tighter, harder skin.

7.4.2. Causes

It is still unclear what causes rheumatic diseases, and the cause can vary greatly depending on the kind of disease. Although there isn't a treatment at this time, many kids will experience remission or sporadic symptoms.

7.4.3. Signs and Symptoms

Rheumatic disease symptoms can fluctuate significantly in a day or a week. "Flares" are times when rheumatic symptoms are especially active.

The specific diagnosis for your child will determine the exact symptoms, which may include some of the following:

- stiffness, edema, and joint pain, especially in the morning.
- persistent fatigue
- muscle weakness
- difficulty sleeping.

Attempt to educate yourself about your child's symptoms and show empathy when they manifest. In order to carry out their regular activities, they will require more rest and assistance than usual if they are ill.

7.4.3.1. Common Emotional Responses

Every child's reaction to their illness will be unique. Common reactions, though, could be:

- social withdrawal
- preoccupation with pain
- anxiety
- fear of joint damage
- self-consciousness.

Typically, rheumatoid arthritis symptoms include pain and discomfort. Since they might not comprehend their condition, children may become fearful and confused by the ongoing pain. Reassure your child that they are not to blame for the pain, and that nothing they have done has caused it.

7.4.4. Diagnosis

A physical examination and a review of your child's medical history are the first steps in the diagnosis process for pediatric rheumatic diseases. Numerous blood tests, as well as other diagnostic procedures like skin and muscle biopsies, X-rays, and medical imaging, may also be requested.

7.4.5. Treatment

Your child's age, overall health, and symptoms will all affect the course of treatment. The objectives of rheumatic disease treatment are to reduce inflammation, manage pain, and enhance quality of life. The majority of treatment regimens combine medication, exercise, and a balanced diet. A combination of medication and therapies administered by a rheumatologist, occupational therapist, and physiotherapist can effectively manage and reduce symptoms.

Strategies for managing pain:

- When necessary, take the prescribed pain relievers.
- Use a diary to look for patterns that lead to "flare-ups."
- Understand the warning signs of pain and create a "pain plan."
- In the morning, promote taking hot showers to help relax your muscles.
- Promote the use of ice or heat packs to help relax muscles and lessen swelling.
- Include energy-saving techniques and rest periods.
- Les principes de protection des joints corrects.

- Splinting hands or fingers to support or limit movement can help protect joints. The splint will be made by an occupational therapist, who will also give advice on where, when, and how to wear it.
- Include methods for distraction and relaxation (music, meditations).

Note: The treatment team for your child should approve all pain management techniques because the methods used will depend on your child's needs (Abdulla, 2011; Berni Canani et al, 2016; Colby, 2017; Murray et al, 2019).

7.5. CARDIOLOGY PROBLEMS

A heart issue, also known as a congenital (present from birth) heart disease, affects about one in every 100 children. Treatment options for heart defects typically include medication, surgery, or other medical procedures. The majority of cardiac tests are easy, quick, and painless. The majority of kids with heart defects lead full, normal lives with very few or no limitations.

7.5.1. Types of Heart Conditions in Children

A heart condition affects approximately one out of every 100 babies born in the US, making it one of the most prevalent birth defects. Heart disorders can be acquired (occurring after birth) or congenital (existing from birth). The most prevalent kind of birth defect is congenital cardiac conditions, which can range in severity from mild to severe. Conversely, acquired heart conditions can strike at any age and stem from a variety of sources, such as infections, underlying medical conditions, and lifestyle choices.

7.5.1.1. Congenital Heart Defects

Congenital heart defects are anatomical abnormalities that exist from birth and can impact the heart's ability to function normally. At around 1% of births, they are the most prevalent birth defect. Congenital heart disease is diagnosed, treated, and managed by the professionals at the CHOC Heart Institute in collaboration with pediatric patients and their families. Several congenital cardiac defects are frequently observed in children.

- **Aortic Stenosis:** a disorder where there is a narrowing or obstruction of the aortic valve, which regulates blood flow from the left ventricle to the aorta, resulting in decreased blood flow.
- **Atrial Septal Defect:** a gap in the wall separating the heart's two upper chambers that permits blood with and without oxygen to mix.
- **Coarctation of the Aorta:** a constriction in the aorta, the primary artery responsible for transporting blood from the heart to the rest of the body.

7.5.1.2. Acquired Heart Conditions

After birth, acquired heart defects can develop and can be brought on by a variety of medical conditions, drugs, and lifestyle choices. Among the prevalent acquired cardiac defects in kids are:

- **Kawasaki Disease:** blood vessel inflammation that may cause harm to the coronary arteries.
- **Rheumatic Heart Disease:** the outcome of heart valves being so severely damaged by rheumatic fever that they may no longer function correctly.
- **Coronary Artery Disease:** Reduced blood flow to the heart results from narrowing or blockage of the coronary arteries, which feed

the organ with oxygen-rich blood. The prevalence of this condition is higher in older kids and teenagers.

- **Cardiomyopathy:** Damage or weakening of the heart muscle results in decreased pumping capacity.

7.5.1.3. Congenital or Acquired Heart Conditions

Children can have cardiovascular diseases that are either inherited or develop during childhood. Among these more typical cardiac ailments are the following:

- **Arrhythmias:** Irregular heartbeats can fall on a spectrum from benign to critical, with potential causes including medical conditions, medications, and lifestyle choices.
- **Pulmonary Hypertension:** high blood pressure in the pulmonary artery, which supplies the lungs with blood from the heart, makes the heart's right-side work harder to pump blood. This may ultimately result in myocardial damage.

A heart condition affects approximately 1 in every 100 children, or 1% of newborns in the United States, making it one of the most common birth defects. Congenital heart defects are anatomical abnormalities that exist from birth and can impact the heart's ability to function normally. They can be minor to severe and may need to be treated with surgery or other medical procedures. In children, acquired cardiac conditions are less common. Children who receive treatment for congenital heart defects are more likely to develop cardiac conditions later in life, such as cardiomyopathy, endocarditis, and arrhythmias.

7.5.2. Risk Factors for Heart Conditions in Children

The chance that a child will receive a heart condition diagnosis can be raised by several risk factors. While some risk factors may develop later in life, others may be present from birth. Congenital heart defect risk factors could include:

- Heart disease in the family history.
- Mother's age (elderly moms are more vulnerable).
- Maternal diabetes
- Substance abuse by mothers, encompassing alcohol, tobacco, and illicit drugs.
- Infections in mothers (like cytomegalovirus or rubella).
- Exposure of mothers to specific drugs or pollutants in the environment.
- Heart defects are related to specific genetic disorders.

Some risk factors for acquired cardiac conditions are as follows.

- Overweight or obesity
- Physical inactivity
- High blood pressure
- High cholesterol
- Diabetes
- Family history of heart disease
- Genetic conditions
- Tobacco use
- Alcohol abuse
- Illegal drug use

A child does not automatically develop a cardiac condition just because they have one or more of these risk factors. There are many kids with heart problems who have no known risk factors. Heart disease can affect children. It may develop later in life or be present from birth. Heart disease is a term used to describe more advanced or severe stages of heart problems; this is the main distinction between heart conditions and heart disease. By contrast, any abnormality or disorder affecting the heart can be referred to as heart conditions. Heart disease may or may not develop from heart conditions.

7.5.3. Prevention

There are several things that parents can do to lower their child's risk of heart disease. Here are a few broad suggestions.

- **Encourage a Healthy Diet:** Maintaining a healthy weight and blood pressure can help prevent heart disease. A diet high in fruits, vegetables, whole grains, lean protein, and low in saturated and trans fats can help achieve this.
- **Encourage Regular Physical Activity:** Frequent exercise can lower the risk of heart disease, enhance cardiovascular health, and help people maintain a healthy weight. Every day, children should engage in moderate-to-intense physical activity for at least 60 minutes.
- **Avoid Tobacco and Smoke Exposure:** Heart disease risk can be raised by using tobacco products and being around secondhand smoke. It is important to teach kids not to use tobacco products and to avoid places where smoking is permitted.
- **Encourage Healthy Habits:** To help maintain good general health and lower the risk of heart disease, parents should encourage their children to brush their teeth twice a day, wash their hands often, and get plenty of sleep.

7.5.4. Symptoms of Heart Conditions in Children

Depending on the particular disorder and how severe it is, children's heart conditions can present with a variety of symptoms. Children with heart conditions may experience the following symptoms frequently:

- **Shortness of Breath:** Breathing problems can arise in children with heart conditions, particularly when they are sleeping or engaging in physical activity.
- **Chest Pain:** Chest pain in children with heart conditions can range in intensity from mild to severe.
- **Rapid or Irregular Heartbeat:** Children who suffer from heart conditions may experience an irregular heart rhythm, leading to rapid, irregular, or erratic heartbeats.
- **Dizziness:** Particularly when standing up or shifting positions, children with heart conditions may experience lightheadedness or dizziness.
- **Fatigue:** Even after resting, children with heart conditions may experience fatigue or weakness.
- **Swelling:** Children with heart problems may develop fluid accumulation that causes swelling in the ankles, feet, legs, or abdomen.
    - **When to See a Doctor for Heart Condition Symptoms:** It's critical to take a child to the doctor for assessment and

treatment if they exhibit any heart-related symptoms. Children's heart conditions frequently manifest as dyspnea, exhaustion, dizziness, rapid or irregular heartbeat, chest pain, and swelling. If a child exhibit any of these symptoms, it's critical to get them checked out by a doctor, especially if they are severe or persistent. Heart conditions can be better managed and complications can be avoided with early diagnosis and treatment.

7.5.5. Screening and Diagnosis for Heart Conditions in Children

Children's heart conditions can be screened for and diagnosed using a variety of techniques. The screening and diagnostic techniques employed may vary based on the child's age, medical background, and symptoms, in addition to their particular heart condition. The following are a few typical screening and diagnostic techniques for assessing cardiac conditions in children.

- **Cardiac Catheterization:** A tiny tube called a catheter must be inserted into an arm or leg blood vessel in order to perform this test. It is then threaded to the heart from there. Cardiac catheterization aids in diagnosing a condition by evaluating heart function.
- **Echocardiogram:** In order to help diagnose heart conditions such as structural abnormalities and problems with the heart valves, sound waves create a detailed image of the heart.
- **CT Scan:** A CT scan employs x-rays to generate precise images of the interior of the body for assessing different conditions in children.
- **Cardiac MRI:** A diagnostic procedure called cardiac magnetic resonance imaging (MRI) uses radio waves and a magnetic field to produce finely detailed images of the heart and its surrounding structures.
- **Electrocardiogram and Cardiac Stress Testing:** An ECG can assess different heart conditions in children, such as arrhythmias and structural abnormalities. A cardiac stress test, a type of ECG done during increased heart activity, measures heart function during physical exertion and aids in diagnosing specific conditions.
- **Holter Monitoring:** A diagnostic procedure called Holter monitoring tracks the electrical activity of the heart over time. It is usually used to assess cardiac conditions that may not show up on a standard electrocardiogram (ECG), such as intermittent or activity-specific arrhythmias (abnormal heart rhythms).

To make sure their hearts are beating properly, children should visit a doctor on a regular basis. Regular check-ups and the monitoring and treatment of any underlying medical conditions that may have an impact on the heart are possible components of these visits (Abdulla, 2011; Berni Canani et al, 2016; Colby, 2017; Murray et al, 2019).

7.6. HEMATOLOGY PROBLEMS

Pediatric hematology is one of the medical specialties that offers children with complex blood disorders hope. Pediatric blood specialists provide consolation and astute assistance to these courageous kids who are coping with various blood problems. Hematology is the study of blood;

it aims to explain how blood functions and the problems that can arise when it is sick. It finds and fixes a number of blood problems. These conditions can include anemia, which is an insufficient supply of blood, autoimmune diseases, which are conditions in which the body attacks itself, and leukemia, a deadly blood cancer. It can be challenging because many blood disorders don't always have any symptoms, so it's critical to identify and treat them as soon as possible.

By bringing this vital area of medicine to children, pediatric hematology guarantees that they receive individualized care that meets their unique needs. A growing number of children receive cancer or leukemia diagnoses each year, a trend that calls for the medical community to respond with compassion.

7.6.1. Common Hematology Problems

Pediatric hematologists treat a wide range of conditions in their daily practice by dealing with blood-related issues, such as:

- **Leukemia:** Both acute and chronic leukemia need to be managed by professionals.
- **Anemia:** For the sake of a child's health, low red blood cell counts must be treated.
- **Lymphomas:** Hematologists who specialize in pediatrics are crucial in the treatment of cancers of the lymphatic system.
- **Myeloma:** This blood cell malignant tumor requires specialized care.
- **Hemophilia:** Handling this bleeding disorder calls for accuracy and knowledge.
- **Cytopenia:** Intervention and close monitoring are necessary in cases of low blood cell counts.
- **Bleeding Disorders:** It's critical to manage diseases like Von Willebrand disease.
- **Werlhof's Disease:** It is also referred to as immune thrombocytopenia and needs to be treated carefully.
- **Neuroleukemia:** This complicated condition necessitates an all-encompassing strategy.

7.6.2. Symptoms

It's critical to determine when your child should see a pediatric hematologist. Some symptoms should give you cause for concern and force you to seek expert care:

- Drowsiness
- Chronic Fatigue
- Numbness of Fingers
- Excessive Sweating
- Enlarged Lymph Nodes
- Dizziness
- Decreased Appetite
- Pale Skin

- Unexplained Bruises or Bruising
- Prolonged Bleeding
- Nosebleeds
- General Malaise
- Dry Skin with Adequate Hydration
- Severe Itching

Furthermore, it is wise to consult a pediatric hematologist if your child has low hemoglobin levels or if a close relative has a history of hematological disorders. Early evaluation is advantageous when the birth weight was below average and artificial feeding was required. A visit to a hematologist in the early years of a child's life is also recommended in cases of maternal anemia during pregnancy, different blood types or Rh factors between the mother and child, or both.

7.6.3. Diagnosing and Treating Pediatric Blood Disorders

Pediatric hematologists effectively treat blood diseases using a variety of diagnostic and therapeutic approaches. Among the diagnostic methods are:

- Blood tests, both biochemical and general.
- Assessments of ferritin and transferrin levels.
- Iron Level Measurement
- Tests for hepatitis and HIV.
- Myelogram (Bone Marrow Smear Test)

To get a complete picture of the condition, more diagnostic techniques like MRIs, X-rays, and ultrasounds might also be suggested.

In the field of pediatric hematology, treatment approaches include:

- Complex Therapy
- Surgical Interventions
- Immunotherapy
- Hormonal Therapy
- Medications
- Chemotherapy

The treatment plan for every child is meticulously tailored, creating a special "protocol" intended to increase the likelihood of a favorable result.

7.6.4. The Significance of Early Diagnosis in Pediatric Hematology

Effective treatment in pediatric hematology/oncology is dependent on an accurate and timely diagnosis. Accurately determining the type of tumor in good time is necessary to start targeted treatment. Raising awareness among medical professionals—general practitioners in particular—is essential for identifying possible childhood oncological pathologies. This knowledge guarantees that young patients are quickly referred to pediatric hematologists, enabling an early diagnosis and course of treatment. Contemporary diagnostic instruments, such as CT, MRI, and ultrasound scans, are essential to this procedure. By assisting in the identification of tumor features and subgroups with various biological behaviors, they facilitate the development of focused and efficient therapeutic approaches. Organizations such as ASEOP provide equipment, training programs, and scholarships to pediatric on cohematology departments in support of their mission to deliver state-of-the-art care to pediatric patients.

Depending on the type of tumor, combinations of chemotherapy, surgery, and radiation therapy are used as treatments. More recently, bone marrow and hematopoietic stem cells from peripheral blood and umbilical cord have also been potentially transplanted. Each of these therapies is combined into a unique therapeutic plan known as a "protocol" for that child. Surgery still plays a vital role in treating pediatric tumors, even though treatment protocols now include it along with chemotherapy and, in certain cases, radiation therapy. This makes it possible for the patient to have surgery when the tumor's volume has already decreased as a result of chemotherapy and/or radiation therapy, increasing the likelihood of a full removal and minimizing the need for invasive procedures on important organs and tissues. For instance, limb amputation procedures related to bone sarcomas are becoming less common, and it is frequently feasible to replace the amputated portion and restore the limb's functionality.

7.6.5. Nurturing Hope for Pediatric Hematology Patients

In the developed world, children with tumors have varying cure rates depending on the pathology; some forms of the disease have cure rates as high as 90%, while other forms have much lower rates. Experts in blood cancer are actively engaged in a global research effort to identify these forms of the disease that are resistant to treatment. A cornerstone of compassionate care for young patients with blood-related issues is pediatric hematology. Numerous children find hope and healing in the hands of pediatric hematologists and new developments in diagnostic technology and treatment approaches. For the upcoming generation of pediatric hematology patients, the future is increasingly promising as awareness and research both flourishes (Abdulla, 2011; Berni Canani et al, 2016; Colby, 2017; Murray et al, 2019).

7.7. ONCOLOGY PROBLEMS

Your child will probably receive treatment from a physician with expertise in pediatric oncology if they have cancer. It is the investigation and management of pediatric cancer. The majority of cancers that commonly affect children differ from those that affect adults. Cancers in newborns, toddlers, and teenagers are the main focus of pediatric oncology. Pediatric oncology physicians have received specialized training in providing your child with the care and comfort they need throughout their treatment.

7.7.1. Types of Childhood Cancer

Childhood cancers fall into three categories: solid tumors, brain tumors, and leukemias and lymphomas. According to estimates from the American Cancer Society, in 2023, 415 out of every 1 million children and teenagers will find out they have one of these cancers.

7.7.1.1. Leukemias

The most common cancer in children is leukemia. According to American Cancer Society estimates, out of every million people, 35 teenagers and 53 children will be diagnosed with leukemia in 2023. In children and teenagers, leukemia comes in two primary forms:

- Acute lymphoblastic leukemia (ALL) is a type of bone marrow and blood cancer that affects children. The blood cells that aid in your child's defense against infection are impacted by ALL.
- **Leukemia Acute Myeloid:** While AML can take many different forms, all of them impact your child's platelets and blood cells.

7.7.1.2. Lymphomas

Cancers in your child's lymphatic system are called lymphomas. Hodgkin lymphoma and non-Hodgkin lymphoma are the two types of lymphomas. An estimated 53 children and 22 teenagers per million will be diagnosed with lymphoma in 2023.

- **Hodgkin Lymphoma:** Although it can affect younger children, the most common cancer diagnosed in teenagers is Hodgkin lymphoma. Hodgkin lymphomas in children are:
    - Hodgkin lymphoma, or nodular sclerosis, usually strikes teenagers.
    - Mixed cellularity Hodgkin lymphoma can impact children who are under the age of 10.
- **Non-Hodgkin Lymphoma:** Adolescents have a higher incidence of non-Hodgkin lymphoma than do children. Among the non-Hodgkin lymphomas in pediatric cancers are:
    - Lymphoblastic lymphoma.
    - Burkitt lymphoma.
    - Diffuse large B-cell lymphoma.
    - Anaplastic large cell lymphoma.

7.7.1.3. Brain Tumors

The most common type of cancer that affects kids and teenagers is brain tumors. Benign (noncancerous) or malignant (cancerous) brain tumors are both possible. Brain tumors can take many different forms. It is projected that one million children and one million teenagers will be diagnosed with malignant brain tumors in 2023.

7.7.1.4. Solid Tumors

Cancerous cells divide, multiply, and eventually bunch up into masses composed of cancerous cells to form solid tumors. Kids and teenagers can get solid tumors all over their bodies. Other prevalent childhood cancers with solid tumors are:

- Neuroblastoma.
- Wilms tumor.
- Retinoblastoma.
- Bone cancer, such as Ewing sarcoma and osteosarcoma.
- Rhabdomyosarcoma.

7.7.2. Diagnosing Childhood Cancer

Your child's medical history, symptoms, and family history of cancer will all be questions your doctor will ask you. A family member's cancer may increase a child's risk of developing cancer. In order to look for any indications of cancer, your doctor may also recommend that your child undergo imaging tests like MRIs or X-rays. They might also recommend that your child have a biopsy. During the test, a sample of your child's tissue is taken by the doctor and sent to a lab to be examined for cancerous cells. Your doctor may inform you of the disease's stage if the tests reveal that you have cancer. Staging helps your doctor determine the best course of action by letting you know how far the cancer has spread. A patient may have stage I, II, III, or IV cancer. A lower stage number indicates that the cancer has not progressed very far throughout your child's body. Should it be greater, the cancer has spread farther.

7.7.2.1. Chemotherapy for Childhood Cancer

Chemotherapy can affect your child's entire body, not just the cancer cells. The specific side effects your child experiences can vary depending on the type of medication they receive. Your doctor may recommend medications or therapies to help alleviate these side effects. In some cases, chemotherapy may also result in lasting adverse effects for your child.

7.7.2.2. Surgery for Childhood Cancer

At times, your child may require surgical intervention to alleviate pain or discomfort associated with cancer. The number of surgeries needed will depend on the type of cancer your child has, with the possibility of either a single surgery or a series of procedures. Surgery may be recommended by the doctor to prevent the spread of cancer, determine its type and stage, as well as provide treatment. Potential side effects of cancer surgery include complications such as bleeding, blood clots, damage to surrounding tissues and organs, as well as the risk of medication reactions or infections.

7.7.2.3. Radiation Therapy for Childhood Cancer

One kind of cancer treatment called radiation uses high-energy waves or particles to destroy cancer cells and reduce tumor size. Before undergoing chemotherapy or surgery, your child might require radiation therapy to reduce the size of the tumor. In other cases, radiation therapy will be administered to your child in place of surgery. Radiation therapy, in contrast to chemotherapy, only harms the cancerous and healthy cells in the targeted area of your child's body. Physicians will ensure that your child receives a safe dose of radiation therapy to target their cancer without seriously harming other organs. Radiation side effects can include fatigue, reduced blood counts, hair loss, skin changes like redness or sensitivity, and mild cell damage.

Cell damage also causes late-onset, long-term effects in certain children. Depending on your child's age, the area of their body that was treated, and the radiation dose, the long-term effects may differ. It is likely that your child will require follow-up appointments with their physician for the rest of their life to monitor any issues that might not surface for years following radiation treatment.

7.7.3. Symptoms of Childhood Cancer

While your child's doctor will likely detect many cancers early, some cancers can be difficult to detect because of their symptoms, which can mimic those of common illnesses and injuries. In order to increase the likelihood of an early diagnosis, you should take your child to the doctor if they exhibit any of the following symptoms.

- Quick weight loss
- Unexpected vision changes
- Constant headaches
- Fevers that do not go away
- Limping
- Ongoing discomfort in a particular body area.
- Easy bleeding or bruising
- Lack of energy
- Unexplained paleness
- A lump or swell that seems unrelated.

Even though your child's symptoms are probably caused by a less serious injury or illness, it's still important to get them checked out by a doctor if any persist.

7.7.4. Getting Support

Every aspect of your family's life is impacted when you learn that your child has cancer. Most doctors will recommend services to support your child so that your family can comprehend and adjust. In order to help your family cope with your child's cancer, your doctor might advise that you and your child see a psychologist or counselor. To make your child feel comfortable while receiving treatment, many pediatric cancer centers provide a welcoming environment. Social workers can frequently assist your child in rearranging their social and academic schedules to accommodate their treatment. Physicians who treat your child for cancer are trained to communicate in a clear, reassuring manner with your family and child about their treatment (Abdulla, 2011; Berni Canani et al, 2016; Colby, 2017; Murray et al, 2019).

7.8. ENDOCRINE PROBLEMS

Hormones are the body's chemical messengers; they enter the bloodstream, travel through particular cell receptors, and then cause a reaction. Numerous physiological functions, such as metabolism, blood pressure control, blood glucose regulation, growth and development, reproduction, the sleep-wake cycle, and mood, are heavily influenced by hormones.

7.8.1. Type 1 Diabetes Mellitus (DM1)

The immune system of the body attacks and destroys beta cells, which are the cells that produce insulin, in type 1 diabetes. Juvenile diabetes is the term for it since it is typically diagnosed in children. Weight loss, polydipsia, polyuria, and polyphagia are the typical symptoms of DM1. Weakness, exhaustion, severe diaper rash, female yeast infections, and mood swings are some additional indications and symptoms. The child may experience decreased LOC, deep, rapid breathing (Kussmaul respirations), and fruity-smelling breath when diabetic ketoacidosis develops. Insulin is used to treat diabetes, and the child will require several daily blood sugar checks. The child will also need to refrain from missing meals and adhere to a diet low in carbohydrates.

It is crucial for parents and older children to be able to identify the symptoms of hypoglycemia and to be aware that low blood sugar levels can be caused by excessive insulin, not eating enough, or exercising. The treatment for hypoglycemia involves giving the person some form of glucose, such as drinking juice or eating something sweet like cake icing, using IM glucagon, or receiving IV dextrose in a medical setting.

7.8.2. Type 2 Diabetes Mellitus (DM2)

Previously known as "adult onset diabetes," Type 2 diabetes is now affecting more children due to the rise in childhood obesity. Aside from being overweight, other risk factors for the development of Type 2 diabetes in children include:

- Inactivity
- A diet heavy in processed foods and red meat.
- A diet heavy in sugar (including sugar-filled drinks).
- Underweight or premature baby born.
- Infants born to diabetic mothers during pregnancy.
- Family history of DM2

Children with type 2 diabetes are treated with pharmacologic interventions in addition to lifestyle modifications such as diet, exercise, and weight loss.

7.8.3. Hyperthyroidism

When the thyroid produces too much thyroid hormone, the condition is known as hyperthyroidism. Triiodothyronine (T-3) and thyroxine (T-4) are the two primary hormones. Thyroid hormones affect every cell in the body and are essential for regulating metabolism, temperature, heart rate, and protein synthesis. The most frequent cause of hyperthyroidism in children is the autoimmune disease Graves' disease, which targets the thyroid gland. Antibodies trigger the thyroid to release too much hormone in Graves' disease. Other potential reasons consist of:

- Growths in the thyroid gland called goiters, or thyroid nodules, have the ability to overproduce thyroid hormone.
- The thyroid leaks excess hormones into the bloodstream when it is inflamed, a condition known as thyroiditis. Usually, this illness gets better on its own.
- Although it is uncommon, neonatal Graves' disease can happen when the mother has the illness and her antibodies affect the fetus' thyroid gland by crossing the placenta.
- An excessive intake of iodine from food, which can come from seaweed consumption or supplements.
- Hyperthyroidism can also result from taking too much thyroid hormone replacement therapy.

In children, tachycardia, hypertension, weight loss, increased appetite, tremors, sweating, heat intolerance, loose stools, hyperactivity, difficulty concentrating, insomnia, and bulging eyes are classic signs and symptoms of hyperthyroidism. When left untreated, hyperthyroidism can be fatal for kids of all ages, but it can also cause cognitive impairments in children under three. Furthermore, children with hyperthyroidism may grow rapidly when they are younger, but this growth usually stops early, resulting in a generally short stature.

7.8.4. Hypothyroidism

A condition known as hypothyroidism occurs when the body does not produce enough thyroid hormones.

- **Congenital Hypothyroidism:** Congenital hypothyroidism results from improper thyroid gland development during pregnancy. Due to the high prevalence of the condition (1 in 2,500–3,000 children), every baby born in the U.S. are examined for this illness. It should be noted that congenital hypothyroidism in infants whose mothers used antithyroid drugs to treat hyperthyroidism during pregnancy can be temporary or chronic. Congenital hypothyroidism can result in severe delays in both physical and mental development if left untreated.

- **Acquired Hypothyroidism:** Usually, an autoimmune condition called chronic lymphocytic thyroiditis—also referred to as Hashimoto's thyroiditis—causes acquired hypothyroidism. It is more prevalent in females and in people who also have other autoimmune diseases like DM1.
- **Iatrogenic Hypothyroidism:** Children who have had their thyroid removed, either completely or partially, or ablated, are susceptible to this type of hypothyroidism.
- **Central Hypothyroidism:** Thyroid stimulating hormone (TSH) deficiency is the result of a pituitary or hypothalamic disorder in central hypothyroidism. The thyroid gland is not stimulated to produce T3 and T4 in the absence of this essential hormone. It is typically associated with radiation therapy for a previous malignant brain tumor or a benign brain tumor known as a craniopharyngioma. Hormone deficiencies in children with central hypothyroidism may include growth hormone, adrenocorticotropic hormone, and antidiuretic hormone.

Fatigue, slowed cognitive functions, bradycardia, weight gain, constipation, dry and thinning hair, intolerance to cold, hoarse voice, facial edema, and goiter are among the indications and symptoms of hypothyroidism.

7.8.5. Growth Hormone Deficiency

A condition known as growth hormone deficiency (GHD) occurs when the pituitary gland fails to produce enough growth hormone. This may be idiopathic or the result of pituitary or hypothalamic underdevelopment or damage. Brain tumors, head radiation therapy, and brain injuries are a few common specific causes of acquired GHD. A child diagnosed with GHD will usually be shorter than five percentile on the growth chart. More specifically, after the child turns three, their growth slows down annually, with a cumulative gain of less than 1/4 inch. Additional signs include delayed puberty, underdeveloped lower jaw, and delayed emergence of permanent teeth. Given that GHD does not impair brain development, children with the illness have normal intelligence. However, because of their diminutive stature, they might struggle academically or emotionally as a result of low self-esteem and people thinking they're much younger than they actually are.

Blood tests and imaging studies are used to diagnose growth hormone deficiency and determine bone age, which is less than calendar age. Children with GHD respond better to early treatment, which entails daily injections of synthetic growth hormone until puberty is reached.

7.8.6. Hyperpituitarism

Hyperpituitarism is rare in children, but it can happen to those who have microadenomas, which are benign pituitary tumors that are small in size. Numerous hormonal disorders, such as hypercortisolism (Cushing's syndrome), hyperthyroidism, hypothyroidism, and acromegaly, can be brought on by the condition. Children with acromegaly have higher levels of growth hormone in their bodies, which can cause abnormally long arms and legs, a maximum height of eight feet, and structural abnormalities in the face, such as enlarged jaw and brow. The goal of hyperpituitarism treatments is to address the child's particular hormonal condition. For instance, a child diagnosed with acromegaly might be prescribed medication to reduce growth hormone levels and have the tumor surgically removed through a procedure known as a transsphenoidal adenomectomy.

7.8.7. Congenital Adrenal Hyperplasia (CAH)

An enzyme that is required to produce aldosterone and cortisol malfunctions in congenital adrenal hyperplasia (CAH). Atypical genitalia, excess androgens (early puberty, acne, hirsuitism), altered growth patterns (early rapid growth but overall shorter stature), cortisol and adrenal insufficiency, and atypical genitalia are all present in children with CAH. When a prenatal diagnosis is made, the mother administers dexamethasone as part of the treatment. Children and infants are given replacement hormones, such as mineralocorticoids to replace aldosterone and corticosteroids to replace cortisol, which also help to maintain potassium and sodium levels (Abdulla, 2011; Berni Canani et al, 2016; Colby, 2017; Murray et al, 2019).

7.9. GENETIC DISORDERS

Genetic abnormalities, which can be inherited from parents or develop spontaneously as a result of genetic mutations, are the root cause of genetic disorders. These abnormalities have the potential to disrupt the structure, function, or regulation of genes, leading to various diseases. Genetic testing and counseling are essential for diagnosing and treating genetic disorders. They also help families make decisions and give important information about the likelihood that future generations will inherit a genetic problem.

7.9.1. Types of Genetic Disorders

The various kinds of genetic disorders are as follows:

7.9.1.1. Single-Gene Disorders

Autosomal Dominant Disorders: Autosomal recessive disorders arise when an individual inherits one copy of the mutated gene from each parent. Autosomal recessive diseases include phenylketonuria (PKU), sickle cell anemia, and cystic fibrosis. These conditions often first show symptoms in childhood and may need lifetime care.

- **Autosomal Recessive Disorders:** Autosomal dominant disorders occur when an individual inherits one copy of the mutated gene from each parent, or two copies in total. Autosomal recessive diseases include sickle cell anemia, PKU, and cystic fibrosis. These disorders may require lifetime care and treatment since they initially manifest in children.
- **X-Linked Disorders:** Mutations in genes on the X chromosome are the cause of X-linked disorders. These disorders are more likely to affect men. X-linked diseases include Duchenne muscular dystrophy, hemophilia, and fragile X syndrome, to name a few. Additionally, females may carry these disorders. Although symptoms and severity can differ, management usually involves a multidisciplinary approach.

7.9.1.2. Chromosomal Disorders

Down Syndrome: The cause of Down syndrome is an extra copy of chromosome 21. Approximately 1 in 700 babies are born with this chromosomal disorder, making it the most common. Oftentimes, children with Down syndrome exhibit distinct physical characteristics, developmental delays, and an increased likelihood of specific medical conditions. Support services and early intervention programs are essential to their wellbeing.

- **Turner Syndrome:** Turner syndrome is a condition that affects females and is brought on by an incomplete or missing X chromosome. About 1 in 2,500 live female births experience it. Physical traits could include ovarian dysfunction, small stature, and possible learning challenges. In order to control symptoms and encourage normal development, hormone therapy and specialized care are frequently offered.
- **Klinefelter Syndrome:** The extra X chromosome that is present in males with Klinefelter syndrome is one of its defining characteristics. It affects roughly 1 in 500–1,000 male babies born. Physical traits include potential learning disabilities, infertility, and tall stature. Managing symptoms and enhancing general health are the main goals of treatment.

There are many different types of genetic disorders; the following is a list of common genetic disorders.

- Cystic Fibrosis
- **Cause:** Mutation in the CFTR gene that impacts the synthesis of a protein required for healthy digestion and lung function.
- **Symptoms:** Digestive issues, breathing difficulties, and recurring lung infections.
- **Diagnosis:** Lung function tests, sweat tests, and genetic testing.
- **Treatment:** Prescription drugs, chest physical therapy, and dietary assistance.
- Sickle Cell Disease
  - **Cause:** A genetic mutation that modifies the structure of hemoglobin and results in aberrant red blood cells.
  - **Symptoms:** Anemia, pain episodes, and organ damage.
  - **Diagnosis:** Blood tests, genetic testing, and newborn screening.
  - **Treatment:** Blood transfusions, pain management, and medication.
- Muscular Dystrophy
  - **Cause:** Genetic changes that impact the proteins in muscles.
  - **Symptoms:** Respiratory issues, motor skill difficulties, and progressive muscle weakness.
  - **Diagnosis:** Muscle biopsy, genetic testing, and physical examination.
  - **Treatment:** Assistive technology, physical therapy, and supportive care.
- Tay-Sachs Disease
  - **Cause:** An enzyme required for the breakdown of specific fatty substances in the brain is absent or malfunctioning.
  - **Symptoms:** seizures, loss of motor skills, vision, and hearing.
  - **Diagnosis:** blood tests, eye exams, and genetic testing.
  - **Treatment:** supportive care for symptom management.
- Phenylketonuria (PKU)
  - **Cause:** insufficiency of an enzyme required for the

phenylalanine amino acid's processing.
- **Symptoms:** Intellectual disabilities, developmental delays, behavioral issues.
- **Diagnosis:** Blood tests, genetic testing, newborn screening.
- **Treatment:** severe dietary limitations and frequent observation.

- Hemophilia
  - **Cause:** changes to the genes that regulate clotting factors in blood.
  - **Symptoms:** Excessive bleeding, joint damage, bruising.
  - **Diagnosis:** blood work, genetic testing, and family history evaluation.
  - **Treatment:** therapy to replace lost clotting factors and control bleeding episodes.
- Fragile X Syndrome
  - **Cause:** a particular gene sequence's expansion that results in decreased protein synthesis.
  - **Symptoms**: behavioral issues, speech and language delays, and intellectual disabilities.
  - **Diagnosis**: Genetic analysis, analysis of family history, and developmental evaluations.
  - **Treatment**: Early intervention, behavioral therapies, and support for education.
- Spinal Muscular Atrophy (SMA)
  - **Cause**: The absence of a protein required for the proper operation of motor neurons.
  - **Symptoms**: respiratory issues, motor skill difficulties, and progressive muscle weakness.
  - **Diagnosis**: muscle biopsy, electromyography (EMG), and genetic testing.
  - **Treatment**: physical therapy, respiratory support, and disease-modifying medication.
- Marfan Syndrome
- **Cause**: a mutation in the connective tissue protein-producing gene.
- **Symptoms**: tall stature, irregular heartbeat, flexible joints, and visual issues.
- **Diagnosis**: Genetic testing, imaging tests, and clinical evaluation.
- **Treatment**: Cardiovascular and musculoskeletal complications: tracking and treatment.
- Neurofibromatosis
  - **Cause**: Tumor growth on nerves caused by genetic mutation.
  - **Symptoms**: tumors, abnormalities of the skin, and learning disabilities.
  - **Diagnosis**: Genetic testing, imaging tests, and clinical evaluation.
  - **Treatment**: routine observation, tumor excision through surgery, and supportive care.

7.9.2. Diagnosis and Management of Genetic Problems

Effective management of genetic issues requires early diagnosis. In order to identify particular genetic mutations, as well as to provide information about the risks and possible treatments associated with them, genetic testing is an important tool. While newborn screening programs aid in the early detection of certain genetic disorders after birth, allowing for early intervention, prenatal testing empowers parents to make educated decisions about their pregnancy. Depending on the particular condition and its symptoms, there are different treatment options for genetic issues. Medications can be used to control symptoms, stop problems from happening, or delay the course of an illness. Surgery can treat complications or rectify physical abnormalities. Physical, speech, and occupational therapies are frequently used to help people with their motor skills, communication, and general quality of life. For people and their families, supportive care—which includes counseling, educational support, and access to support networks—is essential.

Comprehensive management frequently requires a multidisciplinary approach involving medical professionals from different specialties, such as geneticists, pediatricians, therapists, and genetic counselors. Regular monitoring, follow-up appointments, and treatment plan modifications are necessary to ensure optimal outcomes. Children with genetic disorders need to be fully informed about the different kinds, causes, symptoms, and available treatments. Our goal is to enable parents, caregivers, and medical professionals to effectively support children with genetic disorders by increasing awareness and disseminating information about the various types of genetic disorders.

Children with genetic disorders can live happy, fulfilling lives and develop to their full potential if they receive early diagnosis, appropriate care, and access to resources. To ensure the best outcomes for children and their families, it is imperative to seek professional guidance and support when navigating the complexities of genetic disorders (Abdulla, 2011; Berni Canani et al, 2016; Colby, 2017; Murray et al, 2019).

7.10. RENAL AND GENITOURINARY DISORDERS

The kidneys, ureters, urinary bladder, and urethra make up the urinary tract. Dysuria, or pain during micturition, is a common symptom of any disease affecting these structures. Although children tend to pass urine more frequently than adults, this is typically not a medical problem. However, it might be a sign of a urinary disease if it is accompanied by other symptoms. Urinary pathology symptoms include increased frequency of micturition, burning pain during micturition, and pain when the skin surrounding the perineal orifices comes into contact with urine.

7.10.1. Congenital Malformations

One of the most common conditions of this system in children is obstruction of the urinary tract, which can be caused by issues like:

- Vesicoureteral reflux
- Obstruction of the urinary tract, such as a posterior urethral valve obstruction or calculus.
- Fetal hydronephrosis brought on by vesicoureteral reflux or blockage.
- Renal failure is frequently the result of polycystic kidney disease, a condition that is typically inherited and causes fluid-filled cysts to replace the kidneys.
- Multicystic kidney disease, which is typically unilateral and causes big cysts to replace one underdeveloped kidney.
- Renal tubular acidosis is the condition in which the kidneys'

acidification is the cause of renal stones.

- Wilm's tumor is a pediatric renal tumor that typically goes away with treatment and manifests in the first two years of life.
- Urinary tract duplication can manifest as recurrent urinary tract infections that require medication or surgery.
- A horseshoe kidney, where two kidneys are fused at one end, may occasionally obstruct a ureter or other structures, but typically does not require treatment as kidney function is usually normal.

7.10.2. Infections

Acute or chronic renal infections are possible. Among them are:

- Fever, oliguria, edema, hematuria, and pain in the groin region are symptoms of glomerulonephritis, an inflammation of the glomeruli in the kidneys. While some cases quickly go away, others continue and eventually develop into chronic conditions that harm the kidneys over time.
- A condition known as nephrotic syndrome is marked by a significant loss of protein in the urine as a result of renal parenchymal damage. This can manifest as swelling and be caused by immune-related, toxic, or infectious factors. It is typically handled by a doctor.
- The most prevalent urinary illnesses in children are urinary tract infections, which are typically identified by dysuria and frequent urination. They make up the second most common category of pediatric bacterial infections. Fever may be the only indication of infection in very young infants, with no other symptoms showing.

Other symptoms include:

- too little urine
- strongly odorous urine
- dark-colored or bloodstained urine
- refusal to eat
- diarrhea
- irritability and restlessness
- intractable diaper rash

Enteric commensals, like *E. coli*, are a common type of bacteria found in the urinary tract. They could impact the kidneys in cases where infections from the bladder ascend, the bladder itself in cases where bladder infections result from them, or they could spread by blood bacteria.

7.10.3. Acquired Obstruction

This could involve urinary tract strictures as a result of trauma, infection, or surgery. Children who have urinary tract obstructions are more likely to experience urinary infections due to incomplete bladder emptying, which encourages the growth of bacteria. Infancy rates of obstructive urological disease are higher in boys than in girls.

Another significant factor contributing to childhood obstructive uropathy is urinary calculi. These occur when salts and minerals crystallize and accumulate in certain areas of the urinary tract, forming stones. While the majority are small enough to expel on their own, some need to be surgically removed or treated. Changing one's diet is frequently required to stop the formation of stones. The symptoms of calculous disease can include hematuria or pain in the loins.

7.10.4. Urinary Tract Trauma

Urinary tract trauma can result from a blow to the genital or loin region. This can cause symptoms such as renal swelling, pain in the genital or loin region, hematuria, urine retention, or trouble urinating.

7.10.5. Renal Failure

Depending on the mode of onset and length of the condition, renal failure can be either acute or chronic. It explains how the body accumulates toxins due to the kidneys' inability to adequately or quickly eliminate blood waste. Several clinical symptoms result from this, such as hiccups, altered consciousness, pruritus, and edema of the dependent parts. Bacterial infections, trauma, heart failure, muscle deterioration, shock, toxic damage, or drug-induced damage can all result in acute renal failure. In cases like these, dialysis might be required if the underlying cause cannot be corrected. The term "chronic kidney failure" describes the progressive loss of renal function over time, which can lead to hypertension and even death. Chronic renal disease, non-resolving acute renal failure, acquired or congenital kidney defects, and chronic hypertension are possible causes. Early diagnosis is important to allow for the right course of treatment, which could postpone the need for renal transplantation or dialysis. Medication, dietary restrictions, and hypertension control are the methods of treatment.

7.10.6. Diagnosis and Treatment

The symptoms point to urinary issues, which are then investigated further with a thorough medical history and physical examination. Often, there is an increase in blood pressure. Checks should also be made on growth. Numerous tests, such as blood and urine tests, imaging, and renal biopsies, may be performed. The exact ailment and any underlying diseases will determine the course of treatment (Abdulla, 2011; Berni Canani et al, 2016; Colby, 2017; Murray et al, 2019).

7.11. SKIN PROBLEMS

Babies, toddlers, kids, and teenagers can all experience different skin conditions at some point in their lives. Every year, children with skin concerns make over 12 million office visits to healthcare providers. Children's skin conditions can include rashes of all kinds, acne, birthmarks, warts, and hives.

7.11.1. Common Pediatric Skin Conditions

Childhood skin rashes usually resolve on their own and don't require medical attention, so there's usually no need for alarm. Nonetheless, some situations call for additional research and care.

7.11.1.1. Diaper Dermatitis

A collection of skin disorders known as diaper dermatitis or rash involves skin inflammation around the diaper area. The typical skin rash has multiple causes, which include:

- Contact with irritants
- *Candida albicans* yeast overgrowth
- Contact with allergens
- Inflammatory skin diseases, like dermatitis seborrheica.

When the skin comes into prolonged contact with any irritant—such as urine or feces—irritant contact dermatitis develops. It results in a red rash that appears on the skin, potentially swelling and accompanied by blisters. One kind of yeast that is naturally found on the skin in the groin area is called Candida albicans. But in the warm, humid environment of a diaper, it can grow out of control and cause a yeast infection. It appears as bright red spots or bumps on the skin, sometimes with pus visible.

An allergic reaction to any of the diaper's components, including the elastic or adhesive tape, can result in allergic dermatitis. In the specific location where the allergen comes into contact, it results in a red, swollen rash.

- **Eczema:** Eczema, also called atopic dermatitis, is a chronic skin condition that typically first appears in children. It results in skin patches that are dry, red, and itchy and may ooze when scratched. When irritants come into contact with the skin, eczema can get worse. Children with a family history of eczema, asthma, or allergies are more likely to suffer from atopic dermatitis, which is linked to allergies. Oral antihistamine drugs and topical steroid creams are typically used to treat it.
- **Psoriasis:** A layer of scales covers red, flaky skin patches caused by the chronic skin condition psoriasis. While some affected children may not need treatment at all for mild changes, others will require long-term care to manage the condition.
- **Warts:** Children are frequently affected by warts, which appear as hard lumps on the hands and feet. They arise from viral contact, e.g., HPV (human papillomavirus). Warts are treated locally, focusing only on the afflicted area of the skin. There aren't any particular antiviral medications on the market.
- **Cellulitis:** An infection of the skin and underlying tissue known as cellulitis causes the skin to swell and turn red, sometimes turning hot and painful. It can appear anywhere on the body and might need to be treated with antibiotics.
- **Impetigo:** Impetigo, commonly referred to as school sores, is a skin infection that results in blisters and sores. These could be aggressive or not. It is especially prevalent in early school-aged children.
- **Ringworm:** A particular type of fungal infection known as ringworm results in the appearance of a red or silver ring on the skin, which can later become scaly or inflamed. Though it can affect any part of the body, it usually affects the limbs.
- **Scabies:** Tiny mites that burrow into the skin are the cause of scabies, a skin condition. It itch so badly. Usually, it is spread by long-term or frequent skin-to-skin contact between an infected child and another.
- **Slapped Cheek Syndrome:** Young children frequently develop the infectious rash known as "slapped cheek syndrome." It results in a rash that is bright red on the face's two cheeks. The child can return to school once the rash goes away, indicating that the infection is no longer contagious.
- **Erythema Multiforme:** Erythema multiforme is typically a gentle skin rash caused by an allergic response to the herpes simplex virus (HSV). The condition is identified by unique spots featuring a dark-red center encircled by a lighter ring, which

commonly appear on the hands, feet, limbs, and torso.

- **Molluscum Contagiosum:** Clusters of small, firm spots that appear on the skin are the hallmark of the viral skin infection known as molluscum contagiosum. Usually, physical contact is how it spreads from one child to another.
- **Pityriasis Rosia:** Pityriasis rosea is a skin condition that typically affects children and young adults and causes itchy, red, scaly patches to develop.
- **Acne:** Adolescents frequently develop acne, which is brought on by changes in their hormone levels during puberty. When sebum or keratin blocks the pores in the hair follicles, acne develops. If kids have poor hygiene, an unhealthy diet, or a lot of stress, it can get worse. The clogged pore may swell, turn red, and release pus.
- **Other Infections:** A skin rash can result from a number of infections that commonly afflict children.
  - **Hand, Foot and Mouth Disease:** Children who are impacted by this develop mouth ulcers as well as blisters on their hands and feet.
  - **Chickenpox:** All over the body, a rash appears, consisting of red, itchy spots that blister. These soon start to crust over, turn into scabs, and finally fall off.
  - **Measles:** The head, neck, and other parts of the body have reddish-brown spots on them. Because of the widespread use of the measles, mumps, and rubella (MMR) vaccine, it is now uncommon in developed nations.
  - **Scarlet Fever:** This is a rough-to-the-touch, pink rash caused by a bacterial infection.

7.11.2. Causes

Allergies, immune system problems, certain diseases, and genetic makeup can all contribute to skin disorders.

7.11.3. Treating Skin Disorders

Numerous skin conditions are curable. For skin conditions, common treatment options include:

- antihistamines
- medicated creams and ointments
- antibiotics
- steroid injections
- laser therapy
- targeted prescription medications
- biologics

7.11.3.1. Skin Flare-Ups

Certain skin conditions disappear on their own, and not all skin disorders respond to treatment. Individuals who have chronic skin conditions frequently experience excruciating flare-ups of their symptoms. It is occasionally possible to drive incurable illnesses into remission. But most skin conditions have triggers, like stress or illness, that cause them to resurface.

Skin disorders that are temporary and cosmetic can often be treated with:

- medicated makeup
- over-the-counter (OTC) items for skin care.

- good hygiene practices
- small changes in lifestyle, like dietary modifications.

7.11.4. Preventing Skin Disorders

Some skin conditions, such as genetic conditions and skin conditions resulting from other illnesses, cannot be prevented. Certain skin conditions, however, can be avoided.

To avoid contracting infectious skin diseases, heed these tips:

- Frequently wash your hands with warm water and soap.
- Refrain from sharing drinking glasses and cutlery with other people.
- Steer clear of direct contact with the skin of those who are infected.
- Equipment used in public areas, like the gym, should be cleaned before use.
- Share not personal things like hairbrushes, blankets, or bathing suits.
- Every night, get at least 7 hours of sleep.
- Drink plenty of water.
- Try to minimize physical and emotional stress.
- Eat a nutritious diet.
- Vaccinate yourself against contagious skin diseases like chickenpox.

7.11.4.1. Noncontagious Skin Disorders

Certain non-infectious skin conditions, like atopic dermatitis and acne, can occasionally be avoided. The condition determines the different prevention strategies. The following advice can help prevent a few non-infectious skin conditions:

- Every day, wash your face with water and a mild cleanser.
- Use moisturizer.
- Avoid environmental and dietary allergens.
- Steer clear of irritants and harsh chemicals.
- Get at least 7 hours of sleep every night because not getting enough sleep can exacerbate a lot of skin conditions.
- Drink plenty of water.
- Eat a balanced diet.
- Avoid exposing your skin to extreme heat, cold, or wind.

It can be crucial for skin health to understand how to treat skin conditions and how to take good care of your skin. While you can safely treat certain conditions at home, others need to be seen by a doctor. To find the best course of action for treating your symptoms or condition, you should educate yourself and consult a physician (Abdulla, 2011; Berni Canani et al, 2016; Colby, 2017; Murray et al, 2019).

7.12. ORTHOPEDIC PROBLEMS

The Greek root word “ped,” which meaning “child,” refers to the field of orthopedics’ original purpose of treating children (not adults) who were born with or developed musculoskeletal deformities. Physical problems affecting the bones, muscles, joints, tendons, and ligaments are known as orthopedic disorders. These problems are inherited, brought on by illnesses, or the outcome of an incident. Early-onset orthopedic issues may restrict or even forbid children from engaging in physical activity. For this reason, it is best to see an orthopedist as soon as musculoskeletal problems start to show symptoms. Treatments might be able to stop the illness from getting worse or help thwart it.

7.12.1. Pediatric Orthopedic Disorders

The majority of orthopedic disorders in children are inherited or the result of trauma. Since children are still developing, these problems require prompt and appropriate attention. Ignoring these pediatric disorders will harm the child's ability to grow physically. Because the organs and/or tissues are growing in the wrong direction, it could cause anomalies or misalignment of the bones, muscles, and joints. Some of the most typical orthopedic conditions that children see are listed below:

- **Bowlegs:** A disorder known as bowlegs causes the legs to bend excessively outward. Even with the feet together, the knees bend outward when one is standing. Babies frequently have bowlegs because their legs were folded in the womb. When the child starts to walk and put weight on their legs, this condition should be gradually corrected. An orthopedic doctor should be consulted, nevertheless, if the anomaly only affects one leg or if the child is older than two years old and the legs are still bent. The child might have rickets or Blount disease, both of which are curable illnesses.
- **Pigeon Toes:** Another name for pigeon toes is in-toeing. When a baby first stands, it's common for their legs to turn inward for the first 8 to 15 months of life; as they grow, the legs will straighten. On the other hand, the child may have pigeon toes if by the time he or she turns three the legs have not straightened. A qualified orthopedist can handle this.
- **Flatfeet:** A common inherited condition is flatfeet. Flat-footed newborns have flat arches at birth, which can weaken the knees and ankles. This is not regarded as a serious orthopedic issue. Only if the child experiences persistent or frequent foot pain, should they seek medical attention; in that scenario, the physician may recommend orthotics or physical therapy.
- **Knock-Knees:** In contrast to bowlegs, a person with knock-knees has relatively wide ankles spaced apart from their knees when standing. Between the ages of three and six, children frequently develop knock-knees. Kids who have knock-kneeds will probably naturally straighten their legs when they run and walk, as these activities involve bearing weight. But, it's a good idea to take your child to see an orthopedist on a regular basis so the physician can make sure the child's legs are growing appropriately.

7.12.2. Unique Aspects of Orthopedic Care for Kids

Children are sometimes viewed as miniature adults. That is most definitely not the case when it comes to bones, and treating orthopedic problems in children requires special considerations. Youngsters grow, sometimes very quickly, and the growth plate—the region of the bone where growth occurs most quickly—can be injured. A child's bone is also more malleable—it can bend without shattering completely—and can change shape over time. Because of the fast growth that takes place there, healing from a growth plate injury frequently happens very quickly. However, a doctor must make sure the growth plate was not damaged and determine whether it needs to be treated specifically. Growth abnormalities, such as early growth plate closure or aberrant bone growth, can result from undiagnosed injuries to the growth plate. When evaluating treatment options, it's crucial to take into account any age-specific lifestyle concerns or long-term issues associated with a pediatric orthopedic condition.

For example:

- Is it necessary for the child to limit her activities? If yes, how and for how long?
- Should she stay away from running, jumping, or certain sports?
- Will the illness have an impact on future development and growth?
- Is there a chance that the illness will worsen over time or need more care?
- Might this result in any restrictions down the road?

7.12.3. Helping Kids Feel Well

Learning how to support a child with an orthopedic condition is one of the most crucial things parents, relatives, and friends can do for them. Children can experience anxiety and depression as a result of illnesses, injuries, and medical conditions, so it's critical for parents to know how to support their children. Never hesitate to seek assistance from your child's pediatrician or orthopedic specialist. These people should be able to guide you through what is probably unfamiliar ground for you because they have a great deal of experience working with children who have experienced comparable issues.

In the same vein, don't be afraid to discuss with medical staff how you believe your child can benefit. Your child's medical team can better care for your child if they know your child's fears, anxieties, and comforts. You are the one who knows your child the best.

Here are a few direct suggestions to assist a child undergoing orthopedic treatment:

- Encourage your child to ask questions and address those questions seriously
- Praise courageous actions to reinforce them.
- Don't say "it won't hurt" unless it truly won't
- Offer comfort, encouragement, and support; a simple smile and hug can make a big difference.

Nothing makes a parent feel more anxious than when their child is ill or injured. Thankfully, most pediatric orthopedic conditions are just transient annoyances. The skeleton of a child is incredibly resilient; it can recover from trauma, heal from injury, and withstand therapy. The best parents do is to take these illnesses seriously and make sure they receive the proper care. They should also listen to their kids and make sure they have the emotional support they need to get better (Abdulla, 2011; Berni Canani et al, 2016; Colby, 2017; Murray et al, 2019).

7.13. DENTAL PROBLEMS

We are all now aware of the importance of giving children's teeth more consideration thanks to recent advancements in dental treatment. Not too long ago, parents did not want to take their young children to the dentist for routine checkups because they believed that dental issues would be resolved once the kids started getting their permanent set of teeth after their deciduous teeth fell out, with the exception of when the kids were in pain from diseased teeth.

These days, parents are more conscious of the value of good dental health and how it may influence potential dental issues in the future. Children can experience many of the same dental issues as adults, but because children's teeth are more sensitive and softer than an adult's, childhood dental issues have a different effect on children's teeth than adult dental issues do. Additionally, children are undergoing the process of acquiring new teeth, which may be disrupted if there are issues with tooth decay or crowding in the affected children's moth.

7.13.1. Common Dental Problems

These are a handful of the dental issues that kids can have. Knowing about these common dental conditions can help to avoid more serious consequences down the road.

- **Tooth Decay:** Tooth decay is a prevalent dental issue affecting children and adults nationwide and worldwide. In the mouth, a certain type of bacteria grows and resides. On the teeth, these bacteria produce a thin, sticky film known as plaque, which builds up over time. This bacterial film grows on starchy diets. As the sugar breaks down, the bacteria, starch, and sugar combine to produce acid. The tooth enamel, which serves as the tooth's protective layer, is subsequently eroded by this acid. The tooth eventually becomes decayed because the sticky substance continuously allows the acids to come into contact with the enamel. This deterioration is entirely avoidable. Food particles can remain on teeth and in the mouth after consuming a diet high in carbohydrates, such as pasta, bread, rice, and even carbonated drinks, chocolate, and candies. Tooth decay may be avoided if the child is taught to brush and floss on a regular basis, as this would remove any starches from the mouth for bacteria to feed on.
- **Gum Disease:** Periodontal disease is another name for gum diseases. A form of gum disease called gingivitis occurs when tartar and plaque build up at the tooth's base, inflaming the gums. When the child first brushes and flosses, their gums may appear red and inflamed and may even bleed. Gum disease can also be indicated by bad teeth. Maintaining basic dental hygiene is essential to preventing painful gingivitis in the gums.
- **Bad Breadth:** Another name for bad breath is halitosis. Occasionally, the smell of the food being eaten causes poor breadth. However, persistent poor tooth alignment can indicate more serious problems with the gums and teeth. The bacteria that reside in our mouths are the root cause of bad breath. As they break down the carbohydrates, they consume the food particles that are still in the mouth and release hydrogen sulfide. This chemical has a foul odor. Because the bacteria multiply during the night, bad breath is common in both adults and children when they wake up in the morning. However, if this odor is present throughout the day, dry mouth and poor oral hygiene may be to blame. There are numerous

additional reasons for poor breath, such as diabetes, chronic sinusitis, or medications used to treat other illnesses. One of the first steps in ruling out oral bacteria and plaque build-up is to practice good oral hygiene.

- **Sensitive Teeth:** The child's teeth are sensitive and become uncomfortable when exposed to cold or hot foods and beverages. Teeth sensitivity is a sign of a more significant issue. Compared to adults, children's enamel is thinner. Bacteria and plaque quickly wear it down. The teeth get tiny cracks that reveal the gums and nerve endings when the enamel is worn away. Whether eating hot or cold food, these nerve endings are activated. This is a very agonizing circumstance. Tooth sensitivity is frequently a sign of dental decay and cavities. If you practice good dental hygiene, you can avoid this. Sealants are applied to teeth by dentists in order to strengthen the enamel and fill in cracks. Children should be permitted to use soft tooth brushes because hard toothbrushes have the potential to further erode tooth enamel.
- **Thumb Sucking:** A lot of kids have a newborn habit of sucking their thumb or fingers. For a baby or infant, this habit is acceptable because it provides a sense of security and comfort. However, if this behavior persists throughout childhood, it can have a variety of effects on the emergence of permanent teeth. Thumb sucking can disrupt a person's normal dental development, which could have an impact on a moth's roof and tooth alignment. Both temporary and permanent tooth structures may be harmed by forceful and prolonged thumb sucking. If kids continue to thumb-suck well into their fifth year of life, your dentist might offer advice and assistance in helping them kick the habit.
- **Tongue Thrusting:** Certain children have developed the habit of swallowing food by sticking their tongue out while eating. Similar to sucking the thumb, sucking the tongue can also push out the front teeth by applying pressure to them. They become misaligned and have protruding teeth as a result. In addition to misaligned teeth, it could also result in speech issues.
- **Lip Sucking:** An overbite and protruding teeth result from the child's habit of sucking the lip beneath the front upper teeth. The dentist might offer suggestions for breaking the habit if the child still has it by the time they are four years old.
- **Grinding:** Children of school age who grind their teeth frequently have bruxism, as the condition is known. Because the upper and lower teeth are not in alignment, grinding happens. Some kids grind their teeth in reaction to earaches or pain when their teeth are growing in. It might indicate a hyperactive youngster experiencing tension or excitement. As a child gets older, bruxism typically stops. However,

if it continues, it might erode permanent teeth, leading to worn-out enamel and painful, sensitive teeth. The child's teeth grinding can be lessened with the use of a night guard.

- **Sores in the Mouth:** Although they hurt, canker sores or ulcers on the tongue, gums, or mouth are not communicable. They make eating extremely uncomfortable and challenging. Doctors are unable to pinpoint the exact cause of canker sores, although possible causes include allergies, infections, stress or trauma, and diet. The sores might go away in two to three weeks. Right now, soft, mild foods without any spices are helpful. Avoid giving acidic foods as they could exacerbate the sores. Antimicrobial mouthwashes are beneficial.
- **Loss of Baby Teeth:** The first middle tooth in the front usually loosens and falls out around the age of six. It is a painless, natural process that takes five to seven years to complete. By the time the child reaches the age of 13. However, occasionally the tooth does not fall out. When a tooth falls out too soon or does not fall out, it is important to see a dentist. Permanent teeth are also impacted by over retained teeth. It is best to visit a dentist as soon as possible to prevent crowding and misalignment of permanent teeth.

7.13.2. Causes

Your child's oral hygiene is probably the main cause of their poor dental health. Overindulgence in sugar and carbohydrates increases the risk of dental disease in children because these foods promote the accumulation of plaque. When combined with inadequate brushing and flossing practices, cavities are likely to occur more frequently. It's critical that parents instill in their kids proper dental hygiene. Additionally, excessive consumption of candy, fruit juices, soda, cookies, and other sugary foods should be discouraged for children.

7.13.3. Prevent Common Pediatric Dental Problems

Ensuring your children are brushing and flossing correctly, attempting to limit the amount of sugar they eat (and drink, especially for infants and toddlers), and making regular appointments for dental checkups and cleanings are the best ways to safeguard their oral health and reduce their risk of oral health issues. For children in particular, routine dental exams are essential to track their growth and identify any oral health issues early on. Dental sealants and silver diamine fluoride are two preventive pediatric dentistry procedures that can help maintain the health of your children's teeth in addition to orthodontics.

When a child's first tooth erupts, their oral health journey officially begins. Because dental health problems that start in baby teeth don't go away when the teeth fall out, baby teeth should receive the same level of care as permanent teeth. In actuality, having healthy baby teeth is crucial to the optimal health of the permanent teeth as they erupt. Scheduling routine examinations and cleanings allows our pediatric dentists to regularly assess your child's development and oral health. This is the best way to safeguard and preserve your child's dental health and health.

A Closer Look

Hearing Loss

Any age can experience hearing loss. But there is particular concern for hearing impairment that is present from birth or that develops in young children. If not identified and treated at an early age, it may result in developmental difficulties because normal hearing is necessary for understanding spoken language and, eventually, for clear speech production. You should get help right away if your child has hearing loss in their early years of life. Learning spoken language or speech patterns during this period can be extremely difficult for the child, even in the case of a brief but severe hearing impairment.

- Causes of Hearing Impairment in Children

When fluid accumulates in the middle ear as a result of congestion, colds, or ear infections, most children suffer from mild hearing loss. The Eustachian tube, which connects the middle ear to the throat, drains any leftover fluid into the back of the throat, so normal hearing usually returns once the congestion or infection clears up. Approximately 10% of children experience fluid retention in the middle ear after an ear infection due to Eustachian tube abnormalities. Youngsters who have this issue have poorer hearing than typical children. This causes them to occasionally speak slowly. The permanent kind of hearing loss, which always affects normal speech and language development, is far less common. Permanent hearing loss can range in severity from slight to total.

- Types of Hearing Impairment
  - **Conductive Hearing Loss:** A structural anomaly in the middle ear or outer ear canal may be present in a child with conductive hearing impairment. Alternatively, a significant quantity of cerumen, or wax, could be stuck in the ear canal. Fluid in the middle ear that obstructs sound transmission is another potential reason.
  - **Sensorineural Hearing Loss (also Called Nerve Deafness):** An anomaly in the inner ear or in the nerves that transmit sound signals from the inner ear to the brain is the source of this kind of hearing loss. The disability may develop later in life or already exist at birth. The cause of deafness is often genetic, even in the absence of a family history. Parents and other family members are typically unaffected because each parent carries only one copy of the hearing-loss gene. Alternatively, the fetus may have become infected and lost hearing if the birth parent had toxoplasmosis, cytomegalovirus (CMV), rubella (German measles), or another infectious disease that affects the inner ear while they were pregnant. An inner ear malformation could also be the cause of the impairment.

- Diagnosis

It's critical to diagnose hearing impairment in children as soon as possible to prevent delays in language acquisition, which starts the moment they are born. That's the reason the newborn goes through a formal newborn hearing screening before being released from the hospital. But if you or your child's pediatrician suspect that your child has a hearing impairment at any point in their life, make sure that a formal evaluation of their hearing is done right away. A few family physicians, pediatricians, and well-baby clinics offer tests for middle ear fluid and hearing loss. Should a disability be identified, your child might be referred to an otolaryngologist (a specialist in the ears) or an audiologist (a specialist in hearing).

- Types of Hearing Exams for Children
- **Auditory Brainstem & Otoacoustic Emissions Tests:** One of the two tests may be administered to your child if they are younger than six months, exhibit severe developmental delays, are difficult to work with during a hearing examination, or both. These tests are comparable to those carried out during hearing screenings for newborns. They can take five minutes to an hour, and they are painless.
  - The brain's response to sound in deep sleep is measured by the auditory brainstem response (ABR) test. Soft earphones are used to play clicks or tones into the baby's ears, and electrodes are placed on the baby's head to record the brain response. When an infant is younger than three or four months old, ABRs are done while they sleep naturally. Sedation is required for older infants and toddlers to undergo an ABR.
  - The otoacoustic emissions test quantifies the sound waves that the ear produces. When clicks or tones are played into the baby's ear, a tiny probe that is inserted just inside the ear canal measures the baby's reaction. For this quick screening exam, babies and young children typically don't need to be sedated or put to sleep. Any age can participate in it.
- Behavioral Audiometry
  - It is possible to conduct behavioral audiometry, also known as conditioned response audiometry, on a cooperative infant as young as six months old. A combination of visual and auditory stimuli are used in this test. It can assess a child's or toddler's frequency-specific (but not ear-specific) hearing levels.
  - Each ear's eardrum function and hearing levels can be ascertained through formal behavioral audiometry. Soft earphones that project words and sounds into the ear are used for this. Children between the ages of three and five usually tolerate it well.

If these tests reveal that your child might have hearing loss, the diagnosis should be confirmed as soon as possible with a more in-depth hearing assessment. General hearing loss can be impacted by even mild hearing loss, so it is important to get a proper diagnosis and treatment.

- Treatment for Hearing Impairment in Kids

The cause of a hearing impairment will determine how to treat it. The doctor might just advise having your child retested in a few months to determine whether the middle ear fluid has cleared up on its own if the condition is just mild conductive hearing caused by it. Antihistamines, decongestants, and antibiotics are examples of medications that don't work well for clearing middle ear fluid.

- **Ventilating Tubes:** Referral to an ENT specialist may be recommended by the doctor if, after three months, there is still fluid behind the eardrum and no improvement in hearing. The specialist might advise draining the fluid through ventilating tubes if it continues and causes a significant, albeit transient, conductive hearing impairment. These are put in via the eardrum during surgery. This is a quick, minor procedure that takes about 15 minutes, but in order to do it correctly, your child needs to be given a general anesthetic. Infections may recur even with the tubes in place. However, the tubes lessen your child's risk of recurring infections and help reduce the amount of fluid. They will also enhance hearing if the fluid was the only factor contributing to the hearing loss.
- **Hearing Aids:** A hearing aid may help return hearing to normal or nearly normal levels in cases where conductive hearing loss is caused by an abnormality of the outer or middle ear. A hearing aid, however, can only function while it is worn. It is important to always make sure it is turned on and working, especially if the child is very young. When the kid is older, reconstructive surgery might be taken into consideration. Infants with hearing loss should have their hearing aids fitted as soon as possible to help them become aware of language and sound. Early language development benefits greatly from exposure to spoken or visual (sign) language. With the help of hearing aids, most children with mild to moderate sensorineural hearing impairment can acquire normal speech and spoken language.
- **Cochlear Implants:** Your child may be a candidate for cochlear implants if they have profound or severe hearing loss in both ears and receive little to no benefit from hearing aids. For a child whose hearing loss was acquired at birth, getting implants early—ideally by one year of age—rather than later—after the child is older—will increase their chances of developing useful speech and hearing. With early cochlear implant surgery and intensive postoperative therapy, the majority of typically developing children can achieve good to excellent hearing and be supported in a mainstream educational environment. Furthermore, nearly every child who receives a cochlear implant becomes more aware of the sounds around them.
- Learning to Communicate with Hearing Loss

When it comes to their child's ability to learn to speak, parents of children with sensorineural hearing loss typically worry the most. The reason is that while well-timed cochlear implantation increases the likelihood that a person will learn to speak, not everyone will benefit from it. All kids with hearing loss can learn how to communicate, though. While some kids pick up lipreading quickly, others never quite get the hang of it.

- Beyond Spoken Language: Learning to Sign: Remember that speaking is just one way to communicate. Sign language is an additional form of communication that can be learned for kids who didn't get enough improvement from cochlear implants or hearing aids to develop spoken language, or for families who have decided not to pursue it. You and the members of your immediate family need to pick up sign language if your child is learning it. You will be able to instruct, encourage, console, and laugh with them in this way. Urge your loved ones to pick up signing as well. Additionally, written language is essential for success in school and in the future in the workforce.

Summary

- Health issues in children are no different to those of adults. They can suffer from similar diseases, but the severity may differ in some ways. So, for care-giver, it is important to know what to observe more closely as children of different ages will have differing issues.
- While it is normal for children to have indigestion or stomach ache once in a while, if this becomes a recurrent thing and happens often, you should consult a doctor.
- The brain is one of the most important and delicate organs in the human body. Neurological problems are those issues caused by a dysfunction of the brain or nervous system and result in psychological or physical symptoms depending on the area of the brain involved, leading to disorders.
- Pediatric rheumatic diseases refer to a range of musculoskeletal, arthritic, and connective tissue disorders that can develop in childhood. These diseases can affect a child's eyes, joints, skin, muscles and gastrointestinal tract.
- About one in every 100 children has a heart problem, which may also be called a heart defect or congenital (present from birth) heart disease. Heart defects can usually be treated with medicine, surgery or other medical procedures. Most tests for heart problems are simple, quick and not painful. Most children with heart defects live a normal and full life with very few or no restrictions.
- In the world of medical fields, pediatric hematology stands out as a source of hope for kids with tricky blood problems. These brave children, dealing with different blood issues, get comfort and wise help from pediatric blood experts.
- If your child has cancer, they'll likely get treated by a doctor who specializes in pediatric oncology. It's the study and treatment of childhood cancer. There are three groups of childhood cancers: leukemias and lymphomas, brain tumors and solid tumors.
- Hormones are chemical messengers in the body that travel through the bloodstream to specific receptors on cells throughout the body where they elicit a response. Hormones play a key role in many physiologic processes, including metabolism, blood pressure regulation, blood glucose regulation, growth and development, reproduction, the sleep-wake cycle, and mood.
- Genetic disorders arise from abnormalities in an individual's genetic material, which can be inherited from parents or occur spontaneously due to genetic mutations. These anomalies can interfere with the structure, operation, or regulation of genes, which can result in a number of diseases.
- The urinary tract is composed of the kidneys, the ureters, the urinary bladder, and the urethra. Any disease of these structures is usually signaled by symptoms such as dysuria, that is, pain during micturition.
- Various skin conditions can affect babies, toddlers, children and adolescents throughout their lives. Skin conditions in kids may include hives, warts, acne, birthmarks and all sorts of rashes.

- Orthopedic disorders are physical issues that affect the bones, muscles, joints, tendons, and ligaments. These issues are either inherited, caused by diseases, or the result of an accident. Orthopedic problems at a young age may limit or even prohibit children from doing physical activities.
- Children can have more or less the same dental problems as adults but the dental problems during childhood have different repercussions on children's teeth than the adults, because children's teeth are softer and more delicate than that of an adult.

References

1. Abdulla, R. (2011). *Heart Diseases in Children*. Springer US. https://doi.org/10.1007/978-1-4419-7994-0.
2. Becker, P., Carney, L. N., Corkins, M. R., et al. (2015). Consensus statement of the Academy of Nutrition and Dietetics/American Society for Parenteral and Enteral Nutrition: Indicators recommended for the identification and documentation of pediatric malnutrition (undernutrition). *Nutrition in Clinical Practice, 30*(1), 147–161. https://doi.org/10.1177/0884533614557642.
3. Berni Canani, R., Pezzella, V., Amoroso, A., Cozzolino, T., Di Scala, C., & Passariello, A. (2016). Diagnosing and treating intolerance to carbohydrates in children. *Nutrients, 8*(3), 157. https://doi.org/10.3390/nu8030157.
4. Colby, K. (2017). *Corneal Diseases in Children*. Springer International Publishing. https://doi.org/10.1007/978-3-319-55298-9.
5. Goday, P. S., Huh, S. Y., Silverman, A., et al. (2019). Pediatric feeding disorder: Consensus definition and conceptual framework. *Journal of Pediatric Gastroenterology and Nutrition, 68*(1), 124–129. https://doi.org/10.1097/MPG.0000000000002188.
6. Gutierrez, K. (2005). Bone and joint infections in children. *Pediatric Clinics of North America, 52*(3), 779–794. https://doi.org/10.1016/j.pcl.2005.02.005.
7. Korterink, J. J., Diederen, K., Benninga, M. A., & Tabbers, M. M. (2015). Epidemiology of pediatric functional abdominal pain disorders: A meta-analysis. *PLoS ONE, 10*(5), e0126982. https://doi.org/10.1371/journal.pone.0126982.
8. Lee, Y. Y., Annamalai, C., & Rao, S. S. C. (2017). Post-infectious irritable bowel syndrome. *Current Gastroenterology Reports, 19*(11), 56. https://doi.org/10.1007/s11894-017-0595-4.
9. Li, B. U. K. (2018). Managing cyclic vomiting syndrome in children: Beyond the guidelines. *European Journal of Pediatrics, 177*(10), 1435–1442. https://doi.org/10.1007/s00431-018-3218-7.
10. Murray, H. B., Juarascio, A. S., Di Lorenzo, C., Drossman, D. A., & Thomas, J. J. (2019). Diagnosis and treatment of rumination syndrome: A critical review. *American Journal of Gastroenterology, 114*(4), 562–578. https://doi.org/10.14309/ajg.0000000000000060.
11. Perron, A. D., Miller, M. D., & Brady, W. J. (2002). Orthopedic pitfalls in the ED: Pediatric growth plate injuries. *American Journal of Emergency Medicine, 20*(1), 50–54. https://doi.org/10.1053/ajem.2002.30096.

12. Rosen, R., Vandenplas, Y., Singendonk, M., et al. (2018). Pediatric gastroesophageal reflux clinical practice guidelines: Joint recommendations of the North American Society for Pediatric Gastroenterology, Hepatology, and Nutrition and the European Society for Pediatric Gastroenterology, Hepatology, and Nutrition. *Journal of Pediatric Gastroenterology and Nutrition, 66*(3), 516–554. https://doi.org/10.1097/MPG.0000000000001889.

13. Ruffner, M. A., & Spergel, J. M. (2017). Eosinophilic esophagitis in children. *Current Allergy & Asthma Reports, 17*(8), 54. https://doi.org/10.1007/s11882-017-0721-2.

14. Sicherer, S. H., Warren, C. M., Dant, C., Gupta, R. S., & Nadeau, K. C. (2020). Food allergy from infancy through adulthood. *Journal of Allergy and Clinical Immunology: In Practice, 8*(6), 1854–1864. https://doi.org/10.1016/j.jaip.2020.02.010.

15. Snyder, J., Butzner, J. D., DeFelice, A. R., et al. (2016). Evidence-informed expert recommendations for the management of celiac disease in children. *Pediatrics, 138*(3), e20153147. https://doi.org/10.1542/peds.2015-3147.

16. Sorensen, C. J., DeSanto, K., Borgelt, L., Phillips, K. T., & Monte, A. A. (2017). Cannabinoid hyperemesis syndrome: Diagnosis, pathophysiology, and treatment-a systematic review. *Journal of Medical Toxicology, 13*(1), 71–87. https://doi.org/10.1007/s13181-016-0595-z.

17. Sweetser, S. (2019). Abdominal wall pain: A common clinical problem. *Mayo Clinic Proceedings, 94*(2), 347–355. https://doi.org/10.1016/j.mayocp.2018.04.031.

18. Tabbers, M. M., DiLorenzo, C., Berger, M. Y., et al. (2014). Evaluation and treatment of functional constipation in infants and children: Evidence-based recommendations from ESPGHAN and NASPGHAN. *Journal of Pediatric Gastroenterology and Nutrition, 58*(2), 258–274. https://doi.org/10.1097/MPG.0000000000000266.

19. Walker, G. J., Chanchlani, N., Thomas, A., et al. (2020). Primary care fecal calprotectin testing in children with suspected inflammatory bowel disease: A diagnostic accuracy study. *Archives of Disease in Childhood, 105*(10), 957–963. https://doi.org/10.1136/archdischild-2019-317823.

Chapter

PEDIATRIC SURGICAL CONDITIONS

8

Contents

INTRODUCTION

Many medical conditions require surgery, even though the majority of childhood illnesses are typically treated with non-invasive techniques like medication. The medical staff will assess the child's medical history and conduct a physical examination prior to deciding whether to perform surgery. To ascertain whether there are any complications or the severity of the condition, certain imaging studies and laboratory testing might be required. Electrocardiograms (ECGs), blood tests, and x-rays are a few examples of these. If at all possible, the focus should be on non-surgical care. On the other hand, there are circumstances in which surgery is the patient's best option.

Orientation and Directional Terms

Term	Definition	Illustration
Hernia	Inguinal hernias (IH) are one of the most common pediatric surgical problems. Inguinal hernias occur when a piece of intestine or another organ in the abdomen slips through a hole in the abdominal wall. These hernias are most common in preterm male children, but can occur in term infants and females. IH are usually noticed when children cry, cough, or strain and are recognized as a soft bulge underneath the skin in the groin or around the labia. The swelling usually disappears by itself, but occasionally hernias can get incarcerated or 'stuck.'	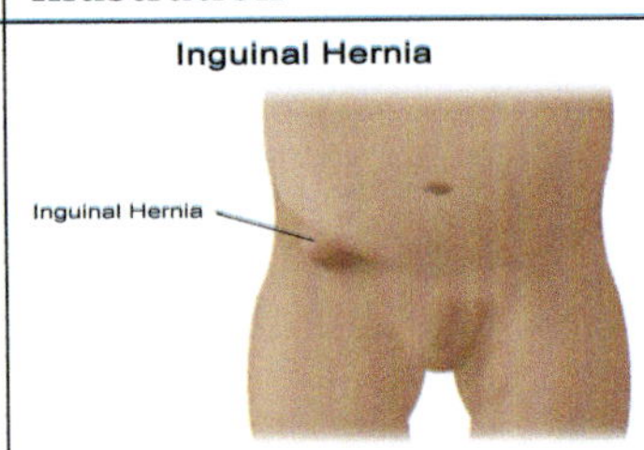
Appendicitis	Acute appendicitis is one of the most common causes of abdominal pain in childhood. This diagnosis must be considered in all age groups but is more common between the ages of 4 and 15 years. The function of the appendix is unknown. However, in rabbits and other animals the cecum is similar in shape to the appendix and plays a role in digestion of food. The middle, inside portion of the appendix may be irregular and somewhat narrow because of the presence of lymph nodes in the wall of the appendix.	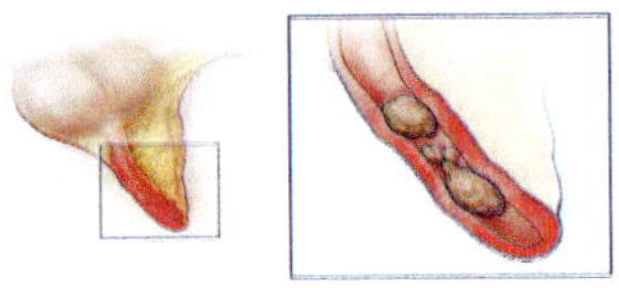
Cholelithiasis	Gallstones are relatively uncommon in blacks (except in sickle cell disease), exceptionally common in groups of Native Americans and Hispanics, and a frequent occurrence in whites. Gallstones currently are being recognized in children with increased frequency. Whether this increase in diagnosis is related to an increase in frequency of the disease or an increase in recognition because of the widespread use of ultrasound for abdominal complaints is unclear. The incidence currently is reported to be 0.15% to 0.22% in children. In comparison, gallstones are found in approximately 10% of adults.	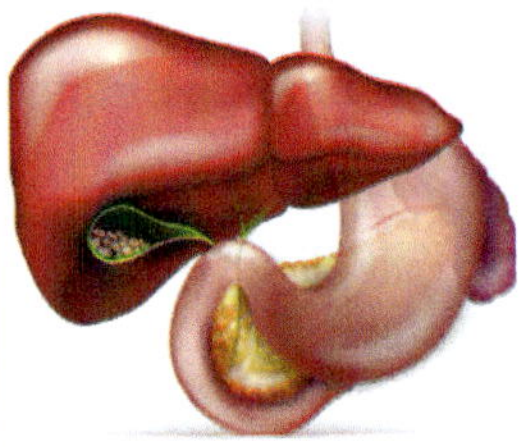
Hyperthyroidism	Grave's disease (hyperthyroidism) is generally diagnosed in adults, but can be seen in children. This can cause enlargement of the thyroid gland (goiter). Although this usually occurs in older children, it can be seen in infants of mother's with Grave's disease. Infants generally respond to medicines (iodine and propylthiouracil) and do not require surgery.	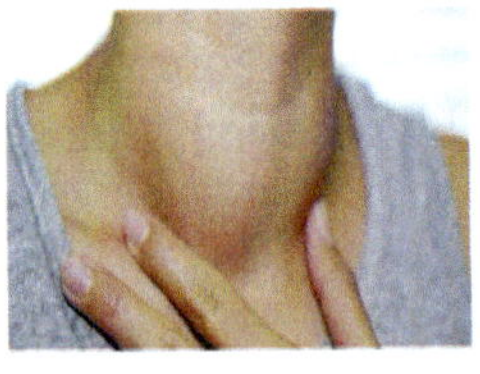

8.1. TYPES OF SURGERY

8.1.1. Major Surgery Versus Minor Surgery

- There are two categories for surgeries: major and minor. Surgeons use a variety of factors to classify procedures; however, there is no definitive definition for these terms. Among them are:
- Type of anesthesia used
- The approximate volume of blood lost.
- The quantity of medical experts required to perform their duties.
- Amount of time required for operation.
- Required specific training to function.
- Requirement for specific gear.
- The existence of additional medical issues that will complicate the procedure.
- Risk of death, or estimated mortality rate.

The head, neck, abdomen, and chest are frequently operated on during major surgery. These are not exclusive to these regions; they also correspond to the thyroid, heart, lung, liver, stomach, and intestines. This category may also include some forms of traumatic injuries. Major surgeries almost certainly need longer operating hours, a great deal of specialized training or equipment, and general anesthesia. To avoid surgical complications, patients may also require closer monitoring and a longer hospital stay. Smaller pathologies or more readily accessible body parts, particularly the skin, are typically the focus of minor surgeries. The majority of biopsies fit into this group. Preferably, local anesthesia is used. Compared to patients undergoing major surgery, patients recover more quickly.

8.1.2. Open Surgery Versus Laparoscopic Surgery

The traditional technique of open surgery involves making an incision through the skin and muscles of the abdomen. Based on the type of procedure, this can be a few centimeters wide or longer. Surgeons perform the procedure and leave the incision open using standard surgical instruments. Conversely, two to four tiny, centimeter-long incisions are made during laparoscopic surgery. Through one of these incisions, a surgical tool called a laparoscope—which holds a tiny camera—is inserted so the surgical team can see the surgical area. The remaining tiny incisions are then used to insert specialized laparoscopic instruments to finish the treatment (Newsome, McKenny and Elkbuli, 2021).

8.2. PREPARATIONS BEFORE SURGERY

Unless the surgery is an emergency or needs to be done quickly, all patients who require surgery should make the necessary preparations beforehand. The patient's clinical condition and circumstances will determine the necessary preparations, some of which may not be strictly necessary. The healthcare team will make this decision. Prematurity, congenital defects, clotting or bleeding disorders, respiratory disorders, heart or lung issues, neurological or behavioral disorders, kidney or liver disease, and organ transplantation are just a few medical conditions that may have an impact on the process. These are also taken into account when choosing the anesthetic to use. In addition, for the patient's safety, any prior use of specific drugs, such as sedatives and opioids, should be taken into account. In the event that a blood transfusion is required due to excessive blood loss, the patient may undergo testing for hemoglobin level and blood type, depending on the nature of the procedure or prevailing medical conditions.

The surgical team usually explains the procedure to the patient's family or companions first, with the exception of surgical emergencies. Families may also discuss their personal or religious preferences or beliefs at this time. Any changes to the process ought to be talked about as well. Patients may be advised not to eat or drink for a few hours prior to major surgeries. This is to avoid any issues following the administration of anesthesia. Imaging and laboratory work that are necessary for the procedure should be completed. Antibiotics and intravenous (IV) fluids are typically given prior to surgery. If you take any maintenance drugs, you should take them exactly as directed. Anesthesia, either general or local, is administered prior to the procedure. Preoperative sedation may be administered prior to surgery to help younger children feel less stressed and anxious. Surgical patients have monitoring devices attached to them that measure their blood pressure, heart rate, respiration rate, temperature, heart trace, and oxygen saturation (Henry, 2011; Daley, 2021; Ahmed and Rufo, 2022).

8.3. COMMON SURGICAL CONDITIONS IN CHILDREN

8.3.1. Appendicitis and Appendectomy

The appendix is a tiny pouch with lymphoid tissue that is joined to the large intestine. The lumen of the appendix can become blocked by foreign objects, tumors, enlargement of the lymphoid tissue, or even parasites that build up inside the organ. This can cause acute appendicitis, an inflammation of the appendix. The most common surgical condition in children, particularly in those aged 10 to 18, is acute appendicitis. Every year, 19–28 out of every 100,000 children are thought to get acute appendicitis. In the majority of cases, surgery is used to remove the entire appendix in order to treat acute appendicitis. Surgeons may select laparoscopic or open surgery based on a number of variables. A standard appendectomy is typically performed on the same day as the diagnosis and is rarely an emergency procedure. The choice to operate may be impacted by a number of circumstances or factors.

8.3.2. Cholelithiasis and Cholecystectomy

Bile from the liver is received by and stored in the gallbladder, an organ shaped like a pear. The liver secretes bile, a greenish fluid, to aid the intestines in using fats. Bile, which is released by the gallbladder, aids in the breakdown of fats in food. These fats shrink, which facilitates their absorption through the intestinal wall. Gallstones may occasionally coexist with acute cholecystitis, which is an inflammation of the gallbladder. Bile that resembles sludge, big gallstones, or inflammation in the gallbladder wall can all obstruct the ducts that carry bile out of the body. Only 4% of cholecystectomies are performed on pediatric patients, making pediatric cholecystitis less common than appendicitis. The preferred surgical procedure for the treatment of cholecystitis is laparoscopic cholecystectomy. Any gallstones in the ducts are removed along with the gallbladder (Shue, 2020).

8.3.3. Thyroid Disorders and Thyroidectomy

Located at the base of the neck, the thyroid is a tiny endocrine gland shaped like a butterfly. It generates thyroid hormone, which plays a role in controlling the body's growth, metabolism, and levels of calcium and protein synthesis. Thyroid removal surgery may be necessary for patients with Graves' disease, a form of hyperthyroidism, or a thyroid mass. Given that the thyroid is situated in the neck, extensive open surgery is required. The diagnosis, medical history, and other factors are taken into account when determining whether or not to remove the thyroid, just like in the case of appendicitis.

8.3.4. Umbilical Hernia and Herniorrhaphy

The placenta and the blood vessels in the umbilical cord carry nutrients and oxygen from the mother to the fetus during pregnancy. The umbilical cord is severed at birth. The portion of the umbilical blood vessels that is still connected to the infant then degenerates and turns into fibrous tissue. A weak abdominal wall can result when this fibrous tissue fails to fully cover or close the space where the umbilical cord once passed through. Consequently, a hernia may develop when certain intestinal segments protrude into this region. This is typical in babies; between 10–30% of kids will get an umbilical hernia. Babies who are born prematurely or with low birth weight are more likely to experience umbilical hernias. Not all hernias of the umbilical cord need surgery. The majority of direct cases are handled with routine monitoring following an assessment by a licensed healthcare professional. Herniorrhaphy, or the repair of an umbilical hernia, is necessary if complications such as incarceration or rupture occur.

8.3.5. Circumcision

Regardless of age, parents may choose to have their boys circumcised. This entails removing the prepuce, or portion of the foreskin that exposes the tip of the penis. The chance of getting infections of the penis or foreskin as well as urinary tract infections is reduced by circumcision.

8.3.6. Trauma Surgery

The most frequent avoidable cause of trauma in children is accidents. An estimated 73% of pediatric injuries are the result of traffic accidents. One of the most frequent causes is falling from a height. Organs that are commonly impacted are the kidneys, spleen, and liver. Abdominal wall hernias, bladder perforations, fractures, neurological issues, and shock can result from severe injuries. Surgical intervention is required in cases of trauma that are moderate to severe. An open surgery is typically carried out because the medical team needs to look into every area of the body that could have been hurt (Hegde et al, 2020).

8.4. MANAGEMENT AFTER SURGERY

Following surgery, patients frequently experience a number of symptoms. These include sore throats from anesthesia, nausea, and post-operative pain. It is possible to treat these symptoms with medication. Depending on the type of surgery, the patient's diet may need to be adjusted by the medical staff during the initial few days. Any wounds from the surgery will be handled and cleaned appropriately. After surgery, the length of confinement is determined by the patient's recovery rate and the type of procedure they underwent. There is no predetermined number of days for this. Follow-up consultations may be recommended following hospital discharge, particularly for patients who have staples or stitches. Monitoring may be done on a regular basis to keep an eye out for potential side effects like bleeding or infection. Additionally, suggestions regarding the kinds of activities the patient can partake in will be given by the medical staff. Until the patient is fully recovered, intense activities are usually avoided. The healthcare team's evaluation may determine whether an individual can attend work or school.

Certain medical conditions in children may necessitate surgical intervention, such as appendicitis, cholecystitis, and physical trauma. Prior to proceeding with surgery, the medical team will assess the patient's medical history, conduct a physical examination, and review relevant lab results. The type and complexity of the surgery will depend on the patient's specific condition, and may be performed using either open or laparoscopic techniques. Proper pre-surgical preparations and post-operative care are essential to the overall success of the procedure (Henry, 2011; Daley, 2021; Ahmed and Rufo, 2022).

A Closer Look

Intussusception

For children under three years old, intussusception is the most common cause of intestinal obstruction. Most pediatric intussusception cases have an enigmatic etiology. Even though adult intussusception is uncommon, when it does occur, it usually stems from an underlying medical condition, like a tumor. With a quick procedure, the intestines can typically be moved back into place in children. In adults, the issue is frequently corrected with surgery.

- Symptoms

When a baby is otherwise healthy, sudden, loud crying due to abdominal pain may be the first indication of intussusception. When an infant cries, they may pull their knees to their chests due to abdominal pain. Initially, intussusception pain usually flares up every 15 to 20 minutes. With time, these excruciating episodes become more frequent and last longer.

Additional signs of intussusception consist of:

- Stool mixed with mucus and blood; because of this, it is sometimes called "currant jelly stool."
- Vomiting.
- A lump in the belly.
- Weakness or lack of energy.
- Diarrhea.

Not every person experiences every symptom. Some babies don't seem to be in any pain. Certain children have a lump in their stomach or don't pass blood. Certain older kids experience pain alone, without any other symptoms.

- Causes

The shape of your intestine is like a long tube. One section of your intestine—typically the small intestine—slips inside an adjacent section when you have an intussusception. Because it resembles the way a collapsible telescope slides together, this is sometimes referred to as telescoping.

Adult telescoping can occasionally be brought on by an intestinal growth known as a lead point, which can be a polyp or tumor. This lead point is grabbed by the intestine's characteristic wave-like contractions, which then pull it and the intestinal lining into the bowel ahead of it. But in most cases, intussusception has no known cause.

The cause of intussusception in children is usually not known. It appears that intussusception happens more frequently in the winter and fall. Additionally, since many of the affected children also exhibit flu-like symptoms, some speculate that a virus may be responsible for the illness.

Occasionally, a lead point can be found to be the source of the illness; the lead point is usually a pouch in the small intestine's lining (Meckel's diverticulum).

- Risk Factors

The following are risk factors for intussusception.

- **Age:** Compared to adults, children, particularly young children, have a significantly higher risk of developing intussusception. It is the most frequent reason for intestinal blockage in kids between the ages of three and six months.
- **Sex:** Boys experience intussusception more frequently.
- **Abnormal Intestinal Development from Birth:** An incorrect development or rotation of the intestine is known as intestinal malrotation. The chance of intussusception rises as a result.
- **Certain Conditions:** Several conditions may raise the chance of intussusception, such as:
  - Cystic fibrosis.
  - Another name for Henoch-Schonlein purpura is IgA vasculitis.
  - Crohn's disease.
  - Celiac disease.
- Complications

The blood supply to the intestine's affected section may be severed due to intussusception. Intestinal wall tissue dies from blood loss if treatment is not received. A rip in the intestinal wall known as a perforation can result from tissue death. Peritonitis, an infection of the lining of the abdominal cavity, may result from this.

A potentially fatal illness, peritonitis necessitates emergency medical care. Peritonitis symptoms include:

- Belly pain.
- Swelling in the belly area.
- Fever.
- Vomiting.

Your child may experience shock due to peritonitis. Shock symptoms consist of:

- Pale or gray skin that feels clammy and cool.
- A quick, weak pulse.
- Breathing that can vary greatly in speed and shallowness.
- Anxiety or agitation.
- Extreme listlessness.

A child experiencing shock could be awake or unconscious. Make sure your child gets emergency medical attention as soon as you suspect they are in shock.

- Diagnosis

The doctor treating you or your child will first ask to see a history of the problem's symptoms. The caregiver might feel a lump in the abdomen that resembles a sausage. Your provider might place the following order to verify the diagnosis:

- **Ultrasound or Other Abdominal Imaging:** A CT (computerized tomography) scan, X-ray, or ultrasound may show intestinal blockage brought on by intussusception. Imaging usually depicts the intestine coiled within the intestine as a bull's-eye. Additionally, abdominal imaging may reveal a torn or perforated intestine.
- Treatment

Intussusception is usually treated as a medical emergency. Emergency medical attention is necessary to prevent infection that can happen when a section of the intestine dies from a lack of blood, as well as severe dehydration and shock.

There are several possible treatments for intussusception.

- **An Air Enema or Water-Soluble Contrast:** This is a treatment as well as a diagnostic process. In most cases, additional treatment is not required if an enema is effective. In fact, 90% of the time, this treatment can correct intussusception in children, negating the need for additional care. This procedure is not applicable if the intestine is torn (perforated).

Up to 20% of cases of intussusception recur, necessitating additional treatment. Consultation with a surgeon is crucial, even in cases where enema treatment is planned. This is due to the tiny chance that this therapy will cause a bowel tear or rupture.

- **Surgery**: Surgery is required if the intestine is torn, if an enema is unable to resolve the issue, or if a lead point is the source. The surgeon will remove any dead intestinal tissue in addition to freeing the trapped portion of the intestine and removing the obstruction. The primary course of treatment for adults and critically ill patients is surgery.

Sometimes intussusception is transient and resolves on its own without medical intervention (Henry, 2011; Daley, 2021; Ahmed and Rufo, 2022).

Summary

- Open surgery is a classical method that utilizes an incision through the skin and abdominal muscles. This is typically a few centimeters wide or longer, depending on the type of procedure. Surgeons use standard surgical instruments to perform the surgery and keep the incision open.
- Laparoscopic surgery creates two to four small incisions that are roughly a centimeter long each.
- All patients who need surgery should have adequate preparations first unless the procedure is an emergency or should be done urgently. The healthcare team will decide the preparations the patient needs; not all are strictly required depending on the clinical condition and circumstances of the patient.
- Depending on the type of procedure or prevalent medical conditions, the patient may be tested for their hemoglobin level and blood type in case excessive blood loss necessitates a blood transfusion.
- Acute appendicitis is the most common surgical condition in children, especially those 10–18 years of age. An estimated 19–28 in 100,000 children develop acute appendicitis yearly.
- Acute cholecystitis is inflammation of the gallbladder, sometimes accompanied by gallstones. The gallbladder ducts through which bile passes may become obstructed because of inflammation in the gallbladder wall, sludge-like bile, or large gallstones.
- The thyroid is a small, butterfly-shaped endocrine gland found at the base of the neck. It produces the thyroid hormone, which helps regulate the body's growth and metabolism, including protein synthesis and calcium levels.
- During pregnancy, an unborn child receives oxygen and nutrients from the mother through the placenta and the blood vessels in the umbilical cord. During delivery, the umbilical cord is cut. Subsequently, the part of the umbilical blood vessels still attached to the baby degenerates and becomes fibrous tissue.
- For boys, parents may opt to have them circumcised regardless of age. This involves removing parts of the foreskin, called the prepuce, which exposes the tip of the penis. Circumcision decreases the risk of developing urinary tract infections and infections of the foreskin or penis.
- Patients often experience several symptoms after surgery. These include post-operative pain, nausea, and sore throat from anesthesia. Medications may be given to ease these symptoms.

References

1. Ahmed, Z., & Rufo, P. A. (2022). Pediatric preoperative management. In *StatPearls* [Internet]. StatPearls Publishing. Available from: https://www.ncbi.nlm.nih.gov/books/NBK559198/ (accessed on 11 September 2024).

2. Daley, B. J. (2021). Considerations in pediatric trauma. *WebMD LLC*. Retrieved from: https://emedicine.medscape.com/article/435031-overview (accessed on 11 September 2024).

3. Diesen, D., & Alaish, S. M. (2021). Thyroid surgery in children. *American Academy of Pediatrics Section on Surgery, American Pediatric Surgical Association, American College of Surgeons*. Retrieved from: https://www.healthychildren.org/English/health-issues/conditions/surgery/Pages/Thyroid-Surgery-in-Children.aspx (accessed on 11 September 2024).

4. Hegde, S., Bawa, M., Kanojia, R. P., Mahajan, J. K., Menon, P., Samujh, R., & Rao, K. (2020). Pediatric trauma: Management and lessons learned. *Journal of Indian Association of Pediatric Surgeons, 25*(3), 142–146. https://doi.org/10.4103/jiaps.JIAPS_35_19.

5. Henry, D. B. (2011). Chapter 112. Perioperative care. In C. D. Rudolph, A. M. Rudolph, G. E. Lister, L. R. First, & A. A. Gershon (Eds.), *Rudolph's Pediatrics* (22nd ed.). McGraw Hill. Available from: https://accesspediatrics.mhmedical.com/content.aspx?bookid=455&sectionid=40310373 (accessed on 11 September 2024).

6. Hollinger, L., & Lee, S. (2021). Appendectomy in children and teens. *American Academy of Pediatrics*. Retrieved from: https://www.healthychildren.org/English/health-issues/conditions/surgery/Pages/Appendectomy-in-Children-and-Teens.aspx (accessed on 11 September 2024).

7. Kliegman, R. M., et al. (2020). Part XVII Digestive system. In *Nelson Textbook of Pediatrics* (21st ed.). Elsevier.

8. Newsome, K., McKenny, M., & Elkbuli, A. (2021). Major and minor surgery: Terms used for hundreds of years that have yet to be defined. *Annals of Medicine and Surgery (2012), 66*, 102409. https://doi.org/10.1016/j.amsu.2021.102409.

9. Poddighe, D., & Sazonov, V. (2018). Acute acalculous cholecystitis in children. *World Journal of Gastroenterology, 24*(43), 4870–4879. https://doi.org/10.3748/wjg.v24.i43.4870.

10. Schwarz, S. M. (2022). Pediatric cholecystitis. *WebMD LLC*. Retrieved from: https://emedicine.medscape.com/article/927340-overview (accessed on 11 September 2024).

11. Shue, E. (2020). Gallbladder removal surgery (cholecystectomy). *American Academy of Pediatrics Section on Surgery, American Pediatric Surgical Association, American College of Surgeons*. Retrieved from: https://www.healthychildren.org/English/health-issues/conditions/surgery/Pages/Gallbladder-Removal-Surgery-(Cholecystectomy).aspx (accessed on 11 September 2024).

12. Troullioud Lucas, A. G., Jaafar, S., & Mendez, M. D. (2022). Pediatric umbilical hernia. In *StatPearls* [Internet]. StatPearls Publishing. Available from: https://www.ncbi.nlm.nih.gov/books/NBK459294/ (accessed on 11 September 2024).

Chapter 9

PEDIATRIC EMERGENCIES

Contents

INTRODUCTION

Children's physiology, anatomy, and developmental stages differ from those of adults, so emergency medical care must be given with special consideration. When treating children in an emergency, there are particular difficulties and factors to take into account. Children's bodies, for instance, are still changing and growing, which affects how they respond to medical treatment, how much medication they take, and other factors. Accurately assessing symptoms in children can be difficult due to their limited communication skills. Healthcare professionals must work closely with parents or legal guardians to obtain informed consent, which can be challenging in some cases, particularly when the child is too young or in distress. Furthermore, since children will likely be feeling scared and confused during emergencies, attending to their emotional needs is essential to ensuring that treatment is successful and reducing psychological trauma.

Pediatric Emergency Medical Technicians (EMTs) are prepared to manage the particular difficulties related to pediatric patients and guarantee that the right care is provided because of these special considerations. One of their specialties is evaluating a child's condition to determine how serious it is and what level of care is needed. Because they are trained to communicate in an age-appropriate manner, pediatric emergency medical technicians can help reduce fear and anxiety. Pediatric EMTs are also capable of handling agitated or uncooperative patients because they are attuned to the emotional needs of children. Better patient outcomes are a result of their capacity to establish rapport and foster trust.

Orientation and Directional Terms

Term	Definition	Illustration
Croup	Croup presents with a barking cough, hoarseness of voice, inspiratory stridor and respiratory distress if severe.	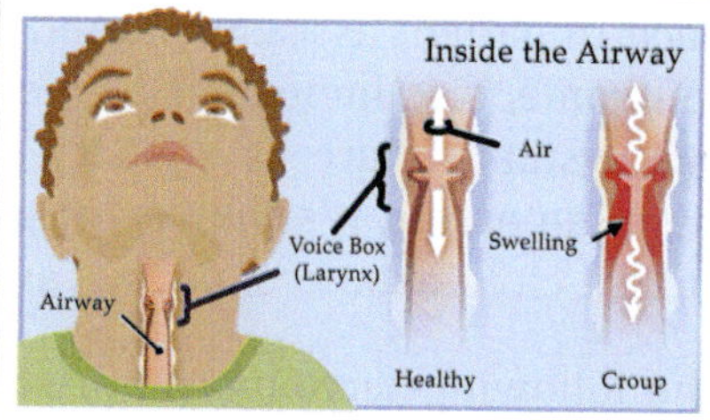
Febrile Seizures	A seizure associated with fever in a child age 6 months – 5 years without evidence of other cause (no evidence of trauma, CNS infection or metabolic cause, and no history of epilepsy).	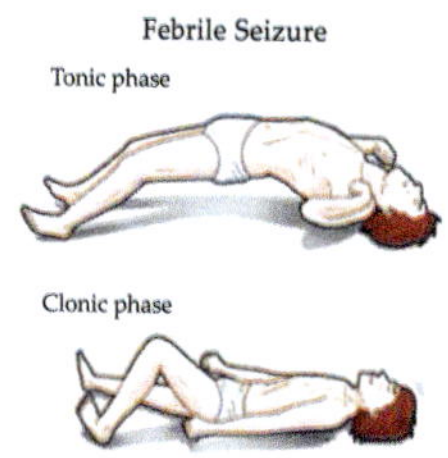
Shock	It is a clinical condition in which tissue perfusion is inadequate to meet metabolic demands. In any form of shock, cardiac output and organ perfusion are inadequate in relative to metabolic needs. It is classified as compensated, uncompensated and irreversible shock.	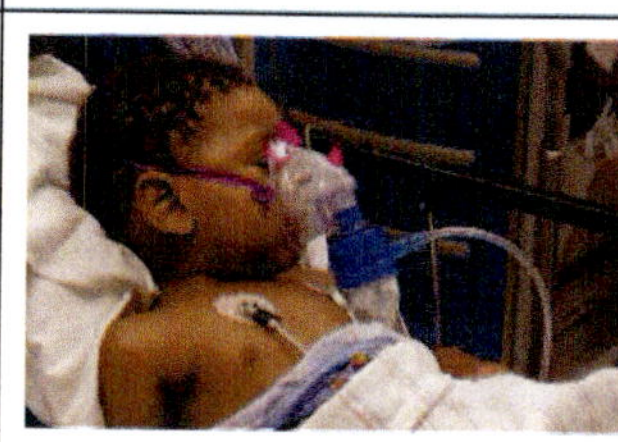
Hypothermia	If the axillary temperature is < 35°C (<95°F) or does not register on a normal thermometer, assume hypothermia. Where a low-reading thermometer is available, take the rectal temperature (<35.5°C or <95.5°F) to confirm the hypothermia.	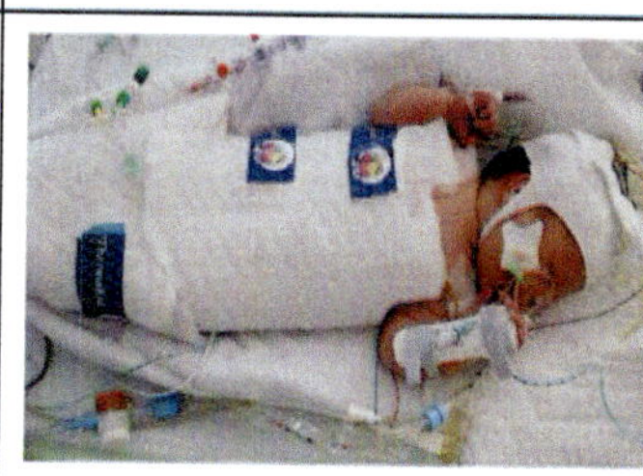

9.1. GENERAL APPROACH TO PEDIATRIC EMERGENCIES

Even the most seasoned clinicians find the case of the critically ill child to be daunting. However, the clinician can identify and treat life-threatening issues methodically by using a calm and structured approach to patient assessment and management. Since cardiac arrest in children generally has a poor outcome, it is important to identify any signs of possible respiratory, circulatory, or central nervous system failure as soon as possible to help stop the situation from getting worse and leading to an arrest. It's important to remember that you are rarely alone in a healthcare setting, so in these circumstances, always ask for assistance as soon as possible.

The following sections comprise the structured approach to the seriously ill child:

- Assessment and resuscitation of the ABCDE primary.
- secondary evaluation and immediate medical attention.
- Stabilization and transfer

9.1.1. Primary ABCDE Assessment and Resuscitation

It should take less than a minute to perform a child's initial fast assessment. Finding life-threatening issues is the goal in order to direct resuscitation. It ought to take under a minute. The elements of the assessment are listed in the Table 9.1.

Table 9.1. Demographic Characteristics and Triage Code Severity of the Pediatric Emergency Department Visits in March–April 2019 (Non-COVID-19 Period) Compared with the Same Period in 2020 (COVID-19 Period)

	2019	2020	*p*-Value
Number of visits, n	3159	1039	
Visits per day, n (SD)	51.62 (10.4)	17.03 (6.8)	<0.001
Sex (n, %)			
Female	1418 (44.9)	437 (42.1)	0.11
Male	1741 (55.1)	602 (57.9)	0.11
Age group (n, %)			
<28 d	78 (2.5)	59 (5.7)	<0.001
28 d–1 y	544 (17.2)	203 (19.5)	0.09
1–3 y	583 (18.5)	241 (23.2)	0.001
3–6 y	860 (27.2)	194 (18.7)	<0.001
6–10 y	436 (13.8)	162 (15.6)	0.15
10–14 y	402 (12.7)	136 (13.1)	0.76
≥14 y	256 (8.1)	44 (4.2)	<0.001
Priority tags at triage			
White (n, %)	1447 (45.8)	364 (35.0)	<0.001

Green (n, %)	1450 (45.9)	574 (55.3)	<0.001
Yellow (n, %)	261 (8.27)	100 (9.6)	0.17
Red (n, %)	1 (0.03)	1 (0.1)	0.41

d = days; y = years.

Source: Silvagni D, Baggio L, Lo Tartaro Meragliotta P, Soloni P, La Fauci G, Bovo C, Ielo S, Biban P. Neonatal and pediatric emergency room visits in a tertiary center during the COVID-19 pandemic in Italy. Pediatric Reports. 2021; 13(2):168–176. https://doi.org/10.3390/pediatric13020023.

9.1.1.1. Airway Assessment

Feel, hear, and look for patency in the airways. When a child or infant is unconscious, use the head tilt chin lift maneuver to open their airway (Figure 9.1). Due to the variations in children's airway anatomy as they grow, the ideal tilt angles for infants and children are neutral and "sniffing" positions, respectively. A jaw thrust may be utilized if this maneuver is not successful in maintaining airway patency.

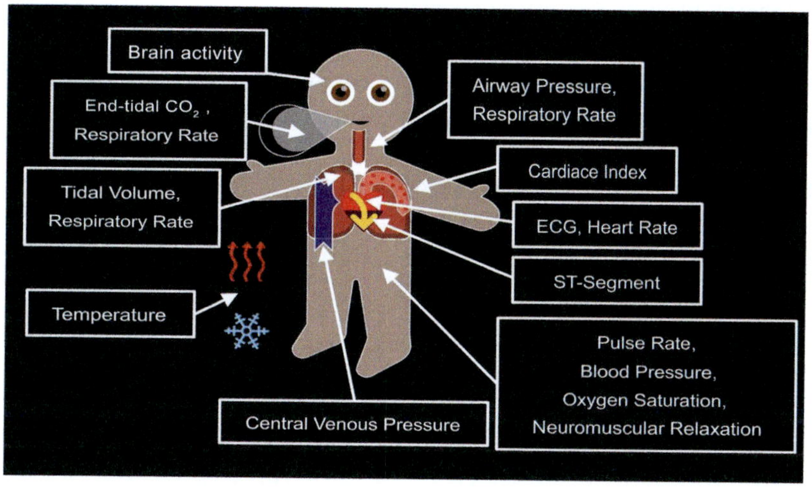

Figure 9.1. *Vital signs.*

Source Lunkiewicz J, Fries D, Milovanovic P, Noethiger CB, Tscholl DW, Gasciauskaite G. Pediatric anesthesia providers' perspective on the real-life implementation of the Philips visual patient avatar: A qualitative study. Children. 2023; 10(12):1841. https://doi.org/10.3390/children10121841.

- **Resuscitation:** Adjuncts like Guedel airways and nasopharyngeal airways may also be useful in an in-hospital setting. Stridor or a hoarse voice in a conscious child can be an indication of a compromised airway, so immediate senior help needs to be sought. Anesthetic assistance must be sought immediately if there is any suspicion that a child's airway is becoming compromised while they are in the hospital.

9.1.1.2. Breathing Assessment

You should evaluate the effect, efficacy, and effort of breathing during this examination.

- **Effort:** 'How much effort does breathing require?'

An elevated respiratory rate can result from a metabolic acidosis (diabetic ketoacidosis, for example) or from lung or airway pathology. Naturally, recognizing a raised respiratory rate necessitates understanding the normal values, which are listed below and on the pediatric early warning score charts (Table 9.2):

Table 9.2. Reasons for Delayed Diagnosis of Pediatric Appendicitis During the COVID-19 Pandemic

1	Public health and social measures
2	Fear of exposure by parents/caregivers/patients/medical staff
3	Telemedicine use
4	COVID-19-positive children with suspected appendicitis
5	Recurrent appendicitis after non-operative management
6	Delayed primary operative management

Source: *Pantalos G, Papachristidou S, Mavrigiannaki E, Zavras N, Vaos G. Reasons for delayed diagnosis of pediatric acute appendicitis during the COVID-19 era: A narrative review.* Diagnostics. *2023; 13(15):2571. https://doi.org/10.3390/diagnostics13152571.*

Grunting, nostril flaring, tracheal tugging, and the use of accessory muscles (intercostal, subcostal, or at the most severe sternal recession) are additional indicators of respiratory distress. A late symptom of severe hypoxia is gasping. Some children will not exhibit any signs of increased respiratory effort in spite of hypoxia. These children are:

- Those who have been fatigued and experiencing serious respiratory issues for a while. One of the pre-terminal symptoms of life-threatening asthma is exhaustion.
- Muscular dystrophy is an example of a neuromuscular disease.
- Respiratory depression caused by elevated intracranial pressure, poisoning, or encephalopathy.
    - **Efficacy:** 'What are they accomplishing in terms of gas exchange and air movement?'

In this case, monitoring oxygen saturation levels along with auscultation for air entry and chest expansion are crucial. The wheeze and decreased air entry of acute asthma can be recognized, as can the asymmetrical air entry and bronchial breath sounds of pneumonia. Take note that a silent chest is a very concerning indication.

- **Effect:** 'What impact does inadequate breathing have on the body as a whole.'

Initially, hypoxia will cause tachycardia; however, if it persists or gets worse, bradycardia, a pre-terminal symptom, will result. Similarly, cyanosis is another late and pre-terminal sign that is evident at saturations lower than 70%. Agitation or sleepiness caused by hypoxia or hypercapnia can manifest as a child refusing to cooperate during an examination and appearing extremely distressed, or it can appear as an unusually quiet and withdrawn child.

- **Resuscitation:** All kids who have hypoxia or respiratory problems should get high flow oxygen (15 liters per minute) via an oxygen mask that has a reservoir bag. If there is insufficient respiratory effort as well, wear a bag-valve mask and, if necessary, consider ventilation and intubation. It is frequently sufficient to encourage coughing in a conscious patient who is choking and appears to be coughing successfully. If coughing is no longer working, try pushing the foreign body out with five back blows and five chest thrusts (or abdominal thrusts in the case of a child). The life support algorithm is applied if they pass out.

9.1.1.3. Circulation Assessment

Take note of the patient's blood pressure, heart rate, capillary refill time, and pulse volume. Since children's bodies are adept at compensating for changes in physiology, hypotension is a late symptom. Examine the impact on other organs of any circulatory insufficiency. These could include decreased urine production, mottled skin with pale, cool peripheries (from inadequate skin perfusion), elevated respiratory rate (from the ensuing metabolic acidosis), or changed mental state.

- **Resuscitation:** Establish venous or intraosseous access quickly and administer a 20 ml/kg bolus of 0.9% sodium chloride if there are indications of circulatory compromise. If more than two boluses are required, further boluses should be determined by reevaluation and inotropic support should be taken into account. Note that because cerebral edema poses a risk in DKA, the initial bolus is 10 ml/kg. In critically ill children, venous access is frequently challenging. Repeated attempts at cannulation should not be used as a justification for delaying fluid bolus administration; instead, intraosseous access is quick, efficient, and should be explored as soon as possible.

9.1.1.4. Disability (Neurological) Assessment

The AVPU score (A is alert, V responds to voice, P responds to pain, and U is unresponsive) or GCS can be used to determine the child's level of consciousness. The AVPU scale responds only to pain and correlates with a GCS score of 8, making it quicker to use. A lot of kids with serious illnesses are clumsy. Severe brain dysfunction is suggested by stiff posturing, such as that seen in decorticate (flexed arms, extended legs) or decerebrate (extended arms and legs). It is important to document pupil size and light-responsiveness. Additionally, blood sugar testing should be done at the patient's bedside (though in practice, this may have been done when gaining access to an IV or IO). Any child who exhibits a low level of consciousness should have their intracranial pressure checked. In these situations, the presence of bradycardia and hypertension signals the impending coning.

- Resuscitation:
  - If a child's conscious level is graded as P or U, consider intubating them to stabilize their airway.
  - To prevent recurrence, treat hypoglycemia with a bolus of 2 ml/kg 10% glucose intravenously or intraocularly, followed by a glucose infusion.
  - Take into consideration mannitol and neuroprotective measures in cases where elevated intracranial pressure is suspected.

9.1.1.5. Exposure Assessment

A quick head-to-toe examination of the child may reveal information about the etiology of the illness; for instance, a purpuric rash that appears only after full exposure or surgical scars that make you think about specific histories are two examples of clues that may be helpful. Take care to recover any exposed areas so the child's dignity is maintained and the temperature is kept under control.

9.1.2. Secondary Assessment and Emergency Treatment

After addressing any immediate life-threatening issues, proceed to a more thorough assessment of the patient. This comprises:

- Reevaluating how the initial resuscitation efforts were received.
- Taking a focused history
- Carrying out in-depth system-based analyzes when necessary.
- Further investigations – Blood tests in the lab, an ECG, radiographs, and other imaging modalities like CT scans can be among them.

A more thorough discussion of a few particular conditions and their emergency care is provided below.

9.1.2.1. Airway and Breathing

The additional clinical characteristics that may be present in a child experiencing respiratory distress are listed in the Table 9.3, along with the diagnoses they may suggest.

Table 9.3. Pulmonary Pathology Features of COVID-19-Associated ARDS (COVID-ARDS) Versus Other Causes of Acute Respiratory Distress Syndrome (ARDS)

Pathology	ARDS	COVID-ARDS
Diffuse Alveolar Damage (DAD)	***Early/Exudative:*** - interstitial/alveolar edema - "hyaline" membranes - neutrophil infiltration - AEC desquamation - pulmonary microvascular thrombosis ***Late/Fibroproliferative:*** - alveolar/interstitial fibrosis - type II AEC hyperplasia	***Similar to ARDS Except:*** - paucity of neutrophils - interstitial/alveolar lymphocytic infiltration - possibly increased pulmonary microvascular thrombi relative to other causes
Other Features	- organizing pneumonia (fibrosis) - alveolar hemorrhage - viral pneumonia	- occasional viral cytopathic changes (multinucleated syncytial cells, atypical enlarged AEC) - viral inclusions in AEC

Abbreviations: AEC, alveolar epithelial cells.

Source: Kassirian S, Taneja R, Mehta S. Diagnosis and Management of Acute Respiratory Distress Syndrome in a Time of COVID-19. Diagnostics. *2020; 10(12):1053. https://doi.org/10.3390/diagnostics10121053.*

9.1.2.2. Circulation

9.1.2.2.1. Congenital Heart Disease

One of the most prevalent kinds of birth defects is this one. Some of those affected initially visit the ED within a few days of birth, even though many are now identified by antenatal scanning or during the newborn baby check. This is because the heart is still changing at this point, transitioning from the circulation of a fetus to that of a newborn. The closure of the ductus arteriosus, which connects the descending aorta and the pulmonary artery, is one of the main structural alterations. This identifies those who depend on this duct to allow blood to mix in order to sustain their pulmonary or systemic circulations. When the duct is beginning to close, the presentation of duct-dependent lesions can range greatly from the faint signs of poor feeding, drowsiness, and slightly rapid breathing to the collapsed baby in cardiogenic shock when the closure is about to occur. Since the decompensated patient with sepsis or an inborn error or metabolism can present very similarly, this can frequently be a challenging diagnosis. IV dinoprostone should be given if a duct dependent lesion is suspected. This helps to maintain the duct open, allowing common mixing to continue until a cardiologist can make a definitive diagnosis and begin treating the patient.

9.1.2.2.2. Supraventricular Tachycardia (SVT)

Supraventricular tachycardia (SVT) is frequently observed in children, with older children usually experiencing palpitations, chest pain, and dizziness. Infants, on the other hand, may show signs of heart failure if prolonged episodes of undetected SVT occur. Treatment for SVT identified on a 12 lead ECG includes attempting vagal maneuvers first, and then administering a rapid IV adenosine bolus or synchronous DC shock based on the child's clinical condition.

9.1.2.3. Disability (Neurological)

9.1.2.3.1. Seizures

One in 20 people will experience a seizure at some point in their lives. The majority of the time, they last less than five minutes, are observed by parents, and involve a stable child who presents to the emergency department. Still, there are instances when seizures are severe and continuing when a patient arrives at the ED, necessitating immediate medical attention. Status epilepticus is defined as continuing seizure activity for 20 minutes or as shorter seizures with insufficient recovery in between. The algorithm for treating status epilepticus is a fairly direct flow chart, but maintaining awareness of the length of the seizure makes it more difficult to determine when to take necessary medication and how much to dose and prepare it. Additionally, benzodiazepines may lead to respiratory depression, necessitating the need for supportive measures.

9.1.2.4. Exposure

9.1.2.4.1. Sepsis

As one of the most frequent causes of severe illness in kids, sepsis should always be taken into account when a kid is either mysteriously ill or stays sick even after receiving the best treatment possible for another ailment. Although hypothermia can happen, fever is not always present, especially in infants. A blood, urine, and CSF culture should ideally be obtained before giving antibiotics (especially in infants or patients exhibiting symptoms of an intracranial infection). Antibiotics should be administered right away, though, if sampling proves to be difficult or the patient is too clinically unstable. Regarding antibiotic selection, each hospital will have its own policy.

9.1.3. Stabilization and Transfer

To provide any sick child with ongoing care, regular reassessment is crucial. The following should be observed in all patients:

- Saturation levels of oxygen (plus CO_2 monitoring if intubated).
- Pulse rate and rhythm
- Blood pressure
- Urine output
- Core temperature

Transfers can occur to the HDU/ICU for continuous care or within the hospital for imaging. Rarely, pediatric patients need an emergency inter-hospital transfer in order to receive life-saving care that cannot wait for stabilization or retrieval and is not easily accessible on-site. An illustration would be a young patient who needs emergency neurosurgical care at the closest pediatric neurosurgical facility due to an expanding intracranial hemorrhage. The ED, anesthesia, children's intensive care, the ambulance service, and radiology must work together as a cohesive team to plan these kids' care and transfer them on time (Silverman, 2006; Tintinalli, 2011).

9.2. NEONATAL EMERGENCIES

While most babies are born healthy, some infants experience neonatal emergencies that require immediate medical attention. These emergencies can occur at birth, during the post-birth period in the hospital, or at home within the first 28 days after delivery. Newborns have a weaker immune system than adults, making them more vulnerable to illnesses caused by bacteria, viruses, and parasites. If a newborn becomes sick, they may need to be hospitalized in the neonatal intensive care unit (NICU) for treatment.

9.2.1. Signs and Symptoms of Neonatal Emergencies

Neonatal emergencies often present with breathing difficulties, poor feeding, skin rash, abnormal body temperature, persistent crying, and irritability. It is advised that you get in touch with your child's physician and seek medical attention if you notice any strange behavior, such as a change in sleeping habits. It is imperative that you keep a close eye out for any symptoms in your child, particularly if they are younger than a month.

9.2.2. Common Types of Neonatal Emergencies

These are the most typical kinds of newborn emergencies.

- **Trauma:** There are two types of trauma: non-accidental trauma and accidental trauma. The majority of unintentional trauma in infants results from motor vehicle accidents, falls, assaults, and child abuse. Seizures, diminished alertness, unconsciousness, no breathing, vomiting, and pale skin are a few mild to severe trauma symptoms. Trauma may be healed by medical interventions, but prevention is always preferable to treatment. A newborn should never be given a violent shake or be held angrily.
- **Cardiovascular Disease:** Heart diseases like heart failure, sudden collapse, and heart murmur are frequently seen in newborns. If you notice your infant having trouble feeding, sweating excessively, or experiencing fluctuations in weight, it could be a sign of a heart condition. These diseases are

generally classified as either Cyanotic or Acyantoic heart disease.

- **Poor Metabolism:** A newborn is said to have poor metabolic function if their body is unable to properly metabolize their food because of a genetic disorder. Toxic substances build up can cause this issue by interfering with the body's natural processes. Seizures, indolence, apnea, altered body temperature, vomiting, and inadequate feeding should all be suspected.
- **Seizures:** Infants frequently experience seizures in the neonatal stage. Since the majority of the time the symptoms of seizures are mild, such as abnormal tongue movements or abnormal eye movements, they are challenging to diagnose.
- **Intestinal Emergencies:** Parents should seek medical attention if their newborn throws up during the neonatal period. Never disregard a problem in a newborn, even if it seems like a minor stomach ache, as it could be a potentially fatal infection.

9.2.3. Complications of Neonatal Emergency

If a newborn's infection isn't treated properly and with immediate attention, it can have fatal consequences in extreme cases. All types of infections cause complications, neurological, cardiac, respiratory, and developmental issues because babies' bodies are delicate and developing quickly. The best course of action for treating and curing the infection is early diagnosis and monitoring.

9.2.4. Prevention

If a pregnant woman with the condition takes preventive measures, the majority of neonatal infections can be avoided. It may lessen the likelihood of transferring it to the new-born. Maternal testing is required for expectant mothers because most infections are treatable with over-the-counter medications. If expectant moms take preventative measures against the diseases in the first place, other neonatal infections can be avoided. This can be avoided by receiving vaccinations and immunizations prior to becoming pregnant against diseases like chickenpox and others. They can also maintain their health by just being hygienic and washing their hands frequently (Silverman, 2006; Tintinalli, 2011).

9.3. POISONING IN CHILDREN

In the U.S, there are more than 24.4 million poisoning incidents reported annually. Since young children frequently put things in their mouths, children under the age of six account for more than half of all poisoning cases.

9.3.1. Poison Prevention

Any substance that can make you sick when consumed, ingested, touched, or inhaled is considered a poison. There are poisons all over the house, and if ingested, even seemingly innocuous objects can turn deadly. Poisons occur on a daily basis. As a result, it's critical for parents to identify poisons, store them safely, and know what to do in the event that a child comes into contact with one. Prevention of poisoning and prompt medical attention are essential to your child's safety.

9.3.2. Common Causes of Poisoning in Children

Cosmetics and goods for personal hygiene.

- Medicine and vitamins
- Products for washing and cleaning, furniture polish, and lamp oil.
- Car fluids – gasoline, windshield wiper fluid, and antifreeze.
- Plants, fertilizer, and insect and weed killers.
- Batteries
- Alcohol
- Carbon monoxide and lead
- Arts and crafts supplies

9.3.3. Treatment

Our emergency physicians may employ various treatments to lessen symptoms and assist in restoring the body's normal functions once they have identified the type of poisoning a child is experiencing.

9.3.3.1. Gastrointestinal Decontamination

Techniques for intestinal decontamination may aid in preventing or minimizing the absorption of harmful substances into the gastrointestinal tract following consumption.

- **Orogastric Lavage:** Orogastric lavage is a procedure a doctor may use in rare cases where it seems a child has been exposed to a toxic substance that has not had time to be fully absorbed into the body and needs to be removed to prevent toxicity. A tube is inserted into the mouth and into the stomach during this procedure. After that, fluid is injected through the tube and removed by suction.
- **Activated Charcoal:** Reducing the quantity of toxin absorbed into the blood can be accomplished by mixing water with an odorless and tasteless black powder called activated charcoal. The activated charcoal solution can be given to a child intravenously orally. Following exposure to specific medications like theophylline, phenobarbital, or aspirin, physicians may administer activated charcoal treatment multiple times.
- **Whole-Bowel Irrigation:** Toxins are "flushed" out of the digestive system during whole-bowel irrigation using an electrolyte solution. The solution can be given to the child to drink, or it can be administered via mouth or nose via a tube that goes straight into the stomach. The process of flushing aids in expelling the body's gastrointestinal contents. Up until clear fluid emerges from the rectum, fluid is passed through the tube.

9.3.3.2. Antidotes

A medicine that counteracts or neutralizes a poison's effects in the body is known as an antidote. While there isn't a remedy for every toxin, there are some that do, including blood thinner warfarin, opioid painkillers, digoxin, acetaminophen, and tricyclic antidepressants like amitriptyline. Usually, antidote drugs are given via an intravenous (IV) line that is placed into the arm. When a child exhibits specific symptoms or when the toxin can be positively identified, doctors administer an antidote. Certain kids who have trouble breathing might need to be sent to a different hospital so they can receive hyperbaric oxygen therapy. With this treatment, blood levels of carbon monoxide are rapidly lowered by administering oxygen under high pressure. For roughly 90 minutes, the child is kept inside a chamber under high pressure while 100% oxygen is given to them. Ipecac syrup is an extract from a plant that makes people throw up and regurgitate. It was once used to treat poisoning victims. It is no longer regarded by the doctors as an effective treatment for pediatric poisoning. It is advised that you discard any bottles containing this substance that are in your home (Table 9.4).

Table 9.4. Common Emergency Antidotes

Formulary Antidotes Before	Formulary Antidotes After	Indication
Acetylcysteine injection	Acetylcysteine injection	Acetaminophen toxicity
NA	Andexanet alfa injection	Reversal of anticoagulation for patients treated with a direct factor Xa inhibitor (apixaban or rivaroxaban)
Atropine injection	Atropine injection	Organophosphate pesticide or nerve agent poisoning, carbamate toxicity
Calcium Chloride 10% prefilled syringe	Calcium Chloride 10% prefilled syringe	Fluoride, calcium channel blocking agent toxicity
NA	Calcium gluconate gel 2.5%	Hydrofluoric acid dermal burns
Calcium gluconate injection 10%	Calcium gluconate injection 10%	Fluoride, calcium channel blocking agent toxicity
Cyproheptadine tablet	Cyproheptadine tablet	Serotonin toxicity
Dantrolene sodium injection	Dantrolene sodium injection	Malignant hyperthermia
Deferoxamine mesylate injection	Deferoxamine mesylate injection	Iron poisoning
Digoxin immune fab injection	Digoxin immune fab injection	Cardiac glycosides toxicity or cardiac steroid toxicity
Dimercaprol injection (BAL in oil) injection	Dimercaprol injection (BAL in oil) injection	Heavy metal toxicity (arsenic, lead, mercury)
NA	Edetate calcium disodium/EDTA ampule	Lead poisoning
NA	Ethanol dehydrated alcohol injection	Methanol or ethylene glycol poisoning
Flumazenil injection	Flumazenil injection	Benzodiazepine toxicity
Fomepizole injection	Fomepizole injection	Methanol or ethylene glycol poisoning

Glucagon prefilled syringe	Glucagon prefilled syringe	β-blocker, calcium channel blocker toxicity
Hydroxocobalamin injection	Hydroxocobalamin injection	Cyanide poisoning
NA	Idarucizumab injection	Reversal of anticoagulant effects of dabigatran
L-carnitine vials	L-carnitine vials	Valproic acid toxicity
Leucovorin calcium vial	Leucovorin calcium vial	Methotrexate or methanol toxicity
Methylene blue injection	Methylene blue injection	Methemoglobinemia, ifosfamide induced encephalopathy
Naloxone injection	Naloxone injection	Opioid toxicity
Octreotide vial	Octreotide vial	Sulfonylurea-induced hypoglycemia
NA	Pentetate calcium trisodium injection (Calcium DTPA)	Internal contamination with plutonium, americium, or curium to increase the rates of elimination
Phentolamine mesylate injection	Phentolamine mesylate injection	Extravasation
Physostigmine injection	Physostigmine injection	Anticholinergic syndrome
Phytonadione injection	Phytonadione injection	Reversal of coumarin-induced coagulopathy
Phytonadione tablet	Phytonadione tablet	Reversal of coumarin-induced coagulopathy
Polyvalanet snake antivenom injection	Polyvalanet snake antivenom injection	Snake envenomation
Polyvalent scorpion antivenom injection	Polyvalent scorpion antivenom injection	Scorpion envenomation
Potassium iodide tablet	Potassium iodide tablet	Thyroid radioiodine protection
Pralidoxime chloride injection	Pralidoxime chloride injection	Organophosphorus poisoning
Protamine sulfate injection	Protamine sulfate injection	Reversal of coagulopathy induced by unfractionated or low-molecular-weight heparin
NA	Prussian blue capsule	Thallium or radiocesium toxicity
Pyridoxine tablet	Pyridoxine tablet	Isoniazid or hydrazine toxicity
Regular human insulin vial	Regular human insulin vial	Beta-blocker toxicity, calcium-channel blocker toxicity
Smoflipid 20% lipid injectable emulsion	Smoflipid 20% lipid injectable emulsion	Local anesthetic systemic toxicity
Sodium bicarbonate injection 8.4% injection	Sodium bicarbonate injection 8.4% injection	Tricyclic antidepressant toxicity, urine alkalization for salicylate toxicity, or cocaine toxicity
NA	Sodium Thiosulphate injection	Extravasation
NA	Succimer DMSA capsule	Heavy metal toxicity (arsenic, lead, mercury)
Sugammadex injection	Sugammadex injection	Reversal of neuromuscular blockade

Thiamine hydrochloride injection	Thiamine hydrochloride injection	Ethylene glycol toxicity, thiamine deficiency associated with chronic alcoholism
Unactivated prothrombin complex concentrates 4 factors II, VII, IX, X, with proteins S and C injection	Unactivated prothrombin complex concentrates 4 factors II, VII, IX, X, with proteins S and C injection	Reversal of anticoagulant bleeding
NA	uridine triacetate 10gram/packet oral granules	Fluorouracil or capecitabine overdose regardless of symptoms or early-onset toxicity

NA: Not available on the formulary

Source: Abu Esba LC, Mardawi G and Al Deeb M (2022) Can't find the antidote: A root cause analysis. Front. Pharmacol. 13:895841. doi: 10.3389/fphar.2022.895841.

Tips for a Safer Home:

- Carefully read the product manual and any warning labels.
- Keep toxic materials out of children's reach and locked up.
- Put safety latches on any cabinets that hold hazardous materials.
- Purchase only medications whose bottles have safety caps on them.
- Empty all pockets, purses, and drawers of medications. Put them in a cabinet that is locked.
- Never call vitamins or prescription drugs "candy."
- Get rid of all leftover prescriptions safely.
- Paints, varnishes, cleaners, and pesticides should all be kept in locked cabinets in their original packaging.
- Poisonous items should never be put in food or drink containers.
- There are some extremely toxic cosmetics. Make sure they are placed in a locked cabinet out of reach and taken out of purses.

Young children should never be left unattended or alone (Silverman, 2006; Tintinalli, 2011).

9.4. FOREIGN BODY ASPIRATION AND INGESTION

Aspirations of foreign bodies are the most common unintentional injury in children under one year old, and they can be potentially fatal situations. Young children are especially vulnerable because they put things in their mouths to explore the world, they eat with great playfulness and energy, and they lack the developed dentition needed to chew food properly. Any age can have a significant increase in morbidity and mortality from a delayed diagnosis. 3,700 people died in the US in 2007 alone as a result of aspirating or ingesting food or other objects that blocked their airways. An urgent medical evaluation is necessary if a child exhibiting respiratory symptoms is suspected of having aspirated a foreign body. The likelihood of secondary complications increases with the length of time after foreign-body aspiration diagnosis. Foods such as peanuts, sunflower seeds, carrots, raisins, grapes, and hot dogs are frequently aspirated by babies and toddlers. Nonfood objects like pen caps, paper clips, coins, and pins are more frequently aspirated by preschoolers.

9.4.1. Presentation

Many stable patients present with aspiration of a foreign body. However, a child who is otherwise healthy and starts coughing and choking suddenly raises serious suspicions about aspiration. When symptoms first appear, they include respiratory arrest, cyanosis, cough, stridor, dyspnea, and stupor. The traditional triad of asymmetric breath sounds, wheezing, and new-onset cough only appears in 16–40% of cases and is neither specific nor sensitive to foreign-body aspiration. Patients who have tracheal foreign bodies typically exhibit dyspnea at presentation, making diagnosis easier. Most aspirations (80–90%) are caused by bronchial foreign bodies, which are more likely to result in decreased breath sounds and a delayed diagnosis in children. Small or partial blockages can complicate the diagnosis and are frequently mislabeled as asthma, bronchiolitis, URIs, or pneumonia. A child's "retained foreign body" should always be considered a differential diagnosis in cases of chronic cough, recurrent pneumonias, persistent croup, or "asthma" that does not respond to conventional medical therapy (Table 9.5).

Table 9.5. Characteristics of the Lower Urinary Tract Foreign Bodies and Their Management

Case	Age (Years)	Clinical presentation	Duration	Location	X-Ray	US	CT	Retrieval method	Characteristics
1	11	Recurrent dysuria and hematuria	2 weeks	Bladder	Not found	Enhanced echoes	Hyperdense lesion	Cystoscopy conversion to open cystotomy	Skipping rope
2	9	Urethral pain	10 h	Urethra	High density shadow	Not done	Strip density shadow	Mosquito forceps	Acne needle
3	11	Lower abdominal pain	1 day	Bladder	High density shadow	Not done	Irregular hyperdense shadow	Cystoscopy conversion to open cystotomy	Multiple magnetic beads
4	13	No symptoms	3 h	Urethra	High density shadow	Not done	Not done	Cystoscopy	Hairpin

Source: Kuang T, Cai W, Qian W and Lin X (2023) Foreign bodies in children's lower urinary tract: A case series and literature review. Front. Pediatr. 10:1095993. doi: 10.3389/fped.2022.1095993.

9.4.2. Evaluation

Typically, chest radiographs are the first diagnostic study requested. While they cannot be used to rule out the diagnosis of foreign body, they can be useful in confirming it. Most aspirated foreign bodies are radiolucent; in over 50% of tracheal foreign bodies, chest radiographs are normal, and in 25% of bronchial foreign bodies, they are normal. When dealing with an older or more cooperative child, end-inspiratory and end-expiratory films can be beneficial. Decubitus radiographs don't really help with diagnosis. Aspiration can be seen in multiple secondary signs on the chest radiograph. As alternatives for diagnosis, CT and fluoroscopy have also been employed; the latter's sensitivity has reached 100%. However, a bronchoscopy is required to rule out a foreign body aspiration if it is clinically suspected (Table 9.6).

Table 9.6. Algorithm for Management of Foreign Bodies in the Lower Urinary tract in Pediatric Patients

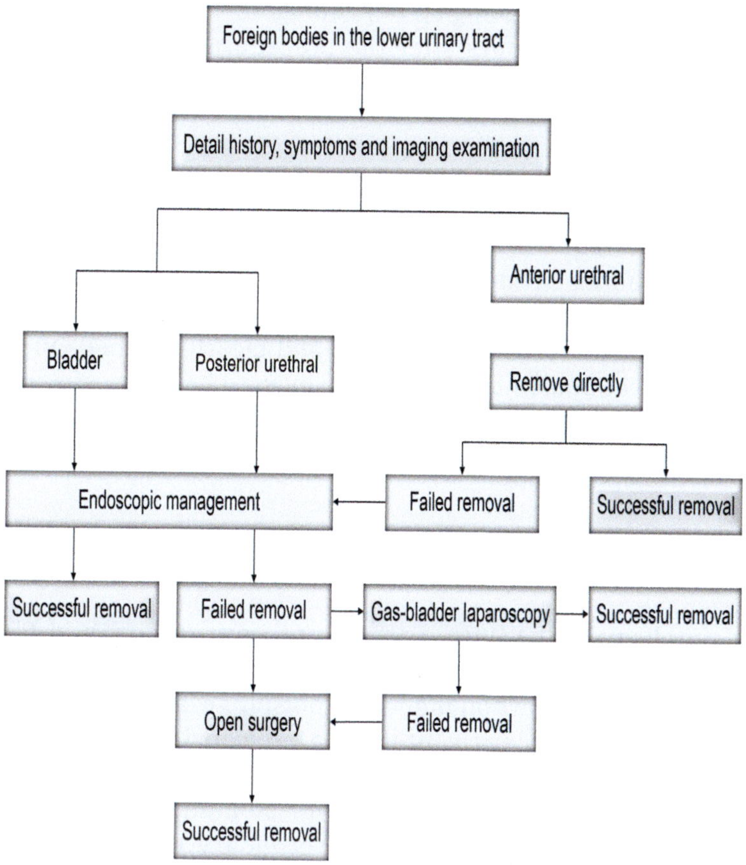

Source: Kuang T, Cai W, Qian W and Lin X (2023) Foreign bodies in children's lower urinary tract: A case series and literature review. Front. Pediatr. 10:1095993. doi: 10.3389/fped.2022.1095993.

9.4.3. Management

To maintain breathing, circulation, and airway integrity, children experiencing respiratory distress need to receive basic life support measures as well as prompt intervention. Swallowing with your mouth openly is not advised. Back strikes and chest compressions are necessary for infants, and abdominal thrusts are necessary for kids older than a year old. Emergency attempts should be made to remove foreign bodies with Magill forceps and perform direct laryngoscopy in cases of severe complete obstruction of the airway. Endotracheal intubation should be done if the foreign body cannot be seen; this procedure may cause the foreign body to become loose and travel farther away. If, despite taking all the necessary precautions, the patient is still unable to breathe, needle cricothyroidotomy may be a life-saving temporary procedure.

Patients who do not have a severe respiratory distress or complete obstruction of their airways should be positioned in a comfortable manner in a quiet room until a rigid bronchoscopy can identify and clear the obstruction. If aspiration of a foreign body is suspected, bronchoscopy should be done even if radiographic studies show no abnormalities. This needs to be done in a controlled environment, like an operating room, under general anesthesia. Bronchoscopy may be carried out by a surgeon, pulmonologist, or otolarnyngologist, depending on the facility. The majority of patients are discharged from the hospital 24 hours after the procedure, and bronchoscopy complications have very low rates, ranging from 1 to 10%.

9.4.4. Complications

The likelihood of secondary complications increases with the length of time after foreign body aspiration diagnosis. The most frequent side effects include post-obstructive pneumonia, atelectasis, and bronchiectasis. Pneumothorax, bronchoesophageal fistula, and airway granulomas are far less common. The desire for a foreign body is the reason behind thousands of ER visits each year. Current management algorithms are well-established and clearly defined, and timely diagnosis is essential. Legislative and educational initiatives have proven to be successful intervention tactics in preventing this frequent pediatric emergency. When appropriate, age-specific anticipatory guidance should be reviewed with caregivers because foreign-body aspiration is a completely preventable event (Ezer, 2011).

9.5. BURNS

Despite the apparent simplicity of the burn diagnosis process, it is critical to acknowledge burn patients as trauma patients and conduct a thorough trauma assessment. Be extremely cautious when it comes to cyanide poisoning, carbon monoxide poisoning, and inhalation injuries. Recognize imminent airway compromise and take early intubation into consideration. Examining for fractures, traumatic brain injuries, thoracic, and abdominal injuries should be part of primary and secondary surveys. Applying cool running water to burn victims for 20 minutes is part of first aid; ice should never be used as it can cause vasoconstriction and secondary tissue damage. If necessary, give tetanus immune globulin and/or a booster shot. Acetaminophen or ibuprofen can be used as an early form of analgesia for mild pain, and fentanyl IN/IV can be used for moderate to severe pain. It's critical to stay warm to avoid hypothermia.

9.5.1. Heat and Cold Injuries

Since they generate and lose heat more quickly than adults, children are far more sensitive to changes in the surrounding temperature. Children tend to ignore their temperature until it becomes an issue because they are too preoccupied playing and having a good time. Ensuring your child is protected from the sun, as well as extreme heat and cold, can prevent them from getting sick or hurt. A medical emergency can be avoided by being prepared for burns and other thermal injuries.

Tending to a thermal burn caused by heat.

- Take the youngster away from the heat source.
- Until the pain subsides or is relieved, cool the affected area with cold compresses or cold water.

- If a blister has formed, do not break it.
- Use a fresh bed sheet or cloth, or a dry, sterile gauze bandage to protect the burn.
- Do not try to remove your child's clothing if it is stuck to the burned area. Rather, make cuts around the garments while preserving the burn area. Seek immediate medical attention.
- Avoid using any sprays, oils, or ointments on the burned area.
- If your child has large-area burns on their hands, feet, faces, eyes, or groin, get medical help right away or call 911 for emergency medical assistance.

Caring for an electrical burn

- A physician should be consulted for any electrical burn. Electrical burns injure areas of the body beneath the skin's surface that are not apparent. In the event of an electrical burn, contact the local emergency department or arrange for someone else to do so on your behalf.
- Turn off the electricity or unplug the appliance or gadget that caused the damage.
- Do not touch the child until you have turned off the source or the circuit breaker if they have come into contact with electrical current.
- Verify the child's breathing continues. Cardiopulmonary resuscitation (CPR) should be started if the child is not breathing. Call the local emergency number or have someone else call it.
- Use a fresh bed sheet or sterile gauze bandage to cover the burned area.
- Don't give your kids any food or liquids.
- Unless there is a suspicion of a neck or back injury, place the child on his or her back. Do not move a child who may have suffered a neck or back injury until emergency medical personnel, such as paramedics, arrive.
- You can lay the child on his or her side if they have puked or if they have a serious injury to their face or mouth.

Use blankets or additional clothing to keep your child warm; do not put them near a heat source (Silverman, 2006; Tintinalli, 2011).

9.6. DROWNING

Submersion or immersion in a liquid medium that causes respiratory distress and/or cardiac arrest is referred to as drowning. Medical professionals are confused about drowning due to the wide variations in definitions. The World Health Organization has established three distinct classes of drowning: drowning death, drowning with morbidity, and drowning without morbidity. This is done to avoid the use of ambiguous and antiquated terminology. The phrases "dry drowning" and "near drowning" are no longer acceptable for use in diagnosing submersion injuries and should be dropped. Even though the great majority of victims of submersion accidents survive, there are a variety of morbidities that can be connected to a drowning incident, ranging from mild, temporary pulmonary symptoms to severe, permanent neurological impairment. Emergency care professionals deal with submersion injury victims on a regular basis, so understanding the pathophysiology, clinical presentation, and treatment is essential.

9.6.1. Risk Factors

An elevated risk of drowning has been linked to several risk factors. The biggest risk factors for children under the age of five are behavioral issues, absence of adult supervision, and undiagnosed dysrhythmic or seizure disorders. It has been demonstrated that poor judgment when it comes to swimming ability and a lack of water safety practices are risk factors linked to an increased risk of drowning in older children. Children who have a tendency to take more risks or who suffer from behavioral disorders are also more likely to drown. When it comes to teens and young adults in particular, the improper use of alcohol and other illegal drugs is arguably the biggest risk factor for drowning globally.

9.6.2. Pathophysiology

When a victim's airways are immersed in a liquid, drowning injuries begin. First, the diving reflex, an inbuilt defensive parasympathetic nervous system activation, is triggered. Bradycardia, hypopnea, peripheral vasoconstriction, and central blood flow shunting are the outcomes of this reflex. It was believed that in patients suffering submersion injuries, this reflex would offer some initial protection. But the sympathetic nervous system's activation and the fight-or-flight response quickly overpower the diving reflex and eliminate its protective qualities. A drowning victim experiences irregular breathing, breath holding, and finally a reflexive inspiratory effort that results in liquid aspiration after the initial diving reflex.

As a result of the liquid being aspirated, surfactant is diluted, changing alveolar surface tension, causing alveolar collapse, and reducing lung compliance. Because these alveoli are not ventilated, this surfactant washout causes a ventilation/perfusion mismatch that eventually results in hypoxemia and intrapulmonary shunting of blood flow. Furthermore, inhaled fluid penetrates the alveoli and airways, resulting in the development of noncardiogenic pulmonary edema. It doesn't matter what kind of water is ingested and causes drowning. It was previously believed that aspirating salt water and its hypertonicity caused water to shift into the pulmonary interstitium and alveolar space, which resulted in hypertonic serum and pulmonary edema. On the other hand, aspirating fresh water or a hypotonic solution was supposed to cause fluid to shift from the alveolar space into the intravascular compartment, resulting in volume overload and electrolyte dilution, including hyponatremia. Given that an individual would need to aspirate between 11 and 22 milliliters per kilogram of body weight in order for there to be a change in electrolytes or blood volume, this distinction is only noticeable in patients who were discovered dead upon arrival, as opposed to nonfatal drowning victims. Less than 3 to 4 mL/kg of fluid are typically aspirated in nonfatal drowning victims, making the difference between fresh and salt water clinically insignificant.

Reflexive laryngospasm is another mechanism that may contribute to the development of hypoxia following submersion injury. A person may experience a reflex laryngospasm after aspirating a liquid medium, which can result in hypoxemia. Aspiration of the liquid into the airways occurs next, which exacerbates the hypoxemia. The mechanism previously believed to be involved in "dry" drowning death was the reflex laryngospasm. This outdated term was created as a result of the autopsy finding that there was no fluid in the lungs. The idea that aspirated fluid is absent has been extensively refuted, and water will always enter the airways in some degree in drowning deaths. It is best to avoid using the phrase "dry drowning." Whatever the initial mechanism causing fluid in the airways, acidemia, hypercapnia, and hypoxia follow. Patients with submersion injuries experience tissue oxygenation deficits, which can lead to end organ damage. The degree of hypoxic end organ damage and, most significantly, the degree of ischemic insult to the central nervous system are related to the ultimate morbidity, mortality, and outcome in submersion injuries (Silverman, 2006; Tintinalli, 2011).

9.6.3. Clinical Presentation

Hypoxemia that results from submersion injuries or drowning with morbidity has a greater impact on the end organs. The respiratory system is the one that is most frequently impacted. Fluid aspiration may cause a clinical presentation similar to any noncardiogenic pulmonary edema etiology or, in certain situations, a clinical presentation of acute respiratory distress syndrome (ARDS). It may lead to respiratory failure, with acute or subacute pulmonary symptoms that may appear suddenly. The patient's symptoms include coughing and dyspnea. Physical examination findings may include wheezing, rhonchi, rales, crackles, increased work of breathing with tachypnea, and/or accessory muscle use.

Hypoxemia can cause cellular damage and neuronal hypoxia in the nervous system. A certain level of cerebral edema, cellular apoptosis, and an elevation in intracranial pressure can result from this cellular damage. An increased risk of long-term morbidity is associated with the estimated 20% of nonfatal drowning victims suffering from some form of hypoxic-ischemic brain injury. Cardiac dysrhythmias may result from hypoxemia from drowning or from possible hypothermia following a nonfatal submersion injury. Atrial fibrillation, ventricular dysrhythmias, and sinus bradycardia are a few examples of these arrhythmias. Renal injury is another common complication seen in patients with a significant submersion injury. When someone drowns, their kidneys are usually injured because of acute tubular necrosis from hypoxemia and/or cardiovascular compromise from shock that may happen as a result of the submersion event. As previously stated, regardless of water tonicity, it is comparatively rare for submersion injuries to result in life-threatening electrolyte disturbances due to the amount of water aspirated in nonfatal drowning victims. Rarely, renal damage from the hypoxemia brought on by the submersion may result in abnormalities of the electrolyte levels. Disseminated intravascular coagulation or consumptive coagulopathy are rare additional complications that drowning victims may experience.

9.6.4. Diagnostic Studies

Chest radiography, such as a plain film chest X-ray, and laboratory tests should be carried out in patients who are exhibiting symptoms of a submersion injury in order to assess for complications arising from pulmonary aspiration and/or hypoxia-related end organ damage. As laboratory tests and/or chest imaging are not indicative of morbidity or the need for hospitalization, they should not be performed on asymptomatic patients. Furthermore, individuals with submersion injuries may have normal initial chest imaging. Patchy airspace opacities, an increase in perihilar markings, cephalization, and/or diffuse pulmonary edema are possible findings on chest imaging. Pleural effusions and/or pneumothorax are uncommon in drowning victims unless they cause complications during their hospital stay. To assess the degree of hypoxic-ischemic brain tissue damage in patients with significant submersion injury who experience significant changes in their mental status, neuroimaging may also be recommended. It should be noted that hypoxic-ischemic brain tissue injury might not be visible on the initial computed tomography (CT) scan done in the ER, necessitating advanced inpatient neuroimaging such as magnetic resonance imaging (MRI) to be performed later.

The assessment of drowning victims can also involve the use of point-of-care ultrasound (POCUS). POCUS doesn't emit any ionizing radiation and is easily accessible. It can be used to keep an eye on a patient while they are being observed in the emergency room or while they are being admitted in order to assess how their pulmonary injury is developing. In particular, the amount and configuration of B lines indicate the severity of pulmonary edema. B lines are typically bilateral and visible in multiple lung zones on POCUS in victims of drowning. B lines, which appear as a vertical beam extending from the proximal pleura (closest to the transducer) to the bottom of the ultrasound screen, are caused by reverberation artifact created by fluid in the alveolar space. On the other hand, normal lung will usually show A lines. Reverberation artifacts can also produce A lines, although these appear as several horizontal lines spaced equally apart from the pleural line. In the clinical context of drowning, diffuse B lines may be secondary to acute respiratory distress syndrome or pulmonary edema. For diffuse B lines, nondrowning differential diagnoses include pulmonary fibrosis and cardiogenic pulmonary edema.

9.6.5. Initial Management

The first step in the management of patients who survive submersion injuries is prehospital care. The goal of prehospital care is to start cardiopulmonary resuscitation as soon as possible. The recommended protocols for basic life support ought to be adhered to. Prehospital care may need to take spinal motion restriction into consideration even though the overall rate of cervical spine injuries among drowning victims is low, particularly if there was a possible associated traumatic mechanism (such as diving, etc.). As well as indications of intoxication. Treatment for concomitant dysrhythmias should follow pediatric advanced life support guidelines.

As drowning victims arrive at the emergency room, their airway needs to be assessed right away. Patients who exhibit symptoms ought to receive continuous cardiac telemetry, end-tidal carbon dioxide monitoring, and oxygen saturation monitoring. Victims of submersion injuries who exhibit hypoxia and/or a Glasgow Coma Scale score of less than 13 should receive additional oxygen and possibly ventilator support. Supplemental oxygen should be administered to patients who are symptomatic but do not need to be intubated right away in order to keep their oxygen saturation level above 94%. Noninvasive positive pressure ventilation (NIPPV), such as continuous positive airway pressure (CPAP) or bilevel positive airway pressure (BiPAP), is one option for oxygenation. In patients with pulmonary edema from a submersion injury, the positive end expiratory pressure (PEEP) attained with NIPPV can enhance oxygenation and reduce ventilation/perfusion mismatch. High-flow nasal cannulas (HFNCs) can be trialed by patients who are unable to tolerate CPAP or BiPAP, though their ability to achieve PEEP is not as great as that of NIPPV.

In the end, tracheal intubation may be necessary for drowning victims. If the patient cannot reach a partial pressure of oxygen of more than 60 mmHg in adults and more than 80 mmHg in children, or if NIPPV is not able to keep the oxygen saturation above 90%, endotracheal intubation should be taken into consideration. Similarly, victims who are obtunded, unable to protect their airway, and/or have significant neurological deterioration should undergo endotracheal intubation. The drowning victim should receive advanced trauma life support as needed, as well as airway and breathing assessment and management, a trauma exam noting any possible traumatic injuries, and other care. It is rare, nevertheless, for a drowning victim to also have a spinal injury or other potentially fatal trauma.

Pediatric advanced life support guidelines should be followed when resuscitation is performed on drowning victims who are in cardiopulmonary arrest and present to the emergency department. A strong attempt at cardiopulmonary resuscitation should be made for victims who were submerged for less than five minutes, who were quickly brought to the emergency department, and who had a higher chance of a favorable neurological outcome. Similar to this, aggressive and possibly prolonged resuscitation efforts should be given to pediatric drowning victims who present in cardiac arrest with concomitant hypothermia from drowning in cold water (icy water) due to the possibility of a favorable neurological outcome.

Hypothermic patients (core temperature <35°C) should be resuscitated while rewarming to a core temperature of 32°C to 35°C. However, pediatric drowning victims who have a prolonged submersion (greater than 15 minutes) and who are normothermic, aggressive emergency department resuscitation may be avoided as there is extremely poor prognosis for an intact neurological outcome in these circumstances. A good neurological outcome is more likely when spontaneous circulation returns within 30 minutes of advanced life support, especially when the drowning incident occurs in winter. In addition, hyperkalemia (> 10 mmol/L) in drowning victims who are hypothermic, it may be appropriate to stop resuscitation. In an attempt to reduce the risk of hypothermia, wet clothing should be removed right away.

9.6.6. Hypothermia Management

Rewarming hypothermic patients should be accomplished through passive (removing damp clothing right away) or active rewarming methods. Different degrees of hypothermia usually manifest with different symptoms. Drowning victims with mild hypothermia (35–32°C) typically shiver, are not experiencing organ dysfunction such as cardiac dysrhythmias, and maintain a normal mental state. Both passive and active external warming, like forced heated air, ought to be applied to them. Patients who suffer from moderate hypothermia (below 32–28°C) are more likely to experience atrial dysrhythmias, such as fibrillation or flutter, and may exhibit altered mental status. Patients with moderate hypothermia should be actively warmed internally. Similar to this, patients experiencing moderate hypothermia may show a J- (Osborn) wave on their electrocardiogram (ECG), with the amplitude of this wave corresponding to the severity of hypothermia. When victims arrive with severe hypothermia (below 28°C), they usually appear obtunded, lack reflexes, and are at risk of asystole and ventricular fibrillation. It should be noted that at temperatures below 32°C, defibrillation and resuscitation medications/antiarrhythmic agents may not work.

Active internal methods for warming hypothermic patients in cardiopulmonary arrest include warm IV fluids (38–42°C), warm water lavage (rectal, gastric, bladder, thoracic, and peritoneal), and the endotracheal tube's delivery of warm, humidified oxygen. When pediatric drowning victims present in cardiac arrest with concurrent hypothermia, extracorporeal membrane oxygenation (ECMO) and extracorporeal rewarming should be considered, if available. With a rate of about 7°C per hour, ECMO has the fastest rate of rewarming. According to a retrospective study, drowning victims who were put on extracorporeal life support during cardiac arrest had a survival rate of 23.4%.

The idea of core temperature after drop is also crucial to understand when treating hypothermic patients. After the patient is taken out of the cold environment, this phenomenon happens as a result of cold blood returning to the core from the periphery. While it is common to experience this ongoing drop in core temperature during the initial resuscitation, it is usually temporary and shouldn't affect rewarming management or resuscitation techniques.

In addition to hypothermia and drowning injuries, pediatric patients may experience hypotension as a result of a condition called "cold diuresis." Peripheral vasoconstriction causes diuresis because it causes the central volume receptors to perceive a hypervolemia. Consequently, this results in an unsuitable diuresis, possible hypotension, and a reduction in the production of antidiuretic hormone. Maintaining volume status in these patients might necessitate intravenous fluid administration. Hypoxia-induced cardiomyopathy, on the other hand, is another possible cause of hypotension in drowning victims and may present as a decompensated cardiogenic shock image. In this situation, giving fluids may worsen the patient's hemodynamic state and even cause cardiopulmonary collapse.

9.6.7. Post-Resuscitation Management

When a patient is admitted to the hospital with symptoms, supportive care is typically provided. Children in the emergency room who need prolonged positive pressure ventilation or cardiopulmonary resuscitation should be admitted to an intensive care unit so they can receive round-the-clock cardiopulmonary monitoring. Maintaining positive pressure ventilation may help to increase oxygenation and draw in fluid-filled alveoli. It's critical to keep an eye out for acute respiratory distress syndrome in these admitted patients. Furthermore, victims of drowning who experienced cardiopulmonary arrest and regained spontaneous circulation (ROSC) might need ongoing epinephrine pressor support.

Antibiotic usage shouldn't be done on a regular basis; instead, it should only be done in cases where there is proof of a pulmonary infection or when the patient has been submerged in highly contaminated water. In these situations, coverage for species like Pseudomonas and/or Aeromonas species ought to be taken into account. When immersed in highly contaminated water, an antipseudomonal beta lactam antibiotic should be chosen. In patients with significant pulmonary involvement following a submersion event, systemic glucocorticoids are frequently administered; however, there is no evidence to support this treatment approach.

Submersion injury has the potential to cause cerebral edema and hypoxic-ischemic brain injury. Attempts to control the related rise in intracranial pressure may involve the use of loop diuretics, mannitol, and/or hypertonic saline. While these efforts to lower intracranial pressure should be taken into consideration, they have not shown a discernible improvement in the long-term neurological impairment of drowning victims. Similarly, there is no evidence that aggressive post-resuscitation care, including induced hypothermia, induced coma or paralysis, and invasive intracranial monitoring, improves the long-term neurological outcomes of pediatric drowning victims.

9.6.8. Admission/Discharge Planning

Individuals who arrive at the emergency room in good mental health and have an oxygen saturation level greater than 95% on room air are deemed to be at low risk for complications and should be kept under observation for a minimum of six to eight hours. The patient may be safely discharged home provided the child has a safe social disposition and suitable adult supervision. If, following this period of observation, the patient remains asymptomatic or minimally symptomatic with a normal pulmonary examination (absence of rhonchi, rales, or wheezing, increased work of breathing, as well as an oxygen saturation above 95% on room air). The occurrence of pulmonary symptoms, such as cough, shortness of breath, fever development, and/or any neurological symptoms, should be discussed along with the strict return precautions. Following the period of observation, if the victim exhibits an oxygen requirement or abnormal findings on a pulmonary exam (rales, rhonchi, increased work of breathing), they should be admitted to the hospital and kept under observation until the hypoxia and/or symptoms go away.

Hospital admission is indicated in the following cases of nonfatal drowning:

- Prolonged submersion (> 5–15 minutes)
- Low mental state, as measured by a Glasgow Coma Scale score of less than 13.
- Persistent complaints like coughing and dyspnea.
- Increased breathing effort or tachypnea.
- Exam results for the lungs included tachypnea, crackles, and/or rales.
- Prolonged hypothermia
- Abnormal chest imaging
- Hypoxia
- Acidosis on blood gasses
- Need for any kind of cardiopulmonary resuscitation, including prehospital lay person basic life support and rescue breathing techniques like chest compressions.
- Social status precludes safe disposition

9.6.9. Prognosis

Due to inadequate data reporting, there are few data available on the survival rate after drowning. Furthermore, there has been significant variation in the incidence of long-term morbidity due to neurological complications. Nonetheless, most patients from submersion incidents who present to the emergency room asymptomatic, with stable vital signs and a normal neurological exam, will survive with little to no long-term disability. In a similar vein, victims of drowning who need to be admitted to the hospital and/or who sustained a submersion injury but did not require cardiopulmonary resuscitation from emergency personnel or first responders usually recover in 48 hours. A delayed acute respiratory distress syndrome, extended hospital stays, severe morbidity, and a higher risk of death are all rare outcomes for submersion victims.

Conversely, the prognosis is not good for drowning victims who need CPR administered on the spot or in the emergency room. Accordingly, it has been demonstrated that patients who arrived at the emergency room in a state of unstable cardiorespiratory status, poor mental status, or stupor, were more likely to experience long-term morbidity and mortality from hypoxic-ischemic central nervous system (CNS) damage. For pediatric patients who need cardiopulmonary resuscitation at the scene of the incident, the mortality rate is about 20%. Of those who do survive, hypoxic-ischemic neurological insult will cause considerable long-term CNS damage in about 5% of cases.

Patients with submersion injuries have been found to have a worse prognosis in correlation with several other prognostic factors. These include being submerged for longer than five minutes, receiving basic life support later than necessary, requiring cardiopulmonary resuscitation in the emergency department, having a Glasgow Coma Scale score of less than five upon presentation, having severe acidosis with an arterial blood pH of less than 7.1 on presentation, and persistent and prolonged apnea. Patients with concurrent suspected drug and/or alcohol abuse have also shown worse outcomes.

Prognostic factors for poorer results in drowning victims include:

- Prolonged submersion (> 5–15 minutes)
- Cardiopulmonary resuscitation is delayed.
- The requirement for CPR performed by bystanders.
- Suspected abuse of alcohol or drugs.
- Metabolic acidosis (pH < 7.1)
- Asystole when she first arrived at the emergency room.
- Glasgow Coma Scale score < 5
- Fixed dilated pupils

Rare case reports of children surviving cardiac arrest after submersion in ice water have been published. The advantages of hypothermia are considered to outweigh this. Cold water is thought to cause CNS cooling before there is noticeable hypoxic tissue damage. Nevertheless, neither in a warm nor a cold liquid medium, the data that are currently available have shown any favorable survival among victims with prolonged submersion longer than 15 minutes. Additionally, case reports have not shown any appreciable survival following a submersion lasting longer than 60 minutes. Furthermore, there hasn't been any evidence of a difference in the survival rates between adult and pediatric victims in relation to water temperature.

9.6.10. Prevention

The majority of pediatric drowning incidents are avoidable. Preventive measures can potentially reduce the incidence of drowning by 80% by keeping children under 4 years old out of bodies of water. These measures include secure fencing and appropriate enclosures/gating of swimming pools. In a similar vein, it's critical that kids wear personal flotation devices and have sufficient adult supervision. In addition, parents must be made aware of the risk of toddler drowning in very shallow water—such as bathtubs, buckets, and toilets—in the event that there is insufficient supervision. (Silverman, 2006; Tintinalli, 2011)

A Closer Look

The Family of a Child in Emergency Care

The illness or injury of the child causes stress for the family both directly and indirectly. Since a child's perception of a sickness or injury is frequently influenced by the attitudes of their parents, taking care of the child necessitates evaluating and working with the family.

Fear and anxiety are the most common emotions felt by parents whose children are being cared for during emergencies. These feelings might get stronger or weaker depending on the past. Parents worry about the potential outcomes listed below:

- Their child might die: The biggest cause of anxiety is this fear, which can exist even in situations where death is improbable, like minor illnesses or injuries. Parents' resentment of healthcare providers is frequently rooted in this anxiety.
- Their child might experience pain. Parents generally make a great effort to shield their kids from harm. For parents, suffering can be difficult to comprehend and accept, even when it is necessary.
- The child might have long-term physical changes. Parents frequently worry that their kids' bodies will change or leave permanent scars.

Another common emotion is parental guilt. There are several reasons why parents might feel guilty:

- They take blame for their child's ailment or injury.
- They are subjecting their kid to an agonizing ordeal.
- They lack the knowledge necessary to decide on their child's care in an informed manner.

Parents may also be concerned about their siblings, finances, work schedules, or other issues, or they may have had bad experiences in the past with healthcare providers.

The specific stressors that affect families during emergencies vary depending on the situation and the family in question. To communicate effectively, the nurse must define the family (e.g., single parent, two parents, grandparent, other caregiver) and identify the decision makers (e.g., family members, religious leaders). When parents experience too many stressors at once, their coping skills may become overworked, leading to feelings of rage, withdrawal, or sadness. Hyperactivity, which includes making a lot of calls, asking the same questions over and over, and involving a lot of people, is another way that stress can show up.

Including family members in their child's upbringing helps foster healthy coping strategies and lessen helplessness. During procedures, nurses ought to assist families in being present and motivate them to support their child. While asking family members to hold or restrain a child during a procedure is inappropriate, they can provide emotional support. Preemptive evaluation and suitable assistance before issues arising are beneficial for healthcare providers as well as the family.

Summary

- The seriously unwell child presents a daunting case, even for the most experienced of clinicians. However, the adoption of a calm and structured approach to assessment and management of the patient, enables the clinician to identify and treat life threatening problems in a methodical manner.
- The initial rapid assessment of a child should take less than a minute. The aim of this is to identify life-threatening problems to guide resuscitation. It should take less than a minute.
- Regular reassessment is essential in the ongoing care of any unwell child.
- While most new-borns enter the world in a healthy state, some infants suffer from neonatal emergencies that require immediate medical treatment. Neonatal emergencies are common problems that affect a human new-born either at the time of birth, during the in-hospital post-birth period, or at home until the neonatal period ends.
- A poison is something that can make you sick if you eat, drink, touch, or breathe it. Poisons can be found everywhere in the home, and even seemingly harmless items can become dangerous if swallowed. Poisonings happen every day. Therefore, parents need to recognize poisons, keep them locked up, and know what to do if a child does come in contact with a poison. Poison prevention and immediate treatment are key to keeping your child safe.
- Foreign-body aspirations are potential life-threatening emergencies and are the leading causes of unintentional injury in children less than one year old. Infants and toddlers are particularly at risk for several reasons: they explore their world by placing objects in their mouths, they are very playful and active when eating, and they do not have developed dentition in order to chew food properly.
- Although the diagnosis of burns seems pretty straight forward, it is essential to recognize that burn patients are trauma patients and perform a complete trauma assessment. Have a high degree of suspicion for inhalational injuries, carbon monoxide, and cyanide poisoning. Anticipate impending airway compromise and consider early intubation. Primary and secondary surveys should include inspection for fractures, traumatic brain injuries, thoracic injuries, and abdominal injuries.
- Drowning refers to the process of submersion/immersion into a liquid medium, which results in respiratory difficulty and/or arrest. The use of point-of-care ultrasound (POCUS) also can be incorporated into the evaluation of drowning victims.

References

1. Arbuthnot, M. K., & Garcia, A. V. (2019). Early resuscitation and management of severe pediatric burns. *Seminars in Pediatric Surgery, 28*(1), 73–78. https://doi.org/10.1053/j.sempedsurg.2019.01.013.
2. Aronoff, D. M., & Bloch, K. C. (2003). Assessing the relationship between the use of nonsteroidal anti-inflammatory drugs and necrotizing fasciitis caused by group A streptococcus. *Medicine, 82*(4), 225–235.

3. Assefa, D. (2007). Use of decubitus radiographs in the diagnosis of foreign body aspiration in young children. *Pediatric Emergency Care, 23*(3), 154–157.
4. Biarent, D., Bingham, R., Richmond, S., et al. (2005). European Resuscitation Council guidelines for resuscitation 2005. Section 6. Paediatric life support. *Resuscitation, 67*(Suppl 1), 97–133.
5. Brierley, J., Choong, K., Cornell, T., et al. (2008). 2007 American College of Critical Care Medicine clinical practice parameters for hemodynamic support of pediatric and neonatal septic shock. *Critical Care Medicine.*
6. Cherry, J. (2008). Clinical practice: Croup. *New England Journal of Medicine, 358*, 384–389.
7. Dellinger, R. P., Levy, M. M., Carlet, J. M., et al. (2008). Surviving Sepsis Campaign: International guidelines for management of severe sepsis and septic shock: 2008. *Critical Care Medicine, 36*, 296–327.
8. Eren, S., Balci, A. E., Dikici, B., et al. (2003). Foreign body aspiration in children: Experience of 1160 cases. *Annals of Tropical Pediatrics, 23*, 31.
9. Ezer, S. (2011). Foreign body aspiration in children: Analysis of diagnostic criteria and accurate time for bronchoscopy. *Pediatric Emergency Care, 27*(8), 723–726.
10. Glaser, N., Barnett, P., McCaslin, I., et al. (2001). Risk factors for cerebral edema in children with diabetic ketoacidosis. *The Pediatric Emergency Medicine Collaborative Research Committee of the American Academy of Pediatrics. New England Journal of Medicine, 344*, 264–269.
11. McWilliams, T. L., Twigg, D., Hendricks, J., et al. (2019). The implementation of an infection control bundle within a total care burns unit. *Burns, 47*(2021), 569–571.
12. Ruiz, F. (2014, August 1). Airway foreign bodies in children. *UpToDate.*
13. Saki, N., Nikakhlagh, S., Rahim, F., & Abshirini, H. (2009). Foreign body aspirations in infancy: A 20-year experience. *International Journal of Medical Sciences, 6*(6), 322–328.
14. Scolnik, D., Coates, A. L., Stephens, D., Da Silva, Z., Lavine, E., & Schuh, S. (2006). Controlled delivery of high vs low humidity vs mist therapy for croup in emergency departments: A randomized controlled trial. *JAMA, 295*, 1274–1280.
15. Sheridan, R. L. (2018). Burn care for children. *Pediatrics in Review, 39*(6), 273–286. https://doi.org/10.1542/pir.2016-0179.
16. Sherry, A., & Levitsky, L. (2008). Management of diabetic ketoacidosis in children and adolescents. *Pediatric Drugs, 10*, 209–215.
17. Silverman, B. K. (2006). Textbook of Pediatric Emergency Medicine. In G. R. Fleisher, S. Ludwig, & F. M. Henretig (Eds.), *Textbook of Pediatric Emergency Medicine* (pp. 2013–2020). Philadelphia: Lippincott Williams & Wilkins.
18. Srivastava, G. (2010). Airway foreign bodies in children. *Clinical Pediatric Emergency Medicine, 11*(2), 67–72.
19. Tan, A., Schulze, A., O'Donnell, C. P., & Davis, P. G. (2005). Air versus oxygen for resuscitation of infants at birth. *Cochrane Database of Systematic Reviews, 18*, D002273.
20. Tintinalli, J. (2011). Pediatrics. In *Tintinalli's Emergency Medicine: A Comprehensive Study Guide* (7th ed., pp. 792–793). New York: The McGraw-Hill Companies

Chapter

10

CHILD HEALTH NURSING IN PICU

Contents

INTRODUCTION

In the pediatric intensive care unit (PICU), the stress level can increase significantly from regular hospital stays for children. You will feel more equipped to support your child if you are familiar with the personnel and facilities in the PICU. Providing sick children with the best medical care possible is the mission of the pediatric intensive care unit (PICU). Like the general medical floors, it is not like other areas of the hospital. Children in the PICU receive close monitoring of vital signs such as blood pressure, respiration, and heart rate, along with intensive nursing care. Therapy that may not be available in other areas of the hospital is another benefit that the PICU offers to medical staff. Some examples of these include medications that should only be taken under strict medical supervision and ventilators, or breathing machines.

When a child's medical needs cannot be satisfied on the hospital's main medical floors and they require critical care, they are admitted to the pediatric intensive care unit (PICU). These may include children with severe asthmatic breathing difficulties, severe infections, some diabetic complications, or children who have been in a serious car accident or have nearly drowned. Children who were stable enough to receive care on the medical-surgical floors of the hospital may occasionally transfer to the PICU if their conditions worsen. Many children receive care in the PICU for several days following major surgery.

Orientation and Directional Terms

Term	Definition	Illustration
Neonatal intensive care units	A neonatal intensive care unit (NICU), also known as an intensive care nursery (ICN), is an intensive care unit (ICU) specializing in the care of ill or premature newborn infants.	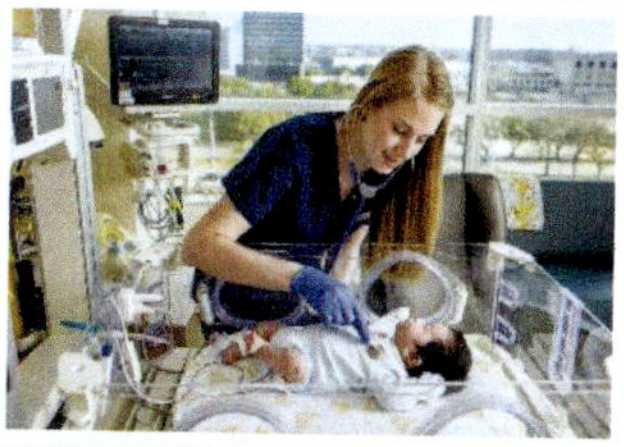
Bronchopulmonary dysplasia	Bronchopulmonary dysplasia (BPD), sometimes called chronic lung disease, is a problem with how a baby's lung tissue develops. Babies who are born very early or who have breathing problems after birth are at risk for bronchopulmonary dysplasia.	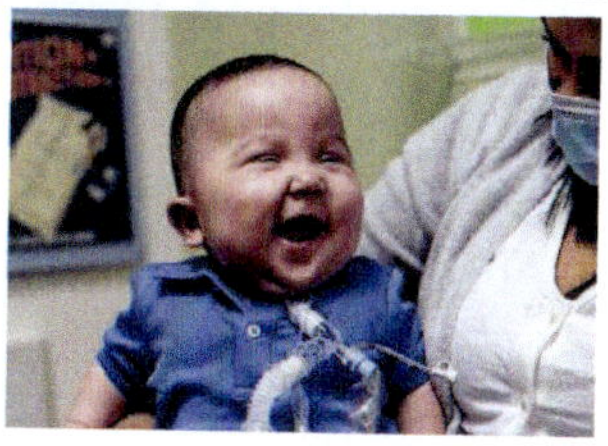
Pulmonary hemorrhage	Pulmonary hemorrhage is the extravasation of blood into the alveoli, that is, bleeding into the lower respiratory tract.	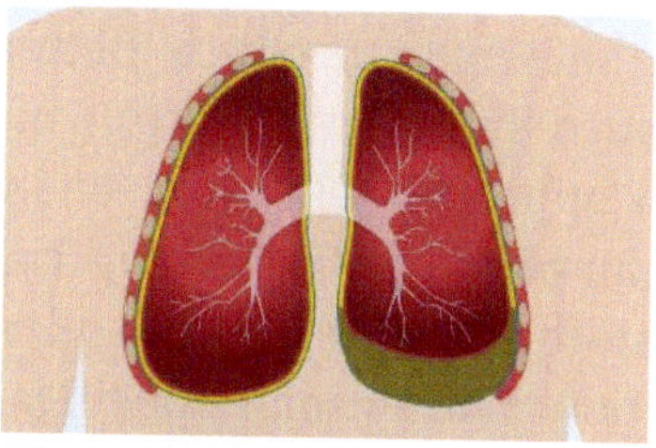
Near infrared spectroscopy	Near-infrared spectroscopy (NIRS) is a spectroscopic method that uses the near-infrared region of the electromagnetic spectrum (from 780 nm to 2500 nm).	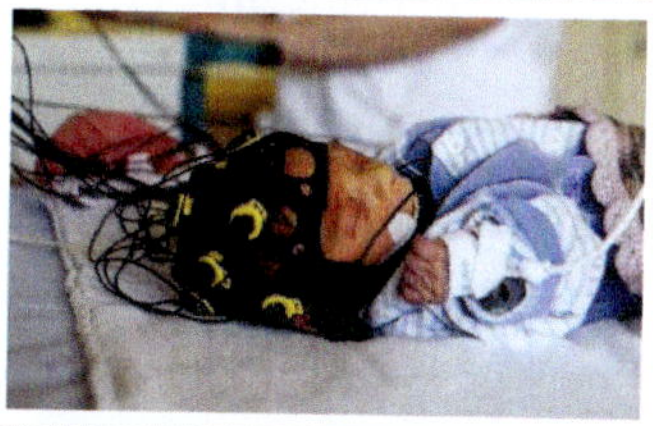
Postextubation atelectasis	Post-extubation atelectasis is a common pulmonary complication of critical neonates who have received long-term, high-setting of mechanical ventilator, resulting in re-intubation, increased morbidity and lengthened hospitalizations.	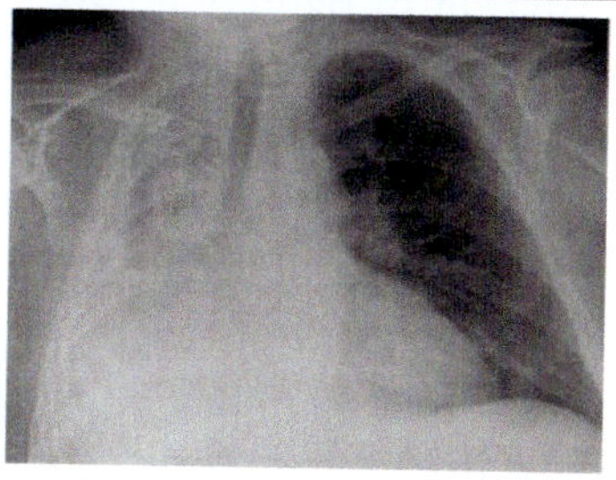

10.1. CARE OF A CHILD ON VENTILATOR

Although the use of noninvasive ventilation techniques is growing in neonatal intensive care units (NICUs), invasive ventilation is still frequently required to treat preterm and term infants with respiratory insufficiency. These days, bronchopulmonary dysplasia (BPD) development is thought to be significantly influenced by prolonged invasive ventilation, and extremely preterm infants are extubated rather quickly.

To maximize mechanical ventilation and avoid ventilator-induced lung injury, a variety of ventilation strategies and modes are available. Volume-targeted ventilation modes have been shown to produce better results than pressure-limited ventilation modes. The use of an appropriately sized endotracheal tube, patient positioning, nursing care, respiratory kinesiotherapy, sedation and analgesia, and infection prevention—specifically, preventing nosocomial infections and ventilator-associated pneumonia—as well as the management of complications like air leaks and pulmonary hemorrhage—are all crucial factors to take into account when ventilating neonates. These days, there is a growing interest in the topic of ventilation in palliative care and in patients receiving extracorporeal membrane oxygenation (ECMO). Echocardiography is now standard in most neonatal units, and monitoring of the ventilated neonate using online pulmonary mechanics and function testing and capnography is becoming more popular. Lung ultrasonography is a new diagnostic tool that can be useful in monitoring the ventilated neonate, and near-infrared spectroscopy (NIRS) is gaining popularity as a means of preventing brain damage. In NICUs, respiratory therapy and individualized nursing care are essential and are being provided more frequently. It has been shown that each baby on mechanical ventilation needs one nurse's care for 60% of the time on average (Foglia et al, 2007; Turton, 2008; Morrow et al, 2009; Chang and Schibler, 2016; Ali et al, 2019).

10.1.1. The Endotracheal Tube

A key component of effective ventilation is the endotracheal tube (ETT), which serves as the basic interface between the patient and the ventilator. The largest inner diameter (ID) tube that can fit through the vocal cords without discomfort and still create a tight enough seal to allow for efficient ventilation is the tube that is the right size. Verifying the presence of a minor leak at maximal inspiratory pressures of less than 20 cm H_2O may aid in avoiding the use of an overly large tube. Poseuille's law states that the resistance increases as the tube ID decreases and is inversely proportional to the fourth power of the tube radius (the tube ID). With less than expected variation between the 3.0, 3.5, and 4 mm tubes, resistance is especially noticeable for tubes with ≤2.5 mm ID. Additionally, longer tubes have more resistance, so they should be cut. It has also been demonstrated that shouldered tubes provide up to 50% less resistance, so they should be taken into consideration, especially for the smaller ID tubes. The first tube size should be chosen using established tables that are based on clinical and experimental research.

The neonatal airway is traditionally characterized as being narrower at the cricoid cartilage than the airways of older children (>8 years) and adults. This anatomical feature has guided years of practice with the use of uncuffed endotracheal tubes (UTT) for small children, infants, and neonates, although recent findings have called into question this practice. Since the invention of cuffed endotracheal tubes (CTT), or high-volume low-pressure (HVLP) cuffs, their use in younger children, newborns, and even neonates has increased. According to a 2016 American Society of Pediatric Anesthesia report,

60% of respondents utilized CTT on full-term neonates more than 50% of the time. As long as cuff pressure is monitored, several short-term reports have concluded that CTT is safe to use in neonates with no higher rates of complications than UTT; however, other reports have found the opposite. There is a dearth of information regarding the effectiveness and safety of using CTT for prolonged ventilation in the NICU, as well as its effect on longer-term outcomes.

There aren't many studies that compare orotracheal and nasotracheal intubation. After nasal intubation, postextubation atelectasis may occur more frequently, especially in neonates with extremely low birth weights (ELBW). Since both routes have comparable rates of complications, none is better than the other. Current resuscitation guidelines recommend a combination of clinical signs (breath sounds under the axillae, thoracic expansion, increased heart rate, and condensation visible on the tube) and exhaled CO_2 monitoring to clinically confirm endotracheal intubation. While they work well in most cases, they need to be used cautiously when considering cardiac arrest.

It's crucial to insert the tube at the proper depth following a successful intubation. Pneumothorax, atelectasis, and/or selective right main bronchus intubation could result from an overly deep insertion. A shallow insertion increases the possibility of an unintentional extubation for the patient. The midtracheal position, often at the T1-T2 level, is the optimal and safe location for the ETT tip. However, in ELBW neonates, the carina level may reach T3, rather than the typical T4, which would result in a slightly higher midtracheal position. Various guidelines and equations have been devised to assist in estimating the optimal tube length. The widely accepted "7–8–9" rule was created by Tochen and, in its most basic version, might be translated as 6+ weight (for orotracheal intubation). This rule assumes that body weight and the appropriate tube length follow a linear relationship (Table 10.1).

Table 10.1. Endotracheal Tube Insertion Depth for Oro- and Nasotracheal Intubation in Neonates

Gestational Age (weeks)	Current Weight (kg)	Endotracheal Tube Length at Lips (cm)	Endotracheal Tube Length at Nostril (cm)
23–24	0.5–0.6	5.5	6.5
25–26	0.7–0.8	6.0	7.0
27–29	0.9–1.0	6.5	7.5
30–32	1.1–1.4	7.0	8.0
33–34	1.5–1.8	7.5	8.5
35–37	1.9–2.4	8.0	9.0
38–40	2.5–3.1	8.5	9.5
41–43	3.2–4.2	9.0	10.0

Source: Rocha G, Soares P, Gonçalves A, Silva AI, Almeida D, Figueiredo S, Pissarra S, Costa S, Soares H, Flôr-de-Lima F, Guimarães H. (2018). Respiratory care for the ventilated neonate. Can Respir J., 13, 7472964. doi: 10.1155/2018/7472964. PMID: 30186538; PMCID: PMC6110042.

The gold standard for confirming appropriate tube placement is still a chest radiograph. While other technical approaches have demonstrated potential (i.e., ultrasonography), they are not as widely available or call for specialized knowledge. The patient's head must be kept in a neutral position and the tube must be fixed to allow for the least amount of movement possible (Foglia et al, 2007; Turton, 2008; Morrow et al, 2009; Chang and Schibler, 2016; Ali et al, 2019).

10.1.2. Positioning the Patient

It has been noted that positions other than the typical supine position—such as the prone position—may enhance respiratory function in neonates receiving mechanical ventilation. Benefits of these positions for critically ill neonates receiving MV are not well defined. Prone positioning is preferred for slightly better oxygenation in neonates receiving mechanical ventilation when the quality is low to moderate. However, no evidence was discovered to support the idea that certain body positions during a neonate's mechanical ventilation are useful in resulting in a long-lasting and clinically significant improvement. Raising the head of the bed a little to enable lung expansion may also be beneficial. To prevent secretions from pooling at the base of the lungs, this position should be adjusted on a regular basis.

Though there is no conclusive solution, preterm infants should lie with their heads in the midline position, at least during the first three days of life, when the risk of hemorrhage is greatest, due to the possibility of germinal matrix-intraventricular hemorrhage and the impact of head position on jugular venous drainage (Figure 10.1).

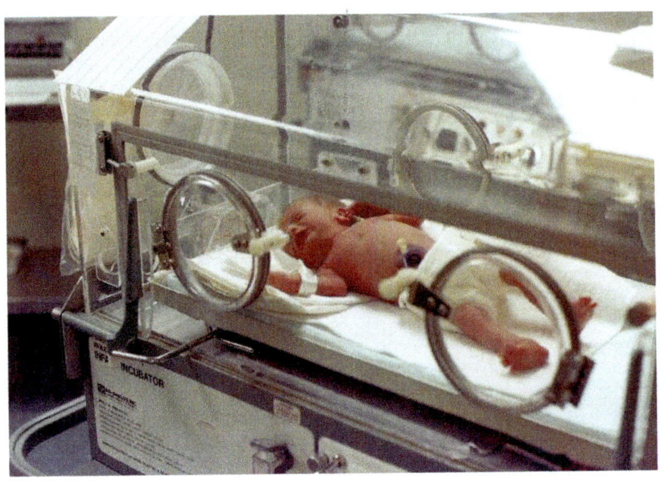

Figure 10.1. *A premature baby in an infant (neonatal) incubator, also known as an isolette. Taken in 1978 in a US hospital. From family archive, scanned from a 35mm negative.*

Source: By Evan-Amos – Own work, Public Domain, https://commons.wikimedia.org/w/index.php?curid=86913279.

10.1.3. Respiratory Kinesiotherapy

The neonatal patient presents with physiological features that include low functional residual capacity, small airway caliber, few collateral airways, compliant chest wall, and difficult airway maintenance and clearance. A tiny amount of mucus can significantly increase airway resistance, which reduces airflow and prevents secretions from being expelled in the absence of expiratory flow. Certain respiratory kinesiotherapy techniques might permit sufficient expiratory flow while preventing airway closure. An endotracheal tube is linked to poor mucociliary function, hampered cough reflex, impaired airway clearance, and possibly increased mucus production. Following extubation, periextubation maneuvers demonstrated a reduction in the incidence of lung atelectasis and an improvement in pulmonary symptoms. Techniques for respiratory kinesiotherapy produce mechanical effects on the lungs, enhance ventilation, and make it easier to get rid of secretions to prevent bronchial blockage, which permits good airway maintenance and makes ventilator weaning easier. Neonates receiving respiratory kinesiotherapy are typically treated with a variety of methods, including suction, postural drainage, vibration, and percussion. Other respiratory rehabilitation methods, like hyperinflation, have been used more recently. It is challenging to pinpoint the precise impact of any given technique because they are typically used in combination and each has indications and contraindications. Chest manipulation in neonates carries some risk and should only be handled by highly skilled and trained professionals. Short sessions ought to come before meals.

10.1.4. Nursing Care

There are various difficulties faced by nurses who care for neonates on mechanical ventilation. Essential elements of nursing care include monitoring the patient and the ventilator, oxygen delivery systems, monitors, and oxygenation. Highly sensitive equipment is useful for patient monitoring. Alarm limits (upper and lower) are established based on the most recent research and the unique standard of care for the NICU for heart rate, respiration, blood pressure, and oxygen saturation. Providing safe and effective nursing care requires a high level of expertise and caution. Thermoregulation, ideal posture, airway clearance, stable hemodynamic status, and sufficient nutrition for maintaining growth and development are essential components of care. To lessen their anxiety, the family must have open and honest communication. The infants in the unit need to be in a safe environment, and nurses are responsible for overseeing the infection control procedures. For nurses working in NICUs, hand washing, isolation, monitoring, and visitor screening are important practices.

10.1.4.1. Heating and Humidification of the Inspired Air

The natural processes of inspired air filtration, humidification, and warming are eliminated by intubation. By the time it enters the pharynx, air inspired to the nose has warmed and become nearly 90% more humid. The application of dry oxygen reduces the water content of the inspired air, and the use of artificial airways avoids the nasopharynx and oropharynx, which are the primary sites for gas humidification.

Ciliary dysfunction, inflammation and necrosis of the ciliated pulmonary epithelium, retention of dried secretions, atelectasis, bacterial infiltration of the pulmonary mucosa, and pneumonia may arise if the humidification of inspired gases is not properly addressed. Using the ventilator circuit's inspiratory line, a humidifier warms and humidifies the gases given to the baby during mechanical ventilation.

If a humidifier has external sources of flow, heat, and water, it is categorized as active. The most common type of humidifiers in NICUs nowadays are bypass models. The gas that travels to the baby crosses the heated water's surface. In the intensive care unit, complex systems made of wires, reservoirs, heating elements, and other components are frequently utilized.

10.1.4.2. Aerosolization and Nebulization

Aerosol therapy has been shown to be a successful drug delivery method. Even with their regular use in NICUs, developing suitable devices and medicinal agents remains a difficult task. Metered dose inhalers (MDIs), holding chambers, and nebulizers (ultrasonic, jet, and vibrating mesh nebulizers, as well as a capillary aerosol generator) are among the tools used for aerosolization of newborns. Among the medications used in critically ill newborns are diuretics, bronchodilators, surfactants, corticosteroids, antiviral agents, and vasoactive agents.

Current recommendations for neonates who are conventionally ventilated (using SIMV, AC, VG, or VC modes) and those on CPAP (continuous positive airway pressure) include cleaning the artificial airways before nebulization, disconnecting the ventilator flow sensor from the wye connector, using a vibrating mesh nebulizer (such as Aeroneb or Pari e-flow) or MDI with a holding chamber, placing the device in the inspiratory limb of the circuit 20 cm from the wye connector, and optimizing breathing support by increasing inspiratory time, decreasing respiratory rate, bypassing the humidifier, and maintaining air flow heating during nebulization.

The current guidelines suggest cleaning the artificial airways before nebulization, removing the ventilator flow sensor from the wye connector, using a vibrating mesh nebulizer (Aeroneb, Pari e-flow) or MDI with holding chamber, placing the device in the inspiratory limb in the circuit 20 cm from the wye connector, and optimizing breathing support (increasing inspiratory time as much as possible, decreasing respiratory rate as much as possible, avoiding the humidifier, and maintaining air flow heating during nebulization).

10.1.4.3. Prevention of Infection

Preventing infection is a major concern for neonatal ventilator patients, especially those with extremely low birth weights. Ventilator-associated pneumonia (VAP) is a common device-associated complication that occurs at a variable rate of 2.3 to 10.9 episodes per 1,000 ventilator days in developed countries. It is defined as a lung infection diagnosed in a patient who has been on a mechanical ventilator for more than 48 hours.

There are no widely recognized standards for diagnosing VAP in the newborn stage. Neonatals younger than 12 months old have been diagnosed with VAP using the Centers for Disease Control's guidelines, which include the following criteria: clinical (presence of tachypnea, apnea, and/or retractions; increased need of supplemental oxygen, respiratory settings to achieve targeted respiratory values, amount of respiratory secretions, incidence of desaturation events); radiological (persistent infiltrates or consolidation in two sequential radiographs after the initiation of mechanical ventilation); and microbiological (isolation of a microorganism obtained by bronchoalveolar lavage or isolation of a microorganism in blood culture without any other focus or histopathological examination). The diagnosis of VAP cannot be made with microbiological analysis of tracheal aspirates because airway colonization cannot be ruled out using this method. Bronchoscopic bronchoalveolar lavage and protected specimen brush are the gold standard for microbiological sampling of the airway; however, due to their invasive nature, they cannot be used universally on neonates intubated with small diameter tubes, for whom blind-protected bronchoalveolar lavage should be administered.

The incidence of VAP has been linked to several risk factors. A recent meta-analysis of observational studies has identified other factors such as low birth weight, prematurity, bronchopulmonary dysplasia, parenteral nutrition, length of hospital stay, enteral feeding, mechanical ventilation, transfusion, and length of hospital stay. However, duration of mechanical ventilation and ELBW infants appear to be the most significant in multivariate analysis. Conversely, there appears to be no effect on the VAP rate when the ventilator circuit changes are lowered from every seven to 14 days.

Gram-negative bacteria, especially *Pseudomonas aeruginosa, Enterobacter* species, and *Klebsiella* species, are the most frequently involved agents in VAP; however, Gram-positive bacteria, such as coagulase-negative staphylococci and *Staphylococcus aureus*, also have a part to play. When tracheal aspirate sampling is used, polymicrobial cultures are often discovered. There is disagreement over how to treat VAP initially. In light of probable causative agents and local patterns of antibiotic resistance, the first empirical treatment should consist of broad spectrum antibiotics that cover both Gram-positive and Gram-negative bacteria.

It has been demonstrated that implementing newborn VAP prevention bundles lowers the rate of VAP in NICUs. Combining multiple evidence-based practices into one bundle has been shown to improve practice more than the benefits of using each practice separately. These should cover head positioning techniques for neonates on ventilators, the use of closed, multiuse suction catheters, how often suctioning systems should be changed, routinely switching breathing circuits, assessing readiness for extubation and carefully evaluating whether reintubation is necessary, using medications that interfere with stomach acidity, using antibiotics for bowel decontamination and oral hygiene, and using separate suctioning equipment for the mouth and trachea. To reduce the incidence of VAP, improving caregiver education and hand hygiene is still crucial, just like it is for other infections linked to healthcare.

10.1.4.4. Sedation and Analgesia

It is now recognized that preterm infants have heightened pain sensitivity compared to older children, and that sedatives and analgesics can alleviate pain and stress due to physiologic changes brought on by intubation and invasive mechanical ventilation. These days, a crucial aspect of clinical practice is the prevention and management of pain and distress. According to a recent study that included 18 NICUs in Europe, only 46% of neonates on invasive ventilation had their continuous pain assessed. Despite the dissemination of national guidelines, another study revealed a generally widespread, but still highly variable, use of analgesia/sedation and pain assessment practices at Italian NICUs, indicating the urgent need to improve routine pain assessment and stress and pain control/ prevention in all infants.

Pain and stress management should be carried out following an accurate assessment of pain. It is necessary to try nonpharmacological interventions like sucrose and nonnutritive sucking. It is necessary to address their use in very preterm, unstable, ventilated neonates. It is not advisable to regularly administer sedation or analgesia to preterm neonates because of safety concerns with pharmaceuticals. However, morphine may be administered to preterm infants who continue to be ventilated. Remifentanil or fentanyl should be used very infrequently.

Neural midazolam worked better in the delivery room than ketamine at sufficiently sedated neonates who needed to be intubated. Both medications had similar effects on breathing and hemodynamics. Although they required ventilation more frequently, preterm infants receiving MIST (minimally invasive surfactant therapy) felt more at ease during sedation. To determine whether the advantages of sedation outweigh the risks of complications, a randomized controlled trial is required. Every NICU ought to have a protocol in place for managing neonatal pain and sedation. It can raise opiate exposure, but it doesn't appear to have an impact on the neurodevelopmental outcomes of very preterm infants. The potential for both short- and long-term adverse reactions must be taken into account, though, just like with any medication. The greatest amount of nonpharmacological therapy ought to be employed. It is not advised to use neuromuscular blocking agents in the NICU. To prevent the hemodynamic effects of deep sedation during quick diagnostic or therapeutic procedures, a transient curarization can be used.

10.1.4.5. Weaning and Extubation

Respiratory drive must be sufficient to maintain alveolar ventilation with a tidal volume of 4 ml/kg after weaning and extubation, which transfers the burden of breathing from the ventilator to the patient. If at all possible, sedation should be tapered off before extubation. FiO_2 should be lowered to below 0.40 as the patient's ventilation improves. Ventilatory parameters can also be lowered in conjunction with normal blood gases, but each should be lowered one at a time, starting with the most harmful one. Methylxanthines are beneficial for preterm newborns, and following extubation, these patients should begin using nasal CPAP or a high flow nasal cannula. After the first week of life, systemic steroids and diuretics may be helpful in extubating preterm infants who are still on ventilation. In certain situations, a hemoglobin level above 15 g/dl is recommended, and anemia may need to be treated. Diaphragmatic excursion can be enhanced and the chest wall stabilized with prone positioning. Generally speaking, unless there is clinical evidence of respiratory distress, a chest radiograph is not required.

10.1.4.6. Tracheostomy

A common necessity for newborns needing prolonged ventilation is a neonatal tracheostomy. Research indicates that early tracheostomy minimizes the risk of subglottic and tracheal stenosis in children undergoing prolonged intubation. It also leads to better comfort, less sedation and systemic corticosteroid use, better nutrition and growth, the capacity to try oral feedings, and, once established, vocalization using a speaking valve. Prolonged mechanical ventilation and occasionally tracheostomy may be necessary for the improved survival of extremely low birth weight and medically complex infants.

Over time, the indications for neonatal tracheostomy have evolved. It has become more prevalent due to the requirement for prolonged ventilation. Chronic medical conditions (cardiac disease, neuromuscular disease, bronchopulmonary dysplasia) and congenital or acquired airway obstruction are common indications for neonatal and infant tracheostomy. When making decisions regarding tracheostomy in neonates, several factors must be carefully taken into account. It is important to take into account factors like mortality, possible short- and long-term effects, chances for home ventilation therapy, and alternatives to tracheostomy.

The specific method for performing a neonatal tracheostomy should be done in the operating room and differs little from a well-executed tracheostomy. There is a chance that tracheostomy will cause severe morbidity. In order to lower the complication rate, surgical skill, experience, and specialized care may be important. However, in neonates, complications are typically minor and don't call for further surgical procedures.

10.1.5. Ventilation in Palliative Care

Some infants whose treatments are harmful, ineffective, or no longer beneficial may have their treatments discontinued after consulting with their family, despite advancements in neonatal medicine and intensive care. Keeping the infant comfortable and assisting the parents in raising their child in accordance with their values and preferences are the two main goals of palliative care.

The process of withdrawal entails informing the parents of what will happen, designating a staff member to remove the endotracheal tube and turn off the ventilator, aspirating the nasogastric tube (which may involve not feeding the child right before extubation), turning off the ventilator and monitor alarms before disconnecting them, suctioning the endotracheal tube before removal, and giving the parents the option to remain with their child during the procedure. If a baby is dying, it may be appropriate to stop providing less intrusive forms of respiratory support, such as nasal continuous positive airway pressure and nasal cannula oxygen, as continuing to do so will only cause the baby's death to be delayed. It is never appropriate to start neuromuscular blocking agents while the ventilator is being turned off. Ideally, the paralytics should have been weaned off hours or days earlier if the newborn had been using them. It is best to titrate sedatives and analgesics to relieve pain. Following extubation, children frequently experience increased pain, agitation, and dyspnea, necessitating higher dosages of medication. There are situations when lowering the ventilation parameters to minimum values—a decrease in oxygen—replaces turning off the ventilator or extubating the newborn. When there are indications of respiratory distress, noninvasive ventilation can help (Foglia et al, 2007; Turton, 2008; Morrow et al, 2009; Chang and Schibler, 2016; Ali et al, 2019).

10.1.6. Care in ECMO

The therapy known as extracorporeal membrane oxygenation, or ECMO, makes it possible to offer cardiorespiratory support. The veno-venous (VV) ECMO achieves this by raising the venous blood's oxygen concentration. By boosting systemic blood flow, veno-arterial (VA) ECMO may offer hemodynamic support in addition to raising blood oxygen content. In the event of pulmonary pathology, this technique ought to facilitate the restoration of pulmonary structure and function, thereby guaranteeing the neonate's survival.

After initiating VA-ECMO, ventilatory parameters can be rapidly weaned. The patient should remain during the treatment (to allow recovery of lung function) with "rest" settings (FiO_2 25–30%, peak inspiratory pressure (PIP) 20–25 cm H_2O; positive end expiratory pressure (PEEP) 4–5 cm H_2O; inspiratory time (Ti) 0.5–1.0 seconds; frequency (F) 20–25 breaths per minute) or even in continuous positive airway pressure (CPAP) with a high PEEP (10–12 cm H_2O) in order to maintain functional residual capacity (FRC) without causing lung injury (volutrauma, barotrauma, or atelectrauma). It is crucial to integrate the presence of two hearts and two lungs operating simultaneously with VA-ECMO. A decrease in arterial oxygen saturation may result from improved native cardiac function, but tissue oxygen delivery may increase.

Weaning off ventilatory and hemodynamic support after starting VV-ECMO should be done gradually and carefully because native lung function still facilitates gas exchanges while oxygen delivery depends on native cardiac function. Cardiac output and pulmonary blood flow can be harmed by using a high PEEP. The same resting parameters as for VA-ECMO will be used, but expired CO_2 should be used to maximize PEEP. Since the technique used ensures ventilation and oxygenation, mild and protective ventilatory strategies can and should be used during ECMO treatment. Severe technical malfunction rescue parameters (e.g., accidental decannulation) must be made evident and promptly adjusted on the ventilator in accordance with the patient's clinical status.

10.1.7. Complications: Air Leaks and Pulmonary Hemorrhage

Air leak syndrome, which encompasses pneumothorax, pulmonary interstitial emphysema, pneumomediastinum, pneumopericardium, pneumoperitoneum, subcutaneous emphysema, and systemic air embolism, is the extravasation of air from the tracheobronchial tree into the lung parenchyma and pleural spaces where it is not normally present. In up to 40% of ventilated newborns, air leaks are a common mechanical ventilation complication. Prematurity, extremely low birth weight, low Apgar score, high peak inspiratory pressure, high tidal volume, high inspiratory time, ventilator-associated pneumonia, aspiration of amniotic fluid, respiratory distress syndrome, and pulmonary hypoplasia are risk factors.

Pneumothorax is the most common type of air leak in neonates on mechanical ventilation. Pneumothorax risk is influenced by various ventilatory strategies; evidence suggests that continuous positive inspiratory pressure is linked to an increased risk of pneumothorax, while high-frequency ventilation, volume-targeted ventilation, and increased PEEP are associated with a decreased risk. Clinical manifestations can vary from mild respiratory distress to severe respiratory distress with progressive symptoms and hemodynamic compromise in cases of tension pneumothorax. A physical examination may show asymmetrical chest rise, muffled or shifted heart sounds, diminished breath sounds over the affected side, and tracheal deviation. Radiography is often used to make the diagnosis. It might be more challenging to identify the classic appearance in neonates, though. 46% of the neonates with pneumothorax had special radiological signs 0–27 hours before they were clinically diagnosed, according to a study assessing the role of special radiological signs in the diagnosis of pneumothorax in neonates. These signs included the double diaphragm sign, the basilar hyperlucency sign, the deep sulcus sign, increased cardio mediastinal sharpness, and basilar hyperlucency. Therefore, in order to make an early diagnosis of pneumothorax in ventilated newborns, these signs should be searched for.

Even before imaging is obtained, a tension pneumothorax needs to be diagnosed and treated right away. Chest transillumination can help in these situations. Conservative management, nitrogen washout with oxygen, needle aspiration, intercostals tube drainage, and pigtail catheter implantation are among the available treatment options. A study that solely involved adult patients found that 1.2% of the hemithorax's volume was spontaneously reabsorbed every 24 hours in cases of pneumothorax. Even in neonates receiving mechanical ventilation, expectant management may be beneficial, but most of the time, intervention is required. By establishing a diffusion gradient, exposing the baby to high oxygen concentrations may speed up the reabsorption of gas in the pleural space. However, the oxygen toxicity and elevated risk of preterm retinopathy in neonates limit the application of this technique. Although it might not always be the best course of action, needle thoracentesis combined with aspiration is the recommended treatment for emergencies like tension pneumothorax. A chest tube inserted via thoracostomy is the most common way of treating a pneumothorax. A recent systematic review, however, discovered insufficient data to assess the safety and effectiveness of intercostal tube drainage vs needle aspiration in the treatment of newborn pneumothorax.

Pigtail catheters have been used more recently to treat newborn pneumothorax; there is evidence that this treatment is safe, effective, and minimizes discomfort during insertion as well as complications, including those that affect preterm neonates. More prospective randomized controlled trials are required to establish the best approach for managing neonatal pneumothorax in patients on mechanical ventilation. Massive bleeding within the lung parenchyma and airways characterizes pulmonary hemorrhage, a rare but serious condition that has a neonatal mortality rate exceeding 50%. Prematurity, respiratory distress syndrome (RDS), exogenous surfactant use, and patent ductus arteriosus (PDA) are the most reliable risk factors for its occurrence. These risk factors are particularly relevant in premature infants born before 28 weeks of gestation and/or with a birth weight of less than 1000 grams. Pneumothorax, pulmonary infection, metabolic acidosis, shock, hypothermia, hypoglycemia, disseminated intravascular coagulation (DIC), ECMO therapy, hereditary coagulation disorders, and airway trauma (particularly after endotracheal intubation) are additional risk factors.

Clinical signs of pulmonary hemorrhage include hypoxia, hypercarbia, the need for higher ventilatory parameters, and a rapidly deteriorating pulmonary function (the rate of setting depends obviously on the magnitude of the hemorrhage). Aspirates taken from the trachea or oropharynx may reveal blood. With metabolic acidosis and shock, a systemic decline is established. A chest X-ray, an echocardiogram (to rule out a PDA), a sepsis work-up, and, if no other risk factors are found, a final screening for inherited coagulation disorders should be part of the investigations. General supportive measures, such as blood, plasma, or platelet transfusions as needed, metabolic acidosis correction, inotropic medication to raise systemic blood pressure, PDA treatment (apart from severe thrombocytopenia), antibiotic treatment, including vancomycin, and coverage for Gram-negative bacteria, should all be part of the treatment plan.

The ventilatory strategy used is essentially observational in nature; no evidence-based recommendations are made. It is advised to increase the positive end expiratory pressure (PEEP), mean airway pressure (Paw), and frequency (F) in conventional ventilatory support. Observational studies indicate that, in comparison to conventional support, high-frequency oscillatory ventilation (HFOV) support can control a greater number of cases of pulmonary hemorrhage, even though there is no proof for this claim. Nebulized epinephrine, repeated endotracheal tube instillations of epinephrine (0.05 mL of a 1:10,000 dilution), and treatment with recombinant factor VIIa (dose, frequency, and consistency of response not yet established in neonatal patients) are additional specific therapeutic measures (Foglia et al, 2007; Turton, 2008; Morrow et al, 2009; Chang and Schibler, 2016; Ali et al, 2019).

10.1.8. Monitoring of the Ventilated Neonate

Ventilation monitoring is crucial for maintaining a healthy oxygenation level and preventing hypercapnia and hypocapnia, which are linked to detrimental effects on both the preterm and term brains, in addition to respiratory care for the ventilated neonate. In the majority of real NICUs, standard procedures include capnography, transcutaneous carbon dioxide measurement, pH and blood gas measurements, and pulse oximetry. In adult and pediatric patients on mechanical ventilation, capnography is a standard tool; however, in neonates, it has limitations related to both physiology and technology. When using side-stream measurements, the high respiratory rate and low tidal volume of neonates necessitate main-stream sensors with quick response times, little dead space, and low suction flow. The measured end-tidal CO_2 (Pet CO_2), which should reflect the alveolar CO_2, is frequently misleading, and capnography is primarily used to assess the trend of Pet CO_2. These technical requirements are challenging to meet in neonates.

Currently, there are useful tools available to support clinical decision making in the management of ventilated infants, such as online pulmonary function and mechanics testing. They serve as a tool for managing infants on ventilators, evaluating therapy, and assessing the condition of the patient. Understanding pulmonary pathophysiology, physiology, and responses to mechanical ventilatory support is further enhanced by familiarity with pulmonary graphics. Such information is now provided by the new ventilators, which physicians ought to be aware of. A useful and often utilized tool in the NICU, neonatal echocardiography can make a significant contribution to the hemodynamic management of the ventilated neonate. It plays a significant role in ruling out a congenital heart defect, managing a patent ductus arteriosus, evaluating pulmonary hypertension, evaluating cases of hypotension or shock, and monitoring the response to therapy.

By monitoring the regional cerebral saturation in oxygen, non-invasive cerebral regional sympatholysis (NIRS) may be able to prevent intraventricular hemorrhage or periventricular leukomalacia in neonates by serving as an early warning system for low cerebral blood flow and oxygenation. Because neonates are particularly sensitive to repeated radiation exposure and because lung immaturity has its own unique pathology, lung ultrasonography is an emerging diagnostic tool that can be useful in monitoring. According to short, neonatal patients have particular physiological traits, and invasive ventilation is frequently required for the treatment of newborns with respiratory insufficiency. Every clinical scenario requires a comprehensive focus on the patient's overall clinical status and related comorbidities. Individualized respiratory care must be tailored to the patient's characteristics, clinical status, coexisting conditions, and overall prognosis (Foglia et al, 2007; Turton, 2008; Morrow et al, 2009; Chang and Schibler, 2016; Ali et al, 2019).

10.2. VENTILATOR-ASSOCIATED PNEUMONIA

In pediatric intensive care units, ventilator-associated pneumonia (VAP) is among the most prevalent infections related to healthcare. A positive lower respiratory tract microbiology result and/or two or more positive clinical signs of pneumonia (signs of inflammation, impaired gas exchange) are combined to form a diagnosis of ventilator-associated pneumonia (VAP). The methods of sampling that are employed determine the positive microbiology results. In tracheal aspirate, $\geq 10^5$ colony-forming units (CFU), $\geq 10^4$ in bronchoalveolar lavage, and $\geq 10^3$ in protective specimen brush culture are considered positive. In ICU patients, ventilator-associated pneumonia (VAP) remains a major cause of morbidity and death despite advances in prevention strategies, therapy, and understanding of the pathophysiology of the disease. A study found that VAP develops in 10% of patients on mechanical ventilation, and in 13% of those cases, it is a fatal complication. The global incidence of ventilator-associated pneumonia (VAP) in pediatric intensive care units (PICUs) ranges from 1 to 63 episodes per 1000 ventilator days. Additionally, VAP is linked to higher hospital stay costs and duration, higher usage of broad-spectrum antibiotics, and significant medical expenses. Thus, it is important to prioritize developing strategies to stop VAP from developing. There has been minimal research on the effects of those bundles on ventilated pediatric patients, despite the fact that a number of interventions have been found to lower the incidence of VAP in adult patients. The majority of the known risk factors for developing VAP include enteral feeding and the use of specific medications, e.g., either histamine-2 receptor blockers or proton pump inhibitors, the latter of which, by reducing acid production, permits nosocomial pathogens to colonize the aero-digestive tract and endotracheal tube. The former frequently causes regurgitation. Maintaining tracheal cuff pressure, avoiding overdistention of the stomach or equipment contamination, and minimizing unnecessary tracheal suction or re-intubation are all important considerations. Furthermore, aspiration risks are higher in patients with genetic syndromes, neurological or cardiovascular conditions that require hospital admission or prolonged mechanical ventilation. The majority of bacteria that are cultured from endotracheal aspirates obtained from VAP patients are also cultured from gastric and naso-oropharyngeal secretions. Considering everything mentioned above, the most popular preventative techniques in pediatric intensive care units involve cleaning hands, rinsing the mouth with an antiseptic solution, and raising the bed to a 30-degree angle. Others include minimizing ventilation days, draining ventilator condensate away from the patient on a regular basis, and only altering the ventilator circuit when necessary.

The prognosis depends heavily on the timely diagnosis. Nevertheless, given the wide range of differential diagnoses for inpatient respiratory declines, this can be challenging despite numerous guidelines. The clinical presentation of symptoms that appear after 48 hours of mechanical ventilation and necessitate adjusting the ventilator's settings serves as the basis for the diagnosis. Many studies concur that the primary evidence for a VAP diagnosis in chest imaging is a new lung infiltrate. In order to isolate the etiological pathogen and customize the antibiotic treatment, a number of tests must be conducted promptly. These include collecting blood and sputum samples for cultures, obtaining PCR-based tracheal sputum (from suctioning or from the BAL procedure), nasopharyngeal swabs, and imaging techniques. The imaging method is still the gold standard for diagnosing VAP (along with the pathogen identification, signs of inflammation, and/or impaired gas exchange). However, a potential change in recent years may be attributed to the rapid diagnosis of pneumonia at the bedside using lung ultrasonography. Chest X-rays and lung computed tomography are still regarded as the gold standard, even with the use of ultrasound.

In terms of therapy, starting broad-spectrum empirical antibiotic therapy is typically the first move. Following confirmation of the causative pathogen, a particular antibiotic treatment—to which the pathogen is susceptible—is selected (e.g., medicine de-escalation). Typically, *Pseudomonas* species are the causative agents. *Staphylococcus aureus* and numerous Gram-negative bacteria; the distribution and prevalence of these pathogenic microorganisms differ amongst pediatric intensive care units worldwide. (Foglia et al, 2007; Turton, 2008; Morrow et al, 2009; Chang and Schibler, 2016; Ali et al, 2019)

10.2.1. Diagnosis

Even though VAP is important for clinical practice, no gold standard for a VAP diagnostic has yet been established. This might negatively affect how quickly VAP management acts. All of the following are necessary for the diagnosis of VAP: fever, productive cough, respiratory decline, and new lung infiltrates on chest imaging.

The likelihood of diagnosing VAP decreases if the imaging shows no new lung infiltrate, and consideration of other possible causes of inpatient respiratory decline must then be given. However, it should be noted that only a few signs of inflammation may be seen on the X-ray in the early stages of pneumonia development, and it should be repeated over time in patients with high clinical suspicion (e.g., sputum production characteristics, cough, and fever). In addition, at least two or three of the following should be present in the standard diagnostic criteria: fever greater than 38°C or hypothermia lower than 36°C; change in sputum volume or character or increased need for suctioning; new or worsening cough; dyspnea, tachypnea, or apnea; breathing difficulties such as rales during pathological pulmonary auscultation; and wheezing, rhonchi, or bronchial breath sounds. Additional criteria include altered hemodynamics (tachycardia or bradycardia), worsening of gas exchange following a period of stability or improvement on the ventilator, and positive serum biomarkers (leukocytosis, procalcitonin, or C-reactive protein).

All of these clinical criteria, which are not unique to pneumonia and have significant overlap with sepsis from other potential etiologies, pose a diagnostic challenge. Many of the above-mentioned signs and symptoms are frequently seen in patients receiving prolonged mechanical ventilation, or they may be the result of other concurrent morbidities. On the other hand, the concurrent medication that is frequently given to critically ill patients may significantly alter the clinical presentation of VAP.

The Centers for Disease Control and Prevention (CDC) listed criteria have been accepted and applied in other contexts for the diagnosis of both adult and pediatric patients. The Clinical Pulmonary Infection Score (CPIS) and the Great Ormond Street Hospital (GOSH) criteria may also be used as additional criteria. The radiographic evidence of pneumonia is what unites all these different approaches to diagnosing ventilator-associated pneumonia (VAP); the variations lie in the clinical criteria and their respective combinations. However, there are challenges in implementing these VAP criteria, primarily related to the reliance on subjective clinical symptoms and the need for radiographic proof of lung infiltrate.

It is advised to obtain blood cultures since they play a crucial role in differential diagnosis by either identifying the pathogen of interest if respiratory cultures are inconclusive or by alerting us to the existence of other infections unrelated to the respiratory tract. The ability of the inpatient to provide a sufficient sample of sputum limits the acquisition of sputum cultures. Simple sputum production by an active cough may not be sufficient for patients unable to produce sufficient samples. Other options include bronchoscopy, bronchoalveolar lavage, or endotracheal aspiration (which is preferred over the other options). Only immunocompromised patients or patients who are not responding to therapy may benefit from invasive and quantitative methods, which have the potential to cause harm and discomfort to patients while offering no advantages.

A crucial step in identifying the causing pathogen is PCR testing. The nasal swab for *Staphylococcus aureus* demonstrates high negative predictive value for methicillin-resistant *S. aures* colonization and can be used as an antibiotic stewardship tool, prompting safe discontinuation of anti-MRSA therapy when negative. The nasopharyngeal swab is another well-known PCR-based test that is used to test the respiratory viral panel. It is especially recommended to use this test during influenza season as it helps determine the appropriate therapy by identifying the viral origin of the infection. PCR testing, also known as tracheal aspirate/BAL, is a fast, dependable technique that has a high sensitivity to bacteria from sputum these days. The high frequency of non-invasive bacterial brands colonizing the airway can lead to false positive results from PCR testing, which may be useful in a few hours. The PCR results were consistently interpreted as numerical results—e.g., indicating the level of bacterial or viral load in the chosen specimen) should be interpreted in conjunction with the clinical status of the patient.

Procalcitonin testing assists in determining the length of therapy, alerts us to coinfection, and helps distinguish between viral and bacterial infections. Antibiotic therapy can be started based solely on clinical judgment, but procalcitonin-guided antibiotic discontinuation has been linked to lower treatment costs and a lower death rate.

Pseudomonas species are frequent etiological agents that cause VAP. several Gram-negative bacteria, including *Staphylococcus aureus*. There is a difference in the percentage of these organisms in the PICUs and ICUs. Furthermore, we are able to distinguish between early and late VAP onset, which have different origins. For early-onset *Staphylococcus aureus*, the usual causative agents are *Streptococcus pneumoniae* and *Haemophilus influenzae*. *Pseudomonas* spp. for late-onset VAP. *Acinetobacter* species. and specific Gram-negative bacteria found in the stomach. When pneumonia develops four days or less after starting mechanical ventilation, it is referred to as early-onset pneumonia; pneumonia that develops more than five days later is referred to as late-onset pneumonia. For instance, these pathogenic organisms—*Acinetobacter*, *Pseudomonas*, *Klebsiella*, *Enterobacter*, and *E. coli* were found to be the most frequently isolated causative agents of VAP in a prospective cohort study conducted in North India.

10.2.2. Management

Given that early empirical antibiotic treatment reduces the risk of sepsis and the ensuing adverse prognosis, it is thought to be essential for the treatment of VAP. On the other hand, patients who received antibiotics quickly after exhibiting symptoms may require longer therapy durations and have a higher mortality rate, most likely as a result of resistant pathogen selection. Individuals with respiratory or hemodynamic instability, immunocompromised individuals, and those for whom it is not possible to adequately sample respiratory tract secretions are among those who may benefit from prompt and aggressive antibiotic treatment, that is, before the sample cultivation results are available.

Empirical ATB therapy ought to be started if it has been decided to treat a patient with suspected VAP. The frequency and resistance of hospital bacteria in the area should be taken into account while selecting a particular antibiotic. We should use empirical coverage of methicillin-susceptible *S. aureus* and Gram-negative bacteria, such as piperacillin–tazobactam, cefepime, levofloxacin, imipenem, and meropenem, if no such institution-specific antibiogram is available. *Pseudomonas aeruginosa* is frequently cultured from patients who have acquired vancomycin-associated pneumonia (VAP) and may be resistant to multiple antibiotic classes. Combination therapy should be started to address all potential causative agents in patients or environments where there is a high likelihood of antibiotic resistance and sepsis-related symptoms. Patients who have recently had intravenous antibiotic treatment, are more likely to die, or are in intensive care units (ICUs), where Gram-negative pathogens are frequently resistant, must receive antibiotics in combination. Antibiotics from two distinct classes ought to be selected, ideally. Antipseudomonal monotherapy patients may experience delays in starting appropriate, effective antipseudomonal medications.

The empirical coverage of MRSA raises additional questions. Not every patient needs to be treated with linezolid or vancomycin. Patients who are at high risk of death, those hospitalized in a unit where the prevalence of MRSA is either unknown or at least 20%, and those who have previously received intravenous antibiotic therapy should not be administered these antibiotics. Certain infections causing VAP may only be sensitive to aminoglycosides or polymyxins when it comes to antibiotic class and mode of administration. It is well known that certain antibiotic classes can cause renal damage, especially when administered intravenously. Inhaled aminoglycosides or colistin should be administered in combination with their intravenous formulations if such a circumstance arises. Furthermore, inhaled versions of the aforementioned antibiotics aid in achieving greater concentrations at the infection site, which enhance clinical cure rates and shorten the need for mechanical ventilation.

The next step in the therapy is to customize the antibiotic treatment based on the pathogen culture cultivation and its resistance, regardless of whether the empiric antibiotic regimen is started or not. Aspiration is known to be a significant risk factor for developing VAP because it frequently results in the colonization of microorganisms. Therefore, the final antibiotic regimen should cover oral and enteric flora, including Gram-negative and anaerobic bacteria, to treat a patient with suspected aspiration. For patients with simple VAP, the course of antibiotic treatment lasts for seven days. The length of therapy is longer and specific to the complication if there are complications like empyema, bacteremia, cases of pneumonia from Pseudomonas or Acinetobacter species, or other pulmonary or extrapulmonary complications. Generally speaking, using cephalosporins or potentiated beta-lactams (e. g., cefotaxime) for VAP with an early onset and piperacillin-tazobactam for VAP with a late onset, along with aminoglycosides in case pseudomonas infection is suspected (Foglia et al, 2007; Turton, 2008; Morrow et al, 2009; Chang and Schibler, 2016; Ali et al, 2019).

10.2.3. Prevention

The primary strategy for prevention is to alter the established VAP risk factors. Table 10.2 lists the VAP risk factors that have been identified.

Table 10.2. Summary of Risk Factors and Preventive Measures Identified in the Literature

Risk Factors	• Enteral feeding • Medication (e.g., proton pump inhibitors, histamine 2-receptor blockers) • Re-intubation • Aspiration of secretions • Use of contaminated equipment • Presence of genetic syndrome or neurological/cardiovascular disease • Duration of mechanical ventilation

Preventive Measures	• Hand hygiene • Mouth rise with antiseptic solution • Maintenance of endotracheal cuff pressure of at least 20 cm H_2O • Semi-recumbent position • Changing of the ventilator circuit only when visibly soiled • Draining ventilator condensate away • Minimizing ventilator days

Source: Antalová N, Klučka J, Říhová M, Poláčková S, Pokorná A, Štourač P. Ventilator-associated pneumonia prevention in pediatric patients: Narrative review. Children (Basel). 2022;9(10):1540. doi: 10.3390/children9101540. PMID: 36291475; PMCID: PMC9600673.

The preventive techniques can be categorized into two easy-to-understand categories: the first is preventive complex care, which entails medical staff members taking care of patients on their own. That would entail practicing good oral and hand hygiene on a regular basis, which the medical staff should adhere to religiously. This group also includes the patient's head positioning, a well-chosen feeding method and how it is administered, and medication. These are all primarily focused on preventing aspiration. The second category would include handling and maintaining the equipment properly, including tubes, suctioning methods, switching out ventilation circuits, and other appropriate procedures related to artificial ventilation.

Maintaining good hand hygiene by medical personnel is crucial to stopping the spread of multi-resistant bacteria and infections linked to healthcare. Therefore, it is highly advised that hand hygiene be included in the VAP bundle. Subsequent research has shown that maintaining good hand hygiene is relevant to lowering VAP. Since poor oral hygiene has been linked to the development of VAP, hospital care should include providing oral hygiene to ventilated patients. Bacteria that colonize the oral cavity also colonize the lungs, the trachea, and the tracheostomy tube, which may facilitate easy access to the lung tissue. Regarding oral hygiene in ventilated patients, there are two primary pillars: the first is mouthwash use, which primarily entails decontaminating the mouth with solutions containing chlorhexidine. This chemical antiseptic has been proposed because it can inhibit the growth of yeast and bacteria, lessen the accumulation of dental plaque, and thereby prevent gingivitis. Therefore, the effects of chlorhexidine mouthwashes may lessen lung exposure to pathogenic bacteria when micro-aspiration of oral secretions occurs, after minimizing the colonization of the oral cavity. Second, dental plaque and debris are removed using foam swabs or oral toothbrushes. However, the recommendation states that dipping these in tap water could contaminate them with pathogenic bacteria, so critically ill patients shouldn't use this as a way to lower their risk of contracting an infection linked to healthcare.

In the ICU setting, medical staff hygiene is crucial for preventing ventilator-associated pneumonia (VAP) and should be strictly enforced as part of inpatient care. One important component of VAP prevention is positioning. Elevating the head of the bed while the patient is in a semi-recumbent position is advised. For neonates, the head of the bed should be elevated between 15 and 30 degrees, and for older children or infants, between 30 and 45 degrees. A clinical randomized cross-over trial showed that patients maintained in the supine position had a higher risk of aspirating stomach content into the airway, even when the endotracheal tube cuff was properly inflated. Furthermore, there was a direct correlation between the duration of a patient's supine position and the rise in aspiration contents. Due to gravitational forces, in the semi-recumbent position, contaminated secretions would cross the tracheal cuff and enter the lower respiratory tract when there is a drop in airway pressure. This movement would be accelerated by suctioning. In addition, secretions cannot be removed from the lower respiratory tract without active suctioning. Comparing patients in the semi-recumbent position against those in the lateral horizontal position, another study discovered that the incidence of aspirating gastric secretions was similar in both groups. More research is required to assess the direct clinical impact of positioning on the incidence of vertical amputation pneumonia (VAP), as there is currently insufficient high-quality evidence of a direct, proven advantage of the semi-recumbent position.

Due to the possibility of regurgitation, enteral feeding is thought to be another significant risk factor for the development of VAP. We can only surmise that putting preventative strategies into practice while keeping in mind everything previously mentioned will enable us to enhance the care given to ventilated patients while lowering the risk of developing VAP. Prophylactics for peptic ulcers (H2 blockers and proton pump inhibitors, or PPIs) elevate the pH of the stomach and may increase the colonization of harmful bacteria in the stomach, raising the risk of developing VAP. The study found that using acid-suppressive medications was associated with a higher incidence of VAP.

Regarding the use of probiotics to prevent VAP, a prophylactic probiotic regimen decreased the incidence of mucolytic agents, like ambroxol, which may be advantageous to ventilated patients in terms of lowering their chance of developing VAP. Moreover, this agent has anti-inflammatory and antioxidant qualities. In addition to these characteristics, ambroxol also modifies the biofilm structure of *P. aeruginosa* and makes antibiotics more permeable through the biofilm. When compared to the control group, the ambroxol-treated patients had substantially lower bacterial counts on the biofilm-covered tubes. Furthermore, when ambroxol was added to the treatment plan, there were less bacterial counts in the lungs as well as milder pathological alterations in the lungs.

Given its potential to reduce aspiration risk and the need for a higher tube exchange rate, the use of cuffed tubes in clinical settings seems reasonable. According to a study that compared the use of cuffed and uncuffed tubes, the tracheal exchange rate was lower when using cuffed tubes—21% versus 30% when using uncuffed tubes. Because one of the main risk factors for VAP is micro-aspirations of oral secretions, using cuffed tubes may help prevent this condition because of the superior tracheal seal's ability to reduce micro-aspirations. All children could safely use the endotracheal high-volume low-pressure cuffed tubes with cuff pressure monitoring.

When cuff pressure is maintained at less than 20 cm H_2O and regular cuff pressure monitoring is carried out with cuff-specific devices, there is no increased risk of post-extubation stridor. The retention of secretion in the subglottic area (over the cuff) may still result in pericuff leak even with appropriate cuff management. Specialized cuffed tubes that allow for secretion clearance (by direct suctioning) from the subglottic area could partially solve this issue (Figure 10.2).

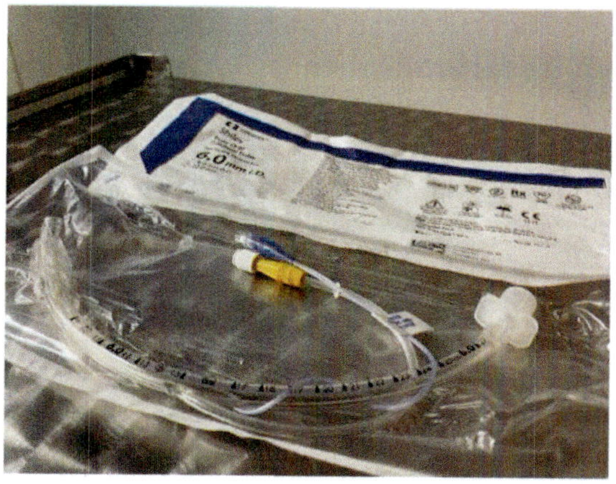

Figure 10.2. *Endotracheal tube with a subglottic suction.*

Source: Antalová N, Klučka J, Říhová M, Poláčková S, Pokorná A, Štourač P. (2022). Ventilator-associated pneumonia prevention in pediatric patients: Narrative review. Children (Basel), 9(10):1540. doi: 10.3390/children9101540. PMID: 36291475; PMCID: PMC9600673.

To avoid contaminating the respiratory system, aseptic techniques must be used when performing endotracheal suction. A study that found a correlation between the bacteria on respiratory equipment and those in the patient's mouth and sputum further supported this. It was discovered that the pathogenic bacteria that colonized the suction tubes during the first 24 hours were comparable to those in the patient's mouth and sputum, based on previously published data. The contrast between open vs. Numerous studies were conducted regarding the incidence of VAP in closed suction systems. Because open-system suctioning procedures can lead to specific complications like hypoxia, cross infections, and environmental contamination, it is preferable to use a closed suction system. Although open suction systems have this clear drawback, neither system was found to have a different VAP incidence.

Re-intubation increases the risk of ventilator-associated pneumonia. Aspiration of stomach contents during the time between extubation and re-intubation may provide an explanation. An alternative theory offered by a different study is that bacteria enter the lungs directly through the endotracheal tube when the ventilator circuit is disconnected. It might be possible to include the frequency of ventilator circuit changes in VAP prevention bundles. To explore and determine the frequency of humidified circuitry replacement, multiple randomized controlled trials were carried out. These studies all provided evidence in favor of the theory that there was no rise in the incidence of ventilator-associated pneumonia (VAP) when the frequency of ventilator circuit changes was decreased.

Studies that have been done on prevention bundles have mentioned evaluating a patient's preparedness for extubation, but they do not advise stopping sedation daily for pediatric patients. The risk of unintentional extubation in young children is taken into account when advising against sedation holidays. Every tactic lowers the risk of aspiration. One intensive care unit created a task force and educational program to increase public awareness of the significance of aspiration and how to prevent it, along with the regular evaluation of compliance with preventive measures. In addition to greatly increasing compliance, the intervention that resulted in the task force and educational plan's creation also reduced the number of ventilation days, reduced VAP by 51%, and saved healthcare costs. The use of aspiration-prevention techniques and educational materials can lower the risk of aspiration and the pneumonia that goes along with it. (Foglia et al, 2007; Turton, 2008; Morrow et al, 2009; Chang and Schibler, 2016; Ali et al, 2019)

A Closer Look

Assessment of the Patient on Admission

To help the nurse plan appropriate care, the patient's overall condition should be evaluated to determine the severity of the illness. For example, nasogastric intubation, positioning, and oxygen administration will be prepared for a child exhibiting abdominal distension and dyspnea.

- **Weighing:** To ensure precise calculations and administration of medications and intravenous fluids, the child needs to be weighed. Sufficient hydration is crucial for the best possible outcome in children undergoing surgery.
- **Nutritional Status:** An evaluation of the child's nutritional status is necessary. An ideal nutritional state will promote a quick recovery and lessen the need for unneeded hospital stays, financial hardships, time missed from school, and morbidity and death.
- Hydration status: Especially in neonates, maintaining adequate hydration will guarantee optimal renal function and a better response to medications.
- **Personal Hygiene:** Maintaining proper personal hygiene lowers the risk of nosocomial infections, including wound infections.
- **Jaundice:** The child needs to be evaluated for jaundice, which can sometimes be a sign of an obstructive illness such as biliary atresia and frequently indicates the 70 of an infectious process.
- **Full Examination:** Additionally, this will highlight any hidden abnormalities that the mother might have overlooked, such as hypospadia, anal stenosis, undescended testicles, and spinal bifida.

Summary

- There is an increasing trend in the neonatal intensive care units (NICUs) to use noninvasive ventilation modes; however, invasive ventilation is still often necessary for treating preterm and term infants with respiratory insufficiency.
- The endotracheal tube (ETT), the fundamental interface between patient and ventilator, is a cornerstone for successful ventilation. The appropriate sized tube could be defined as the one with the largest possible inner diameter (ID) that will comfortably pass through the vocal cords providing a sufficient seal for effective ventilation.
- In neonates undergoing mechanical ventilation, it has been observed that positions other than the standard supine position, such as the prone position, may improve respiratory performance.
- The neonatal patient has physiological characteristics such as difficult airway maintenance and clearance, smaller airway caliber, few collateral airways, compliant chest wall, poor airway stability, and lower functional residual capacity.
- Nurses caring for newborns receiving mechanical ventilation face several challenges. Observing the monitor, ventilation devices, oxygen delivery systems, and patient's oxygenation along with the patient himself are essential components of nursing care.
- Despite advances in neonatal medicine and intensive care, there are some infants whose treatments are harmful, are not or are no longer beneficial, and may be discontinued after discussion with the family. Palliative care aims to keep the baby comfortable and to support the parents in caring for their baby according to their wishes and beliefs.
- ECMO (extracorporeal membrane oxygenation) is a treatment that allows to provide cardiorespiratory support. The veno-venous (VV) ECMO does so by increasing the oxygen content in the venous blood. Veno-arterial (VA) ECMO, in addition to increasing blood oxygen content, may provide hemodynamic support by increasing systemic blood flow. This technique, in the presence of pulmonary pathology, should allow the recovery of pulmonary structure and function to ensure the survival of the newborn.
- Air leak syndrome refers to the extravasation of air from the tracheobronchial tree into the lung parenchyma and pleural spaces where it is not normally present, and includes pneumothorax, pulmonary interstitial emphysema, pneumomediastinum, pneumopericardium, pneumoperitoneum, subcutaneous emphysema, and systemic air embolism.
- Along with respiratory care for the ventilated neonate, ventilation monitoring is of great importance for good oxygenation avoiding hypercapnia and hypocapnia, both associated with deleterious effects not only on preterm but also on the term brain.
- Ventilator-associated pneumonia (VAP) is one of the most common healthcare-associated infections in pediatric ICUs. VAP is defined as a new infiltrate chest X-ray together with positive microbiology findings from the lower respiratory tract and/or two or more positive clinical signs of pneumonia (signs of inflammation, gas exchange impairment).

References

1. Beardsley, A. L., Nitu, M. E., Cox, E. G., & Benneyworth, B. D. (2016). An evaluation of various ventilator-associated infection criteria in a PICU. *Pediatric Critical Care Medicine, 17*, 73–80.
2. Bickenbach, J., & Marx, G. (2013). Diagnosis of pneumonia in mechanically ventilated patients: What is the meaning of the CPIS? *Minerva Anesthesiologic, 79*, 1406–1414.
3. Bradley, J. (2010). Considerations unique to pediatrics for clinical trial design in hospital-acquired pneumonia and ventilator-associated pneumonia. *Clinical Infectious Diseases, 51*, S136–S143.
4. Brierley, J., Highe, L., Hines, S., & Dixon, G. (2012). Reducing VAP by instituting a care bundle using improvement methodology in a UK pediatric intensive care unit. *European Journal of Pediatrics, 171*, 323–330.
5. Chang, I., & Schibler, A. (2016). Ventilator associated pneumonia in children. *Pediatric Respiratory Reviews, 20*, 10–16.
6. Chomton, M., Brossier, D., Sauthier, M., Vallières, E., Dubois, J., Emeriaud, G., et al. (2018). Ventilator-associated pneumonia and events in pediatric intensive care: A single center study. *Pediatric Critical Care Medicine, 19*, 1106–1113.
7. Citak, A., Karaböcüoğlu, M., Uçsel, R., Uğur-Baysal, S., & Uzel, N. (2000). Bacterial nosocomial infections in mechanically ventilated children. *The Turkish Journal of Pediatrics, 42*, 39–42.
8. Cocoros, N. M., & Klompas, M. (2016). Ventilator-associated events and their prevention. *Infectious Disease Clinics of North America, 30*, 887–908.
9. da Silva, P. S. L., de Aguiar, V. E., de Carvalho, W. B., & Machado Fonseca, M. C. (2014). Value of clinical pulmonary infection score in critically ill children as a surrogate for diagnosis of ventilator-associated pneumonia. *Journal of Critical Care, 29*, 545–550.
10. Ericson, J. E., McGuire, J., Michaels, M. G., Schwarz, A., Frenck, R., Deville, J. G., et al. (2020). Hospital-acquired pneumonia and ventilator-associated pneumonia in children: A prospective natural history and case-control study. *The Pediatric Infectious Disease Journal, 39*, 658–664.
11. Foglia, E., Meier, M. D., & Elward, A. (2007). Ventilator-associated pneumonia in neonatal and pediatric intensive care unit patients. *Clinical Microbiology Reviews, 20*, 409–425.
12. Gionfriddo, A., Nonoyama, M. L., Laussen, P. C., Cox, P. N., Clarke, M., & Floh, A. A. (2018). Retrospective application of new pediatric ventilator-associated pneumonia criteria identifies a high-risk population. *Pediatric Critical Care Medicine, 19*, 507–512.
13. Jacobs Pepin, B., Lesslie, D., Berg, W., Spaulding, A. B., & Pokora, T. (2019). ZAP-VAP: A quality improvement initiative to decrease ventilator-associated pneumonia in the neonatal intensive care unit, 2012–2016. *Advances in Neonatal Care, 19*, 253–261.
14. Joy, B. F., & Brilli, R. J. (2016). Is the new really better than the old? *Pediatric Critical Care Medicine, 17*, 95–96.
15. Kabak, E., Hudcova, J., Magyarics, Z., Stulik, L., Goggin, M., Szijártó, V., et al. (2019). The utility of endotracheal aspirate bacteriology in identifying mechanically ventilated patients at risk for ventilator-associated pneumonia: A single-center prospective observational study. *BMC Infectious Diseases, 19*, 756.

16. Karakuzu, Z., Iscimen, R., Akalin, H., Kelebek Girgin, N., Kahveci, F., & Sinirtas, M. (2018). Prognostic risk factors in ventilator-associated pneumonia. *Medical Science Monitor, 24*, 1321–1328.

17. Karandikar, M. V., Coffin, S. E., Priebe, G. P., Sandora, T. J., Logan, L. K., Larsen, G. Y., et al. (2019). Variability in antimicrobial use in pediatric ventilator-associated events. *Infection Control & Hospital Epidemiology, 40*, 32–39.

18. Klompas, M. (2010). Prevention of ventilator-associated pneumonia. *Expert Review of Anti-Infective Therapy, 8*, 791–800.

19. Kobayashi, H., Uchino, S., Takinami, M., & Uezono, S. (2017). The impact of ventilator-associated events in critically ill subjects with prolonged mechanical ventilation. *Respiratory Care, 62*, 1379–1386.

20. Lauzier, F., Ruest, A., Cook, D., Dodek, P., Albert, M., Shorr, A. F., et al. (2008). The value of pretest probability and modified clinical pulmonary infection score to diagnose ventilator-associated pneumonia. *Journal of Critical Care, 23*, 50–57.

21. Lodha, R., & Kabra, S. K. (2011). Diagnosis of ventilator-associated pneumonia: Is there a simple solution? *Indian Pediatrics, 48*, 939–940.

22. Mohd Ali, N. A., Jauncey-Cooke, J., & Bogossian, F. (2019). Ventilator-associated events in children: A review of literature. *Australian Critical Care, 32*, 55–62.

23. Morrow, B. M., Argent, A. C., Jeena, P. M., & Green, R. J. (2009). Guideline for the diagnosis, prevention and treatment of pediatric ventilator-associated pneumonia. *South African Medical Journal, 99*, 255–267.

24. Morrow, B. M., Mowzer, R., Pitcher, R., & Argent, A. C. (2012). Investigation into the effect of closed-system suctioning on the frequency of pediatric ventilator-associated pneumonia in a developing country. *Pediatric Critical Care Medicine, 13*, e25–e32.

25. Mourani, P. M., Sontag, M. K., Williamson, K. M., Harris, J. K., Reeder, R., Locandro, C., et al. (2021). Temporal airway microbiome changes related to ventilator-associated pneumonia in children. *The European Respiratory Journal, 57*, 2001829.

26. Niederman, M. S. (2010). Hospital-acquired pneumonia, health care-associated pneumonia, ventilator-associated pneumonia, and ventilator-associated tracheobronchitis: Definitions and challenges in trial design. *Clinical Infectious Diseases, 51*, S12–S17.

27. Osman, S., Al Talhi, Y. M., AlDabbagh, M., Baksh, M., Osman, M., & Azzam, M. (2020). The incidence of ventilator-associated pneumonia (VAP) in a tertiary-care center: Comparison between pre- and post-VAP prevention bundle. *Journal of Infection and Public Health, 13*, 552–557.

28. Peña-López, Y., Pujol, M., Campins, M., González-Antelo, A., Rodrigo, J. Á., Balcells, J., et al. (2016). Implementing a care bundle approach reduces ventilator-associated pneumonia and delays ventilator-associated tracheobronchitis in children: Differences according to endotracheal or tracheostomy devices. *International Journal of Infectious Diseases, 52*, 43–48.

29. Prinzi, A., Parker, S. K., Thurm, C., Birkholz, M., & Sick-Samuels, A. (2021). Association of endotracheal aspirate culture variability and antibiotic use in mechanically ventilated pediatric patients. *JAMA Network Open, 4*, e2140378.

30. Pugin, J. (2002). Clinical signs and scores for the diagnosis of ventilator-associated pneumonia. *Minerva Anesthesiologic, 68*, 261–265.

31. Ramirez-Estrada, S., Peña-Lopez, Y., Kalwaje Eshwara, V., & Rello, J. (2018). Ventilator-associated events versus ventilator-associated respiratory infections: Moving into a new paradigm or merging both concepts, instead? *Annals of Translational Medicine, 6*, 425.

32. Rello, J., Ramírez-Estrada, S., Romero, A., Arvaniti, K., Koulenti, D., Nseir, S., et al. (2019). Factors associated with ventilator-associated events: An international multicenter prospective cohort study. *European Journal of Clinical Microbiology & Infectious Diseases, 38*, 1693–1699.

33. Robinson, S., & Westrope, C. (2019). Ventilator associated pneumonia UHL Children's Intensive Care Guideline. (Report No.: C43/2016). University Hospital of Leicester, NHS.

34. Rogerson, C. M., Beardsley, A. L., Nitu, M. E., & Cristea, A. I. (2020). Health care resource utilization for children requiring prolonged mechanical ventilation via tracheostomy. *Respiratory Care, 65*, 1147–1153.

35. Sachdev, A., Chugh, K., Sethi, M., Gupta, D., Wattal, C., & Menon, G. (2011). Clinical pulmonary infection scores to diagnose ventilator-associated pneumonia in children. *Indian Pediatrics, 48*, 949–954.

36. Schurink, C. A. M. (2022). Clinical Pulmonary Infection Score (CPIS) for Ventilator-Associated Pneumonia (VAP). MDCalc. Retrieved from: https://www.mdcalc.com/clinical-pulmonary-infection-score-cpis-ventilator-associated-pneumonia-vap#next-steps (accessed on 11 September 2024).

37. Shein, S. L., Karam, O., Beardsley, A., Karsies, T., Prentice, E., Tarquinio, K. M., et al. (2019). Development of an antibiotic guideline for children with suspected ventilator-associated infections. *Pediatric Critical Care Medicine, 20*, 697–706.

38. Stover, B. H., Shulman, S. T., Bratcher, D. F., Brady, M. T., Levine, G. L., & Jarvis, W. R. (2001). Nosocomial infection rates in US children's hospitals' neonatal and pediatric intensive care units. *American Journal of Infection Control, 29*, 152–157.

39. Tarquinio, K. M., Karsies, T., Shein, S. L., Beardsley, A., Khemani, R., Schwarz, A., et al. (2022). Airway microbiome dynamics and relationship to ventilator-associated infection in intubated pediatric patients. *Pediatric Pulmonology, 57*, 508–518.

40. Turton, P. (2008). Ventilator-associated pneumonia in pediatric intensive care: A literature review. *Nursing in Critical Care, 13*, 241–248.

41. van der Meer, S. B., Figaroa, G., van der Voort, P. H. J., Nijsten, M. W., & Pillay, J. (2021). Ventilator-associated pneumonia in critically-ill patients with COVID-19 in a setting of selective decontamination of the digestive tract. *Critical Care, 25*, 445.

INDEX

Q

R

S

T

U

V

W

Y

Printed and bound by CPI Group (UK) Ltd, Croydon, CR0 4YY

18/09/2026

14965061-0008